T0189121

CLINICAL REASONING
AND CARE COORDINATION
IN ADVANCED PRACTICE NURSING

RuthAnne Kuiper, PhD, RN, CNE, ANEF, is a professor of nursing in the School of Nursing at the University of North Carolina at Wilmington. She earned a PhD in nursing from the University of South Carolina, Columbia; a master's of nursing degree as a clinical nurse specialist in cardiopulmonary nursing from the University of California, Los Angeles; a BSN from Excelsior College, Albany, New York; and a diploma in nursing from Mountainside Hospital School of Nursing in Montclair, New Jersey. Dr. Kuiper's research interests include clinical reasoning, metacognition, self-regulated learning, and technological innovation in nursing education. Dr. Kuiper has been the primary investigator for numerous studies related to nursing education and has authored many data-based publications based on this work. She has been a grant reviewer for the National League for Nursing, Sigma Theta Tau International, International Nursing Association for Clinical Simulation, and the U. S. Department of Health and Human Services. She is on the editorial board for *Clinical Simulation in Nursing* and is a reviewer for multiple other professional journals. She is a member of Sigma Theta Tau International and has held multiple leadership positions in local chapters. She holds an alumnus status from the American Association for Critical-Care Nurses for CCRN certification and has been a National League for Nursing certified nurse educator since 2007. In 2011, Dr. Kuiper was inducted into the Academy of Nursing Education Fellows. Dr. Kuiper was also included in the top 20 list of medical and nursing professors in North Carolina in 2013, based on being chosen as one of the top 100 nursing professors in the East by the Louise H. Batz Patient Safety Foundation. Dr. Kuiper's instructional and clinical expertise is in the area of adult health, specifically, critical care nursing. She continues to teach nurse educator classes, nurse practitioner classes, supervise nurse educator practicums, and mentor graduate students across the country on master's and dissertation research projects. She has received a number of teaching awards in her professional career and is sought out as a mentor by her colleagues. Most recently, Dr. Kuiper has been a faculty mentor for the past two classes in the Nurse Faculty Leadership Academy, cosponsored by Sigma Theta Tau International and the Elsevier Foundation.

Daniel J. Pesut, PhD, RN, PMHCNS-BC, FAAN, is a professor of nursing in the Nursing Population Health and Systems Cooperative Unit of the School of Nursing at the University of Minnesota, and director of the Katherine J. Densford International Center for Nursing Leadership. He holds the Katherine R. and C. Walton Lillehei Chair in Nursing Leadership. Dr. Pesut has an international reputation and is known for his ability to inspire and support people as they create and design innovative practices with a desired future in mind. Dr. Pesut is a master teacher and has devoted his academic nursing career to developing learning innovations for nursing education. He is best known for his work in creativity and metacognition and the development and testing of the Outcome-Present State-Test model of reflective clinical reasoning. Dr. Pesut earned a PhD in nursing from the University of Michigan; a master's degree in psychiatric mental health nursing from the University of Texas Health Science Center in San Antonio, Texas; and a BS degree with a major in nursing and a minor in psychology from Northern Illinois University, DeKalb, Ilinois. He has completed certificates in management development from Harvard Institute for Higher Education, core mediation skills training from the International Association of Dispute Resolution (IARD), and integral studies from Fielding Graduate University. He is a certified coach of the Hudson Institute of Santa Barbara and a past president (2003–2005) of the Honor Society of Nursing, Sigma Theta Tau International. He is a fellow in the American Academy of Nursing and the recipient of many awards, including an Army Commendation Award earned while on active duty (1975–1978) in the U.S. Army Nurse Corps; the Honor Society of Nursing, Sigma Theta Tau International Edith Moore Copeland Founder's Award for Creativity; the American Assembly for Men in Nursing Luther Christman Award; as well as a number of other distinguished alumni, teaching, mentoring, and leadership awards.

Tamatha E. Arms, DNP, RN, PMHNP-BC, NP-C, is an assistant professor of nursing in the School of Nursing in the College of Health and Human Services at the University of North Carolina at Wilmington. During her professional career she specialized in critical care and nephrology. After obtaining her master's degree with concentration as an adult/geriatric nurse practitioner from the University of North Carolina at Greensboro, she specialized in geriatrics. She later obtained her doctorate of nursing practice degree with concentration as a family psychiatry–mental health nurse practitioner from the College of Nursing at the University of Tennessee Health Science Center. She currently maintains a specialized clinical practice in geropsychiatry. Dr. Arms is a member of Sigma Theta Tau International Nu Omega Chapter, North Carolina Nurses Association, American Academy of Nurse Practitioners, and she serves on the gerontology/psychiatric focus group of the Gerontological Advanced Practice Nurses Association. As a full-time assistant professor of nursing, Dr. Arms coordinates the undergraduate prelicensure gerontology/end-of-life course, teaches clinical psychiatric–mental health courses, lectures in the graduate family nurse practitioner program, and is a guest speaker across health care disciplines. Her research areas focus on geropsychiatry and interprofessional education. She has delivered presentations of scholarly work to the U.S. Preventive Health Services, at interprofessional conferences, the Sigma Theta Tau International 43rd Biennial Convention, and the Southern Nursing Research Society. Dr. Arms is passionate about mentoring students, which has resulted in two of her students being recognized for the National Gerontological Nursing Association Leadership award in 2014.

CLINICAL REASONING AND CARE COORDINATION IN ADVANCED PRACTICE NURSING

RuthAnne Kuiper, PhD, RN, CNE, ANEF
Daniel J. Pesut, PhD, RN, PMHCNS-BC, FAAN
Tamatha E. Arms, DNP, RN, PMHNP-BC, NP-C

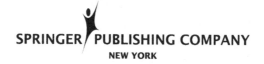

SPRINGER PUBLISHING COMPANY
NEW YORK

Springer Publishing Company, LLC
11 West 42nd Street
New York, NY 10036
www.springerpub.com

Acquisitions Editor: Margaret Zuccarini
Composition: Newgen KnowledgeWorks

ISBN: 978-0-8261-3183-6
e-book ISBN: 978-0-8261-3184-3
Instructor's Manual: 978-0-8261-3208-6
Student Study Guide: 978-0-8261-3209-3

Instructors' Materials: Qualified instructors may request supplements by e-mailing textbook@springerpub.com

Student supplements are available from springerpub.com/kuiper.

16 17 18 19 / 5 4 3 2 1

The author and the publisher of this Work have made every effort to use sources believed to be reliable to provide information that is accurate and compatible with the standards generally accepted at the time of publication. The author and publisher shall not be liable for any special, consequential, or exemplary damages resulting, in whole or in part, from the readers' use of, or reliance on, the information contained in this book. The publisher has no responsibility for the persistence or accuracy of URLs for external or third-party Internet websites referred to in this publication and does not guarantee that any content on such websites is, or will remain, accurate or appropriate.

Library of Congress Cataloging-in-Publication Data
Names: Kuiper, RuthAnne, author. | Pesut, Daniel J., author. | Arms, Tamatha E., author.
Title: Clinical reasoning and care coordination in advanced practice nursing / RuthAnne Kuiper, Daniel J. Pesut, Tamatha E. Arms.
Description: New York, NY : Springer Publishing Company, LLC, [2016]
Identifiers: LCCN 2016000337 | ISBN 9780826131836 | ISBN 97808261-31843 (e-book)
Subjects: | MESH: Nursing Process | Patient-Centered Care | Clinical Competence | Judgment | Models, Nursing | Advanced Practice Nursing—methods
Classification: LCC RT51 | NLM WY 100.1 | DDC 610.73—dc23
LC record available at http://lccn.loc.gov/2016000337

Printed in the United States of America by McNaughton & Gunn.

CONTENTS

PREFACE

The purpose of this book is to introduce an innovative model of care coordination clinical reasoning that builds on past work with the Outcome-Present State-Test (OPT) model of reflective clinical reasoning (Pesut & Herman, 1999). It includes contemporary knowledge, skills, and abilities required to work effectively as a member of an interprofessional care team in the current health care arena.

The OPT model has been described as a third-generation nursing process model that responds to the need for patient-centered nursing care coordination challenges. The OPT model provides a structure and process for using standardized nursing terminology and supports the development of critical, creative systems and complex-thinking skills. The OPT model reinforces the need for clinical thinking to move away from a traditional problem-solving nursing process and focus on outcome specification and the development of clinical judgments. The model supports the development of a systems-thinking mind-set related to the complexities associated with caring for patients and families with multiple competing health care needs.

In this text the fundamental aspects of the OPT model of clinical reasoning are explained and linked to care coordination challenges at several levels—those related to patient-centered care planning, team-centered negotiation, and service or health care system considerations. In Part I, we set the stage and argue that care coordination clinical reasoning is a derivative of contemporary policy, practice, and competency expectations. We underscore the importance and value of knowledge complexity and nursing knowledge work and relate the use of standardized terminology to care coordination clinical reasoning efforts.

In Chapter 1, we discuss the social and practice changes in nursing that influence the thinking strategies and skills that are needed for competent practice in interprofessional teams for care coordination. Chapter 2 reviews nursing informatics, topics of knowledge complexity, and standardized nursing terminology as foundational to clinical reasoning and evidence-based practice. In Chapter 3, we trace the history and evolution of the nursing process and describe some of the essential thinking strategies associated with effective clinical reasoning. In Chapter 4, we introduce readers to the Care Coordination Clinical Reasoning (CCCR) model and discuss some of the distinctions, system dynamics, and relationship issues that emerge when health care team members have different points of view with regard to care coordination. Navigating and negotiating competing values and understanding the value exchange between and among members of the health care team provide insights and strategies related to care coordination efforts. Realizing that clinicians filter, frame, and focus on different disciplinary perspectives helps the advanced practice clinician understand how diagnoses and nursing care issues are related. In Chapter 5, we build on the development of the CCCR model and propose ways to master the self-regulating thinking skills that enable effective care coordination.

Advanced practice clinicians will find Part II to be of interest. In this section, a series of case studies illustrates how the CCCR model is activated and applied across the life span and in a number of health care contexts. Cases across the health care continuum related to primary care, acute care, rehabilitative care, and long-term care are presented with patient scenarios that are in need of care coordination. Each case unfolds with attention to the distinction and relationships between nursing care domains and International Classification of Diseases (ICD)-10 medical diagnoses. Patient-centered, team-centered, and service-centered systems thinking clinical reasoning skills are illustrated with reasoning webs that help pinpoint keystone issues and frame important care coordination dynamics among members of the interprofessional team as these relate to practice issues, interventions, outcomes, and value exchange. Through the use of CCCR model webs, team members can visualize important relationships between and among the essential elements of the CCCR model: needs assessment, medical care services and testing, coaching, and education. As the team engages in activity planning, members are able to attend to an individualized plan of care that focuses on monitoring safety needs and evaluating the capacity, resources, and skills that patients need in service of self-management.

Part III summarizes the benefits of the CCCR model and suggests future evolution and development of the model. The need for health care team members to develop competencies related to ongoing innovations is discussed. The value of data science to support future developments in nursing knowledge work is proposed. The trends and models discussed in this book imply that ongoing analysis and evaluation are in place to determine whether outcomes are being achieved by both the advanced practice nurse who is coordinating care and the patient who is the recipient of that care. Potential research questions related to the ongoing study of the CCCR model are recommended. The authors believe that advanced practice nursing clinicians and nurse educators will find value in the CCCR model as nurses continue to lead and influence care coordination activities into the future.

Qualified instructors may request supplements to this book in the form of a PowerPoint presentation and Instructor's Manual by e-mailing textbook@ springerpub.com. Student supplements are also available from springerpub .com/kuiper.

RuthAnne Kuiper
Daniel J. Pesut
Tamatha E. Arms

REFERENCE

Pesut, D., & Herman, J. (1999). *Clinical reasoning: The art and science of critical and creative thinking*. New York, NY: Delmar.

ACKNOWLEDGMENTS

We admire and appreciate the clinical practice, insights, and wisdom of the following nurse practitioners and educators who added to the development of the case study chapters in this book.

Deborah Adams-Wingate, MSN, RN, NP-C
Carolyn W. Jones, PhD, RN, NNP-BC
Michelle McEwen-Campbell, DNP, RNC-OB, CNE, FNP, LNC
Brandy Mechling, PhD, RN, PMHCNS-BC
Rand Pennington, MSN, FNP-C, AGACNP-BC
Stephanie Turrise, PhD, RN, BC, APRN, CNE
Andrew Weaver, MSN, FNP-BC
Patricia H. White, MSN-Ed, RNC-NI, CNE

PART I

CARE COORDINATION CLINICAL REASONING FOUNDATIONS

CHAPTER 1

CARE COORDINATION CLINICAL REASONING: CONTEMPORARY COMPETENCY EXPECTATIONS

The contributions of nurses are vital in meeting 21st-century health care challenges (Institute of Medicine [IOM], 2010). In spite of advancements in disease prevention and health promotion, a need exists to educate people about healthy lifestyles and provide care for and counsel people if and when they do become ill, disabled, or unable to care for themselves.

As health care systems become more complex, the economic, technical, and social forces that shape the nature of health care experiences shape the nurses' role. Nurses have to collaborate on care coordination with other members of the health care team across systems and contexts of care. Clinical reasoning challenges multiply as the advanced practice clinician thinks about patient-centered care issues from the perspective of a health care provider, and then considers those issues in terms of the dynamics and competing values of health care teams. Add the complexity of working between and among specialty clinics and services across continuums of care and it becomes quickly evident that new models and strategies for clinical reasoning and interprofessionality (D'Amour & Oandasan, 2005) are needed to maximize care coordination that yields safe, high-quality, cost-effective health care (Lamb, 2013).

LEARNING OUTCOMES

After completing this chapter, the reader should be able to:

1. Define and explain why care coordination clinical reasoning is an essential nursing skill needed to support 21st-century health care demands
2. Describe contemporary policies and competency expectations for advanced practice nurses
3. Define the term "interprofessionality"
4. Explain the core competencies nurses are expected to have to support interprofessional practice, teamwork, and care coordination
5. Describe selected characteristics that support and enhance a clinical reasoning mind-set

This book contributes a new model of care coordination clinical reasoning that builds on previous research and development of the Outcome-Present State-Test (OPT) model of reflective clinical reasoning (Pesut, 2001, 2002, 2004, 2006, 2008; Pesut & Herman, 1992, 1998, 1999). There is an art and a science to clinical reasoning. Nurses develop clinical reasoning skills based on analysis and understanding of individual patient stories. Each patient encounter presents opportunities to reason. Every time nurses reason about a patient story, they add to their repertoire of understanding and resources so that they can reason more effectively. Patient-centered clinical reasoning in the context of care coordination is only one aspect of the care coordination process.

Reasoning about specific patients in the context of 1:1 care is quickly being superseded by the challenges of reasoning with teams and considering large numbers of patients and populations of care. Clinical reasoning in the context of teamwork that involves negotiation of competing values in multiple systems and contexts of care is especially challenging. The complexities and challenges of teamwork and multiple contexts of services require the provider to reason from different perspectives simultaneously (D'Amour & Oandasan, 2005).

Each discipline has a particular filter through which it frames and then focuses on patient-care goals. Each member of the health care team views and processes information differently. This results in a team that approaches information from multiple perspectives, which challenges traditional methods and techniques of reasoning. Clinical reasoning on a case-by-case basis is the foundation of diagnostic thinking. Nonetheless, it is evident that an interprofessional health care team's work and reasoning with regard to multiple competing patient-care issues require the development of team- and systems-centered thinking skills and concurrent consideration of different levels of filtering, framing, and focus. Thus, new models of care coordination clinical reasoning are needed to support the education, training, and professional development of contemporary health care providers and clinicians.

Patients who present multiple issues require the application and use of several types of thinking skills: critical, creative, reflective, systems, and complex thinking. The OPT model of clinical reasoning (Pesut & Herman, 1998, 1999), developed in the late 1990s, provides tools and resources to help clinicians think about their thinking and gain insight into how multiple problems combine and relate. Attending to the complexity of the interrelationships of problems and taking a systems-thinking perspective often reveal a keystone issue that represents the core of the system dynamic and provides a leverage point for intervention that shifts the patient system from a present problem-oriented state to a specified desired-outcome state.

There is evidence that the OPT model and its associated teaching–learning strategies positively influence the development of clinical reasoning skills in nursing students. Using an OPT model worksheet analysis and synthesis tool helps students master the clinical reasoning associated with complex patient-care scenarios. The worksheets were tested and evaluated by researchers using the clinical and simulation experiences of nursing students, and with personal assistant devices (Kuiper, 2008; Kuiper, Heinrich, Matthias, Graham, & Bell-Kotwall, 2008; Kuiper, Pesut, & Kautz, 2009). The OPT model worksheets provide structure, strategies, and scaffolding for the analysis, synthesis, and organization of data; for use of standardized nursing language; and care planning and reflection on outcomes. Evidence suggests that students who used the OPT model and methods strengthened their thinking skills, and realized differences in how they thought about patient-centered problems (Kuiper et al., 2009). The structure and process of OPT guarantee that nursing care outcomes are well defined, and promote new ways to think about the role of interventions in achieving and making judgments about outcomes in complex patient-care situations. In addition, clinical reasoning self-efficacy is strengthened as the advanced practice clinician focuses on associations and cause-and-effect relationships concerning patient-care needs, issues, and challenges.

Given the shift to care coordination, the authors built on previous research and have developed a model of clinical reasoning for care coordination that extends from the foundation of the OPT model's strategies and methods, and evolves the application of the model to interprofessional team dynamics and service/organizational considerations. The need to articulate and expand clinical reasoning expectations at the care coordination level is influenced by traditional policies, disciplinary perspectives, and current competencies and role expectations.

CONTEMPORARY POLICIES AND COMPETENCY EXPECTATIONS

A profession is distinguished from other occupations by several criteria. A profession has an orientation toward service within the context of a code of ethics. A profession uses a developed knowledge base. A profession systematically uses theory to guide actions. In a profession, there are standards of practice. A profession provides for the education and socialization of its members. A profession is autonomous and self-regulating. Professional self-regulation is the process by which nursing ensures that its members act in the public interest by providing the unique service with which society has entrusted them (American Nurses Association [ANA], 1995, 2010, 2015).

The social context of nursing is discussed in the ANA document *Nursing's Social Policy Statement* (ANA, 1980, 1995, 2010, 2015). *Nursing's Social Policy Statement* is used by nurses as a framework for understanding nursing's social contract and relationship with society and nursing's obligations to those who receive nursing care (ANA, 2015). *Nursing's Social Policy Statement* provides a definition of nursing; explains the knowledge base for nursing practice; explains the differences between basic and advanced nursing practice; and discusses the professional, legal, and self-regulated governance of nursing practice for the benefit of society. The statement provides clues about the importance of thinking and reasoning for professional nursing practice.

In 1980, the statement defined nursing as "the diagnosis and treatment of human responses to actual or potential health problems" (ANA, 1980, p. 6). This definition capitalized on advances nurses made in practice, research, and knowledge development. This definition clarified that nurses deal with the human response to health care issues and underscored the importance of nursing diagnostic reasoning. In 1995, the statement was revised. Of particular interest are descriptions of nursing through time, which was included in the revised document. The document begins describing how Florence Nightingale (1859/1946) defined nursing as those things nurses do "to put the patient in the best condition for nature to act upon him" (p. 75). About a hundred years later, Virginia Henderson (1961) stated that the purpose of nursing is

> To assist the individual, sick or well, in the performance of those activities contributing to health or its recovery (or to a peaceful death) that he would perform unaided if he had the necessary strength, will, or knowledge and to do this in such a way as to help him gain independence as rapidly as possible. (p. 5)

Both of these definitions focused on nursing actions and what nurses do to promote health and healing. In recent times, the definition of nursing and especially the definition of advanced practice nursing, continues to evolve and change. In fact, scope of practice for advanced practice nursing may be different in each state and or country. Readers are advised to know the definition of nursing in their state and what the scope of practice definitions are with regard to state laws and regulations and be familiar with the Advanced Practice Registered Nurse (APRN) Consensus model for regulation that is currently sponsored by the National Council of State Boards of Nursing (2008, 2012).

NURSING ART AND SCIENCE

Nursing science involves the use of logic to understand and solve patient problems. Research and the scientific method are the ways people use logic to generate knowledge that nurses use in patient care. The scientific method is a problem-solving approach in which a problem is identified, possible solutions to the problem are hypothesized, and experiments are designed to test a solution to the problem. Based on the evidence from the experiment, potential solutions are identified. This is a step-by-step process that follows specific rules. The step-by-step process is guided by logic and reasoning. There are three kinds of nursing science: basic nursing science, applied nursing science, and practical science.

Basic nursing science refers to knowledge that is developed purely for the sake of knowing. This knowledge adds to our sense of understanding about people. It is generally understood that the knowledge may be useful one day. *Applied nursing science* is knowledge that is used to care directly for patients. Both basic and applied nursing science serves as the foundation for clinical reasoning. Johnson (1991) argues for a third type of science, which she calls practical science. *Practical nursing science* combines the science and art of nursing. In nursing, more attention is often paid to the topic of science rather than art. However, "science alone will not solve all the problems of nursing" (Johnson, 1994, p. 1). Johnson (1994) theorized that art in nursing means (a) the ability to grasp meaning in patient encounters,

(b) the ability to establish a meaningful connection with patients, (c) the ability to skillfully perform nursing activities, (d) the ability to rationally determine an appropriate course of action, and (e) the ability to morally conduct nursing practice. The art of nursing is based on caring and respect of human dignity and a compassionate approach to patient care that embraces spirituality, healing, empathy, mutual respect, and partnership (ANA, 2015).

A challenge for future nurses is to figure out how to combine the science and art of nursing into a practical science. Although the science of nursing is important, the art of nursing is equally significant. The art and science of nursing are nurtured and developed in education programs that provide essential knowledge, skills, and abilities to achieve the goals and ideals of the profession. Contemporary policies and competency expectations provide the context for the professional practice of nursing.

ESSENTIAL EDUCATION REQUIREMENTS

The American Association of Colleges of Nursing (AACN) is the national voice for university and 4-year college education programs in nursing. This organization has published a series of documents that outlines fundamental education requirements for those wishing to pursue a career in nursing. For example, the "Essentials of Master's Education in Nursing" (AACN, 2011) identifies the necessary curricular elements and frameworks required of master's programs. The document delineates the core knowledge and skills that all master's-prepared graduates, regardless of focus, major, or intended practice setting, should acquire in nine foundational areas:

1. Sciences and humanities
2. Organizational and systems leadership
3. Quality improvement and safety
4. Translating and integrating scholarship into practice
5. Informatics and health care technologies
6. Health policy and advocacy
7. Interprofessional collaboration for improving outcomes
8. Clinical prevention and population health
9. Master's-level nursing practice

Consistent and aligned with the educational foundations for practice, the National Organization of Nurse Practitioner Faculty (NONPF, 2015) has outlined the core competencies expected of nurse practitioners. These competencies are related to several of the AACN essentials in regard to scientific foundations for practice, leadership, knowledge, and skills related to quality assurance, practice, systems understanding, health information and technology, ethics, as well as skills related to independent practice and policy.

Another advanced practice role that aligns practice competencies with the AACN essentials is that of clinical nurse leader (CNL). Although the practice setting for the CNL may vary, the core of responsibility is accountability for patient-care outcomes while applying evidence to design, implement, and evaluate patient-care processes and models of care delivery (National Transitions of Care Coalition [NTOCC], 2008). This care coordination role occurs across health care systems. The NONPF and CNL competencies can be reviewed in Table 1.1. To what degree have you mastered these core competencies?

Try this exercise. Using a scale from 1 to 10 (1 = "I have yet to master this competency" and 10 = "I have totally mastered this competency") review and rate yourself on each of the competencies listed in Table 1.1.

Consider your ratings. What competency areas are strengths for you? What areas need attention? How specifically will you create a professional development plan to master the skill set you need based on these national standards and expectations? If you are currently in an educational program, how specifically is your curriculum preparing you to master the knowledge, skills, competencies, and abilities you will need in reference to the national AACN and NONPF or CNL standards and expectations? If you are not getting the experiences or knowledge you need what will you do to activate your learning in order to master the competencies? The profession of nursing has unique contributions to make to the diagnosis, treatment, and care of individuals, families, groups, and communities. However, nurses are part of a larger team of health care providers, all of whom have contributions to make in regard to health and healing. Care is influenced and achieved through the interprofessionality of a cohesive health care team.

INTERPROFESSIONALITY

Nurses have a professional responsibility to advance the science and practice of the discipline; however, the care of patients, families, and communities requires cooperative partnerships with other members of the health care team. There is a movement underway to understand more about the nature of interprofessional health care education and practice.

The National Center for Interprofessional Practice and Education was recently created at the University of Minnesota in the United States to coordinate research and scholarship on the topic of interprofessional health profession work in health care. The center has established a resource exchange (https://nexusipe.org/resource-exchange) and creates forums for people to come together to communicate with and learn from each other about the complexities and challenges of interprofessionality. The future success of care coordination depends on interprofessionality.

Danielle D'Amour and Ivey Oandasan (2005) define interprofessionality as "the development of a cohesive practice between professionals from different disciplines. It is the process by which professionals reflect on and develop ways of practicing that provide an integrated and cohesive answer to the needs of the patient/family/population" (p. 9). They further note that interprofessionality is a preoccupation among professionals used to reconcile differences and opposing views in service of continuous interaction and knowledge sharing that invites and optimizes partnership with patients. Interprofessionality is possible when professionals commit to sharing goals and visions as they embrace the complex task of addressing patient-care

TABLE 1.1 Comparison Table of Clinical Nurse Leader (CNL) and Nurse Practitioner Competencies

AACN ESSENTIALS[a]	CNL COMPETENCIES[b]	NONPF COMPETENCIES[c]
ESSENTIAL 1: BACKGROUND FOR PRACTICE FROM SCIENCES AND HUMANITIES		
1. Integrate nursing and related sciences into the delivery of advanced nursing care to diverse populations. 2. Incorporate current and emerging genetic/genomic evidence in providing advanced nursing care to individuals, families, and communities while accounting for patient values and clinical judgment. 3. Design nursing care for a clinical or community-focused population based on biopsychosocial, public health, nursing, and organizational sciences. 4. Apply ethical analysis and clinical reasoning to assess, intervene, and evaluate advanced nursing care delivery. 5. Synthesize evidence for practice to determine appropriate application of interventions across diverse populations. 6. Use quality processes and improvement science to evaluate care and ensure patient safety for individuals and communities. 7. Integrate organizational science and informatics to make changes in the care environment to improve health outcomes. 8. Analyze nursing history to expand thinking and provide a sense of professional heritage and identity.	1. Interpret patterns and trends in quantitative and qualitative data to evaluate outcomes of care within a microsystem and compare to other recognized benchmarks or outcomes, e.g., national, regional, state, or institutional data. 2. Articulate delivery process, outcomes, and care trends using a variety of media and other communication methods to the health care team and others. 3. Incorporate values of social justice to address health care disparities and bridge cultural and linguistic barriers to improve quality outcomes. 4. Integrate knowledge about social, political, economic, environmental, and historical issues into the analysis of and potential solutions to professional and health care issues. 5. Apply concepts of improvement science and systems theory.	1. Critically analyze data and evidence to improve advanced nursing practice. 2. Integrate knowledge from the humanities and sciences within the context of nursing science. 3. Translate research and other forms of knowledge into practice to improve practice processes and outcomes. 4. Develop new practice approaches based on the integration of research, theory, and practice knowledge.

(continued)

TABLE 1.1 Comparison Table of Clinical Nurse Leader (CNL) and Nurse Practitioner Competencies *(continued)*

AACN ESSENTIALS[a]	CNL COMPETENCIES[b]	NONPF COMPETENCIES[c]
ESSENTIAL 2: ORGANIZATIONAL AND SYSTEMS LEADERSHIP		
1. Apply leadership skills and decision making in the provision of culturally responsive, high-quality nursing care, health care team coordination, and the oversight and accountability for care delivery and outcomes.	1. Demonstrate working knowledge of the health care system and its component parts, including sites of care; delivery models; payment models; and the roles of health care professionals, patients, caregivers, and unlicensed professionals.	1. Assume complex and advanced leadership roles to initiate and guide change.
2. Assume a leadership role in effectively implementing patient safety and quality-improvement initiatives within the context of the interprofessional team using effective communication (scholarly writing, speaking, and group interaction) skills.	2. Assume a leadership role for an interprofessional health care team with a focus on the delivery of patient-centered care and the evaluation of quality and cost-effectiveness across the health care continuum.	2. Provide leadership to foster collaboration with multiple stakeholders (e.g., patients, community, integrated health care teams, and policy makers) to improve health care.
3. Develop an understanding of how health care delivery systems are organized and financed (and how this affects patient care) and identify the economic, legal, and political factors that influence health care.	3. Use systems theory in the assessment, design, delivery, and evaluation of health care within complex organizations.	3. Demonstrate leadership that uses critical and reflective thinking.
4. Demonstrate the ability to use complexity science and systems theory in the design, delivery, and evaluation of health care.	4. Demonstrate business and economic principles and practices, including cost–benefit analysis, budgeting, strategic planning, human and other resource management, marketing, and value-based purchasing.	4. Advocate for improved access, quality, and cost-effective health care.
5. Apply business and economic principles and practices, including budgeting, cost-benefit analysis, and marketing, to develop a business plan.	5. Contribute to budget development at the microsystem level.	5. Advance practice through the development and implementation of innovations incorporating principles of change.
6. Design and implement systems change strategies that improve the care environment.	6. Evaluate the efficacy and utility of evidence-based care delivery approaches and their outcomes at the microsystem level.	6. Communicate practice knowledge effectively both orally and in writing.
7. Participate in the design and implementation of new models of care delivery and coordination.		7. Participate in professional organizations and activities that influence advanced practice nursing and/or health outcomes with a population focus.

7. Collaborate with health care professionals, including physicians, advanced practice nurses, nurse managers, and others, to plan, implement, and evaluate an improvement opportunity.
8. Participate in a shared leadership team to make recommendations for improvement at the micro-, meso-, or macro-system levels.

ESSENTIAL 3: QUALITY IMPROVEMENT AND SAFETY

1. Analyze information about quality initiatives recognizing the contributions of individuals and interprofessional health care teams to improve health outcomes across the continuum of care.
2. Implement evidence-based plans based on trend analysis and quantify the impact on quality and safety.
3. Analyze information and design systems to sustain improvements and promote transparency using high reliability and just-culture principles.
4. Compare and contrast several appropriate quality-improvement models.
5. Promote a professional environment that includes accountability and high-level communication skills when involved in peer review, advocacy for patients and families, reporting of errors, and professional writing.
6. Contribute to the integration of health care services within systems to affect safety and quality of care to improve patient outcomes and reduce fragmentation of care.

1. Use performance measures to assess and improve the delivery of evidence-based practices and promote outcomes that demonstrate delivery of higher value care.
2. Perform a comprehensive microsystem assessment to provide the context for problem identification and action.
3. Use evidence to design and direct system improvements that address trends in safety and quality.
4. Implement quality-improvement strategies based on current evidence, analytics, and risk anticipation.
5. Promote a culture of continuous quality improvement within a system.
6. Apply just-culture principles and the use of safety tools, such as failure mode effects analysis (FMEA) and root cause analysis (RCA), to anticipate, intervene, and decrease risk.

1. Use best available evidence to continuously improve quality of clinical practice.
2. Evaluate the relationships among access, cost, quality, and safety and their influence on health care.
3. Evaluate how organizational structure, care processes, financing, marketing, and policy decisions impact the quality of health care.
4. Apply skills in peer review to promote a culture of excellence.
5. Anticipate variations in practice that are proactive in implementing interventions to ensure quality.

(continued)

TABLE 1.1 Comparison Table of Clinical Nurse Leader (CNL) and Nurse Practitioner Competencies *(continued)*

AACN ESSENTIALS[a]	CNL COMPETENCIES[b]	NONPF COMPETENCIES[c]
7. Direct quality-improvement methods to promote culturally responsive, safe, timely, effective, efficient, equitable, and patient-centered care. 8. Lead quality-improvement initiatives that integrate sociocultural factors affecting the delivery of nursing and health care services.	7. Demonstrate professional and effective communication skills, including verbal, nonverbal, written, and virtual abilities. 8. Evaluate patient handoffs and transitions of care to improve outcomes. 9. Evaluate medication reconciliation and administration processes, to enhance the safe use of medications across the continuum of care. 10. Demonstrate the ability to develop and present a business plan, including a budget, for the implementation of a quality-improvement project/initiative. 11. Use a variety of data sets, such as Hospital Consumer Assessment of Healthcare Providers and Systems (HCAHPS), nurse-sensitive indicators, National Data Nursing Quality Improvement (NDNQI), and population registries, appropriate for the patient population, setting, and organization, to assess individual and population risks and care outcomes.	
ESSENTIAL 4: TRANSLATING AND INTEGRATING SCHOLARSHIP INTO PRACTICE		
1. Integrate theory, evidence, clinical judgment, research, and interprofessional perspectives using translational processes to improve practice and associated health outcomes for patient aggregates.	1. Facilitate practice change based on best available evidence that results in quality, safety, and fiscally responsible outcomes. 2. Ensure the inclusion of an ethical decision-making framework for quality improvement.	1. Provide leadership in the translation of new knowledge into practice. 2. Generate knowledge from clinical practice to improve practice and patient outcomes.

12

2. Advocate for ethical conduct in research and translational scholarship (with particular attention to the protection of the patient as a research participant).
3. Articulate to a variety of audiences the evidence base for practice decisions, including the credibility of sources of information and the relevance to the practice problem confronted.
4. Participate, leading when appropriate, in collaborative teams to improve care outcomes and support policy changes through knowledge generation, knowledge dissemination, and planning and evaluating knowledge implementation.
5. Apply practice guidelines to improve practice and the care environment.
6. Perform a rigorous critique of evidence derived from databases to generate meaningful evidence for nursing practice.

3. Implement strategies for encouraging a culture of inquiry within the health care delivery team.
4. Facilitate the process of retrieval, appraisal, and synthesis of evidence in collaboration with health care team members, including patients, to improve care outcomes.
5. Communicate with the interprofessional health care team, patients, and caregivers about current quality and safety guidelines and nurse-sensitive indicators, including the endorsement and validation processes.
6. Apply improvement science theory and methods in performance measurement and quality-improvement processes.
7. Lead change initiatives to decrease or eliminate discrepancies between actual practices and identified standards of care.
8. Disseminate changes in practice and improvements in care outcomes to internal and external audiences.
9. Design care based on outcome analysis and evidence to promote safe, timely, effective, efficient, equitable, and patient-centered care.

3. Apply clinical investigative skills to improve health outcomes.
4. Lead practice inquiry, individually or in partnership with others.
5. Disseminate evidence from inquiry to diverse audiences using multiple modalities.
6. Analyze clinical guidelines for individualized application into practice.

ESSENTIAL 5: INFORMATICS AND HEALTH CARE TECHNOLOGIES

1. Analyze current and emerging technologies to support safe practice environments and to optimize patient safety, cost-effectiveness, and health outcomes.

1. Use information technology, analytics, and evaluation methods to:
   a. Collect or access appropriate and accurate data to generate evidence for nursing practice

1. Integrate appropriate technologies for knowledge management to improve health care.

(continued)

TABLE 1.1 Comparison Table of Clinical Nurse Leader (CNL) and Nurse Practitioner Competencies *(continued)*

AACN ESSENTIALS[a]	CNL COMPETENCIES[b]	NONPF COMPETENCIES[c]
2. Evaluate outcome data using current communication technologies, information systems, and statistical principles to develop strategies to reduce risks and improve health outcomes.	b. Provide input in the design of databases that generate meaningful evidence for practice	2. Translate technical and scientific health information appropriate for various users' needs.
3. Promote policies that incorporate ethical principles and standards for the use of health and information technologies.	c. Collaborate to analyze data from practice and system performance	a. Assess the patient's and caregiver's educational needs to provide effective, personalized health care.
4. Provide oversight and guidance in the integration of technologies to document patient care and improve patient outcomes.	d. Design evidence-based interventions in collaboration with the health professional team	b. Coach the patient and caregiver for positive behavioral change.
5. Use information and communication technologies, resources, and principles of learning to teach patients and others.	e. Examine patterns of behavior and outcomes	3. Demonstrate information-literacy skills in complex decision making.
6. Use current and emerging technologies in the care environment to support lifelong learning for self and others.	f. Identify gaps in evidence for practice	4. Contribute to the design of clinical information systems that promote safe, quality, and cost-effective care.
	2. Implement the use of technologies to coordinate and laterally integrate patient care within/across care settings and among health care providers.	5. Use technology systems that capture data on variables for the evaluation of nursing care.
	3. Analyze current and proposed use of patient-care technologies, including their cost-effectiveness and appropriateness, in the design and delivery of care in diverse care settings.	
	4. Use technologies and information systems to facilitate the collection, analysis, and dissemination of data, including clinical, financial, and operational outcomes.	
	5. Use information and communication technologies to document patient care, advance patient education, and enhance accessibility of care.	

6. Participate in ongoing evaluation, implementation, and integration of health care technologies, including the electronic health record (EHR).
7. Use a variety of technology modalities and media to disseminate health care information and communicate effectively with diverse audiences.

ESSENTIAL 6: HEALTH POLICY AND ADVOCACY

1. Analyze how policies influence the structure and financing of health care, practice, and health outcomes.
2. Participate in the development and implementation of institutional, local, and state and federal policy.
3. Examine the effect of legal and regulatory processes on nursing practice, health care delivery, and outcomes.
4. Interpret research, bringing the nursing perspective, for policy makers and stakeholders.
5. Advocate for policies that improve the health of the public and the profession of nursing.

1. Describe the interaction between regulatory agency requirements (such as The Joint Commission [TJC], Centers for Medicare & Medicaid Services [CMS], or Healthcare Facilities Accreditation Program [HFAP]), and quality, fiscal, and value-based indicators.
2. Articulate the contributions and synergies of the CNL with other nursing and interprofessional team member roles to policy makers, employers, health care providers, consumers, and other health care stakeholders.
3. Advocate for policies that leverage social change, promote wellness, improve care outcomes, and reduce costs.
4. Advocate for the integration of the CNL within care delivery systems, including new and evolving models of care.

1. Demonstrate an understanding of the interdependence of policy and practice.
2. Advocate for ethical policies that promote access, equity, quality, and cost.
3. Analyze ethical, legal, and social factors influencing policy development.
4. Contribute in the development of health policy.
5. Analyze the implications of health policy across disciplines.
6. Evaluate the impact of globalization on health care policy development.

(continued)

TABLE 1.1 Comparison Table of Clinical Nurse Leader (CNL) and Nurse Practitioner Competencies *(continued)*

AACN ESSENTIALS[a]	CNL COMPETENCIES[b]	NONPF COMPETENCIES[c]
ESSENTIAL 7: INTERPROFESSIONAL COLLABORATION FOR IMPROVING PATIENT AND POPULATION HEALTH OUTCOMES		
1. Advocate for the value and role of the professional nurse as member and leader of interprofessional health care teams.	1. Create an understanding and appreciation among health care team members of similarities and differences in role characteristics and contributions of nursing and other team members.	1. Apply knowledge of organizational practices and complex systems to improve health care delivery.
2. Understand other health professions' scopes of practice to maximize contributions within the health care team.	2. Advocate for the value and role of the clinical nurse leader as a leader and member of interprofessional health care teams.	2. Effect health care change using broad-based skills, including negotiating, consensus building, and partnering.
3. Employ collaborative strategies in the design, coordination, and evaluation of patient-centered care.	3. Facilitate collaborative, interprofessional approaches and strategies in the design, coordination, and evaluation of patient-centered care.	3. Minimize risk to patients and providers at the individual and systems levels.
4. Use effective communication strategies to develop, participate, and lead interprofessional teams and partnerships.	4. Facilitate the lateral integration of health care services across the continuum of care with the overall objective of influencing, achieving, and sustaining high-quality care.	4. Facilitate the development of health care systems that address the needs of culturally diverse populations, providers, and other stakeholders.
5. Mentor and coach new and experienced nurses and other members of the health care team.	5. Demonstrate a leadership role in enhancing group dynamics and managing group conflicts.	5. Evaluate the impact of health care delivery on patients, providers, other stakeholders, and the environment.
6. Function as an effective group leader or member based on an in-depth understanding of team dynamics and group processes.	6. Facilitate team decision making using decision tools and convergent and divergent group-process skills, such as SWOT (strengths, weaknesses, opportunities, threats) analysis, Pareto analysis, and brainstorming.	6. Analyze organizational structure, functions, and resources to improve the delivery of care.
	7. Assume a leadership role, in collaboration with other interprofessional team members, to facilitate transitions across care settings to support patients and families and reduce avoidable recidivism to improve care outcomes.	7. Collaborate in planning for transitions across the continuum of care.

1. Synthesize broad ecological, global, and social determinants of health; principles of genetics and genomics; and epidemiologic data to design and deliver evidence-based, culturally relevant clinical prevention interventions and strategies.
2. Evaluate the effectiveness of clinical prevention interventions that affect individual- and population-based health outcomes using health information technology and data sources.
3. Design patient-centered and culturally responsive strategies in the delivery of clinical prevention and health-promotion interventions and/or services to individuals, families, communities, and aggregates/clinical populations.
4. Advance equitable and efficient prevention services, and promote effective population-based health policy through the application of nursing science and other scientific concepts.
5. Integrate clinical prevention and population health concepts in the development of culturally relevant and linguistically appropriate health education, communication strategies, and interventions.

1. Demonstrate the ability to engage the community and social service delivery systems that recognize new models of care and health services delivery.
2. Participate in the design, delivery, and evaluation of clinical prevention and health-promotion services that are patient-centered and culturally appropriate.
3. Monitor the outcomes of comprehensive plans of care that address the health-promotion and disease-prevention needs of patient populations.
4. Apply public health concepts to advance equitable and efficient preventive services and policies that promote population health.
5. Engage in partnerships at multiple levels of the health system to ensure effective coordination, delivery, and evaluation of clinical prevention and health-promotion interventions and services across care environments.
6. Use epidemiological, social, ecological, and environmental data from local, state, regional, and national sources to draw inferences regarding the health risks and status of populations, to promote and preserve health and healthy lifestyles.
7. Use evidence in developing and implementing teaching and coaching strategies to promote and preserve health and healthy lifestyles in patient populations.

1. Integrate ethical principles in decision making.
2. Evaluate the ethical consequences of decisions.
3. Apply ethically sound solutions to complex issues related to individuals, populations, and systems of care.

(continued)

TABLE 1.1 Comparison Table of Clinical Nurse Leader (CNL) and Nurse Practitioner Competencies (continued)

AACN ESSENTIALS[a]	CNL COMPETENCIES[b]	NONPF COMPETENCIES[c]
	8. Provide leadership to the health care team to promote health, facilitate self-care management, optimize patient engagement, and prevent future decline, including progression to higher levels of care and readmissions.	1. Function as a licensed independent practitioner.
	9. Assess organization-wide emergency preparedness plans and coordination with the local, regional, and National Incident Management System (NIMS).	2. Demonstrate the highest level of accountability for professional practice.
		3. Practice independently, managing previously diagnosed and undiagnosed patients.
	ESSENTIAL 9: MASTER'S-LEVEL NURSING PRACTICE	a. Provide the full spectrum of health care services to include health promotion, disease prevention, health protection, anticipatory guidance, counseling, disease management, and palliative and end-of-life care.
1. Conduct a comprehensive and systematic assessment as a foundation for decision making.	1. Conduct a holistic assessment and comprehensive physical examination of individuals across the life span.	
2. Apply the best available evidence from nursing and other sciences as the foundation for practice.	2. Assess actual and anticipated health risks to individuals and populations.	b. Use advanced health assessment skills to differentiate among normal, variations of normal, and abnormal findings.
3. Advocate for patients, families, caregivers, communities, and members of the health care team.	3. Demonstrate effective communication, collaboration, and interpersonal relationships with members of the care delivery team across the continuum of care.	
4. Use information and communication technologies to advance patient education, enhance accessibility of care, analyze practice patterns, and improve health care outcomes, including nurse-sensitive outcomes.	4. Facilitate modification of nursing interventions based on risk anticipation and other evidence to improve health care outcomes.	
5. Use leadership skills to teach, coach, and mentor other members of the health care team.	5. Demonstrate the ability to coach, delegate, and supervise health care team members in the performance of nursing procedures and processes with a focus on safety and competence.	
6. Use epidemiological, social, and environmental data in drawing inferences regarding the health status of patient populations and interventions to promote and preserve health and healthy lifestyles.		

7. Use knowledge of illness and disease management to provide evidence-based care to populations, perform risk assessments, and design plans or programs of care.
8. Incorporate core scientific and ethical principles in identifying potential and actual ethical issues arising from practice, including the use of technologies, and in assisting patients and other health care providers to address such issues.
9. Apply advanced knowledge of the effects of global environmental, individual, and population characteristics to the design, implementation, and evaluation of care.
10. Employ knowledge and skills in economics, business principles, and systems in the design, delivery, and evaluation of care.
11. Apply theories and evidence-based knowledge in leading, as appropriate, the health care team to design, coordinate, and evaluate the delivery of care.
12. Apply learning and teaching principles to the design, implementation, and evaluation of health education programs for individuals or groups in a variety of settings.
13. Establish therapeutic relationships to negotiate patient-centered, culturally appropriate, evidence-based goals and modalities of care.
14. Design strategies that promote lifelong learning of self and peers and that incorporate professional nursing standards and accountability for practice.

6. Demonstrate stewardship, including an awareness of global environmental, health, political, and geo-economic factors, in the design of patient care.
7. Facilitate the lateral integration of evidence-based care across settings and among care providers to promote quality, safe, and coordinated care.
8. Facilitate transitions of care and safe handoffs among health care settings, providers, and levels of care.
9. Evaluate the effectiveness of health teaching by self and others.
10. Facilitate the implementation of evidence-based and innovative interventions and care strategies for diverse populations.
11. Design appropriate interventions using surveillance data and infection-control principles to limit health care–acquired infections (HAI) at all points of care.
12. Advocate for patients within the health care delivery system to affect quality, safe, and value-based outcomes.
13. Collaborate in the development of community partnerships to establish health-promotion goals and implement strategies to address those needs.
14. Evaluate the care of at-risk populations across the life span by identifying and implementing programs that address specialized needs.

  c. Employ screening and diagnostic strategies in the development of diagnoses.
  d. Prescribe medications within scope of practice.
  e. Manage the health/illness status of patients and families over time.
4. Provide for patient-centered care recognizing cultural diversity and the patient or designee as a full partner in decision making.
  a. Work to establish a relationship with the patient characterized by mutual respect, empathy, and collaboration.
  b. Create a climate of patient-centered care to include confidentiality, privacy, comfort, emotional support, mutual trust, and respect.
  c. Incorporate the patient's cultural and spiritual preferences, values, and beliefs.
  d. Preserve the patient's control over decision making by negotiating a mutually acceptable plan of care.

(continued)

TABLE 1.1 Comparison Table of Clinical Nurse Leader (CNL) and Nurse Practitioner Competencies *(continued)*

AACN ESSENTIALS[a]	CNL COMPETENCIES[b]	NONPF COMPETENCIES[c]
15. Integrate an evolving personal philosophy of nursing and health care into nursing practice.	15. Engage individuals and families to make quality-of-life decisions, including palliative and end-of-life decisions. 16. Assess an individual's and group's readiness and ability to make decisions, as well as to develop, comprehend, and follow a plan of care. 17. Assess the level of cultural awareness and sensitivity of health care providers as a component of the evaluation of care delivery. 18. Demonstrate coaching skills, including self-reflection, to support new and experienced interprofessional team members in exploring opportunities for improving care processes and outcomes. 19. Use coaching techniques to assist individuals in developing insights and skills to improve their current health status and function.	

AACN, American Association of Colleges of Nursing; NONPF, National Organization of Nurse Practitioner Faculty.

[a] American Association of Colleges of Nursing (2011, 2015a).

[b] National Transitions of Care Coalition (2008).

[c] National Organization of Nurse Practitioner Faculty (2015).

challenges in organizations and governance structures that are committed to high-quality clinical outcomes for both patients and providers.

Interprofessional work requires attention to insight, understanding, and negotiation of competing values (Quinn, Bright, Faerman, Thompson, & McGrath, 2015). Every member of the health care team has to attend to issues of collaboration, creation, competition, and control. In terms of collaboration, this requires understanding self and others, communicating honestly and effectively, and mentoring and facilitating the development of others while attending to team dynamics. Creating change requires innovation and brokering skills that use power ethically and effectively while remaining open to creative thinking and negotiating agreement and commitment to new ideas. Control is about monitoring, coordination, working productively, and managing time and stress while simultaneously paying attention to performance and quality. Competition is managing execution; driving for results through communication of vision, goals, and objectives; and motivating self and others.

There are many models of care coordination; however, the authors believe that the clinical reasoning model presented in this book provides strategies and insights into the complexities of care coordination models and strengthen the nature of core interprofessionality competencies. The model suggests that there are several levels of reasoning that are required in care coordination activities: patient-centered clinical reasoning, team-centered clinical thinking, and service/systems-of-care–centered reasoning. Working on or with an interprofessional team requires attention to yet another set of competencies.

The Interprofessional Educational Collaboration Expert Panel (2011) outlined and described four domains of interprofessional practice: values and ethics, roles and responsibilities, communication, and teams and teamwork. Review the competencies in Table 1.2 and rate yourself on your degree of mastery of the competency. Using a scale from 1 to 10 (1 = "I have yet to master this competency" and 10 = "I have totally mastered this competency"), consider how each of these competencies is related to the negotiation and navigation of the competing values of creating and controlling and competing and collaborating.

CLINICAL REASONING MIND-SET

With the aforementioned competencies in mind and the professional obligations, mandates, and responsibilities outlined by the ANA (2015) *Nursing: Scope and Standards of Practice*, it is important to reinforce the need for nurses to develop a clinical-reasoning mind-set that transcends and includes perspectives related to patients, teams, and services. The prerequisite skills of clinical reasoning include an understanding of how knowledge in nursing is represented and how this knowledge helps nurses filter, frame, and focus patient-care planning. Such understanding of knowledge work requires an appreciation and valuing of contemporary issues related to nursing informatics. Understanding, valuing, and insight are gained through purposeful reading, understanding clinical terminology, knowing the facts, putting facts together in meaningful ways, using facts, recognizing patterns, and deciding about the usefulness of facts for a particular situation. Nurses as well as other health care professionals filter information and use filtered information to

TABLE 1.2 Domains of Interprofessional Practice

VALUES AND ETHICS INTERPROFESSIONAL CORE COMPETENCIES	ROLES AND RESPONSIBILITIES INTERPROFESSIONAL CORE COMPETENCIES
• Place the interests of patients and populations at the center of interprofessional health care delivery. • Respect the dignity and privacy of patients while maintaining confidentiality in the delivery of team-based care. • Embrace the cultural diversity and individual differences that characterize patients, populations, and the health care team. • Respect the unique cultures, values, roles/responsibilities, and expertise of other health professions. • Work in cooperation with those who receive care, those who provide care, and others who contribute to or support the delivery of health prevention and health services. • Develop a trusting relationship with patients, families, and other team members. • Demonstrate high standards of ethical conduct and quality of care in contributions to team-based care. • Manage ethical dilemmas specific to interprofessional patient/population-centered care situations. • Act with honesty and integrity in relationships with patients, families, and other team members. • Maintain competence in the profession appropriate to scope of practice.	• Recognize limitations in skills, knowledge, and abilities. • Engage diverse health care professionals who complement one's own professional expertise, as well as associated resources, to develop strategies to meet specific patient care needs. • Explain the roles and responsibilities of other care providers and how the team works together to provide care. • Use the full scope of knowledge, skills, and abilities of available health professionals and health care workers to provide care that is safe, timely, efficient, effective, and equitable. • Communicate with team members to clarify each member's responsibility in executing components of a treatment plan or public health intervention. • Forge interdependent relationships with other professions to improve care and advance learning. • Engage in continuous professional and interprofessional development to enhance team performance. • Use unique and complementary abilities of all members of the team to optimize patient care.
INTERPROFESSIONAL COMMUNICATION CORE COMPETENCIES	**TEAMS AND TEAMWORK INTERPROFESSIONAL CORE COMPETENCIES**
• Choose effective communication tools and techniques, including information systems and communication technologies, to facilitate discussions and interactions that enhance team function. • Organize and communicate information with patients, families, and health care team members in a form that is understandable, avoiding discipline-specific terminology when possible.	• Describe the process of team development and the roles and practices of effective teams. • Develop consensus on the ethical principles to guide all aspects of patient care and team work. • Engage other health professionals—appropriate to the specific care situation—in shared patient-centered problem solving.

(continued)

TABLE 1.2 Domains of Interprofessional Practice *(continued)*

INTERPROFESSIONAL COMMUNICATION CORE COMPETENCIES	TEAMS AND TEAMWORK INTERPROFESSIONAL CORE COMPETENCIES
• Express knowledge and opinions to team members involved in patient care with confidence, clarity, and respect, working to ensure common understanding of information and treatment and care decisions. • Listen actively, and encourage ideas and opinions of other team members. • Give timely, sensitive, instructive feedback to others about their performance on the team, responding respectfully as a team member to feedback from others. • Use respectful language appropriate for a given difficult situation, crucial conversation, or interprofessional conflict. • Recognize that uniqueness, including experience level, expertise, culture, power, and hierarchy within the health care team, contributes to effective communication, conflict resolution, and positive interprofessional working relationships. • Communicate consistently the importance of teamwork in patient-centered and community-focused care.	• Integrate the knowledge and experience of other professions— appropriate to the specific care situation—to inform care decisions while respecting patient and community values and priorities/preferences for care. • Apply leadership practices that support collaborative practice and team effectiveness. • Engage self and others to constructively manage disagreements about values, roles, goals, and actions that arise among health care professionals and with patients and families. • Share accountability with other professions, patients, and communities for outcomes relevant to prevention and health care. • Reflect on individual and team performance for individual, as well as team performance improvement. • Use process-improvement strategies to increase the effectiveness of interprofessional teamwork and team-based care. • Use available evidence to inform effective teamwork and team-based practices. • Perform effectively on teams and in different team roles in a variety of settings.

Source: Interprofessional Education Collaborative Expert Panel (2011).

frame issues associated with patient-care stories to then focus on discipline-specific problems that can be transformed into an outcome and influenced by an intervention. In addition to an understanding about the importance of knowledge work in nursing, clinical reasoning is influenced by intention, mind-set, and perspective taking. The prerequisite attitudes that you need for clinical reasoning are (a) intention, (b) reflection, (c) curiosity, (d) tolerance for ambiguity, (e) appreciation of perspectives, (f) self-confidence, and (g) professional motivation.

Hawkins, Paul, and Elder (2010) advise that all clinical reasoning has a purpose and is an attempt to figure something out, to settle some question, or to solve a problem. These critical thinking experts also caution that all clinical reasoning is based on assumptions and is done from a point of view. Furthermore, all clinical reasoning is based on data, information, and evidence. And all clinical reasoning is expressed through and informed and influenced by concepts and theories. Finally, all clinical reasoning involves inference and interpretations, which lead to conclusions that have consequences.

Good thinking does not happen by accident. It happens by intention. With intention, you have an idea about the end result you expect your actions to achieve and how you are going to organize your thinking to get there. Intention means that you have a deliberate plan of thinking and reason with a purpose in mind. The ability to have intention requires that you understand the importance and differences between your action self and reflective self. *Reflection* is the ability to see yourself thinking and doing. For some people, reflection is the ability to talk themselves through a situation. Whether you see yourself or talk to yourself, you really have two selves: an action self and a reflective self. The action self engages in activity while the reflective self watches or comments about the action self. People who have well-developed skills in clinical reasoning are able to have both selves functioning simultaneously. An aspect of reflection is the ability to appreciate and value different levels of perspective involved in reasoning efforts. Patient-centered, team-centered, and service/organization-centered perspectives are necessary for care coordination.

This text is designed to support the development of the advanced practice clinician's reflective self and make explicit the different levels of perspective required in care coordination. Clinical reasoning develops best when a person can cycle through four phases of the experiential learning cycle: concrete experience, reflective observation, abstract conceptualization, and active experimentation (Kolb & Kolb, 2012). Clinical reasoning also develops when you are skilled enough to reflect while you are acting or doing. One way to develop expertise at reasoning is to look back on what you did and ask yourself questions about how and why you did what you did. Conducting a reflection check means you self-monitor your actions and thinking after an encounter with a patient or think about your own thinking. Reflection is the way you become aware of what you are thinking (the content of your thinking) and how you are thinking (the process of thinking).

Having curiosity means you are eager to ask and acquire information or knowledge. The origin of this word is from the Latin word *cura*, which means "to care" (American Heritage Dictionary, 1985). Reflection and curiosity go hand in hand. Nursing is curiosity (care) with a purpose. The greater your curiosity, the more tolerant of ambiguity you become. The more curious you are about the ways in which people think, act, and believe, the less likely you are to be judgmental. The greater your curiosity, the more compassion you are likely to possess.

Tolerance for ambiguity is the ability to feel comfortable when the situation is unclear and the outcome is undefined. This is referred to as cognitive dissonance, when a situation or information that is encountered is not familiar to you. Encounters with patients are often ambiguous. You do not know what the patient is going to say or do, you do not know what is going to happen, and you do not know how you are going to react. Most people believe that situations have right answers. But right answers are seldom evident. For example, in some instances, the advanced practice clinician is forced to choose between two goals. If you were forced to choose between truth and loyalty, which choice would you make? If you were to decide between a short-term and long-term gain for some project, which decision would you favor? The degree to which the advanced practice clinician can tolerate ambiguity is often a matter of self-confidence.

Self-confidence is belief in yourself, affirming yourself, and knowing that you are capable of thinking on your feet and responding appropriately. Part of self-confidence is knowing your strengths and weaknesses and obtaining the experiences you need to develop the necessary competencies. Self-confidence also involves knowing that you possess the personal qualities and characteristics of a professional nurse.

Professional motivation involves commitment to the vision, values, and mission of a profession. Taking on these values means that you will behave in a different way. One of these ways is that you shall become your own judge. An individual's commitment to a professional vision and mission requires skill in self-judgment. None of us is perfect and we all make mistakes in thinking and acting. A professional recognizes mistakes made and develops a plan of corrective action. You use your reflective self to make judgments about your professional behavior.

In addition to the aforementioned attitude and habits of mind, it is vital that health care providers develop systems-thinking skills in order to function in the complex health care environment of the 21st century. As noted earlier, there are multiple levels of perspective involved in care coordination clinical reasoning. First, providers and clinicians have to focus on the patient so that reasoning is patient centered. Second, the conclusions derived from an individual provider analysis and synthesis of the patient's needs then need to be processed in the context of the health care team dynamics, so that team-centered thinking is required. Finally, the contexts and organizations that provide care also need to be factored into care coordination clinical reasoning efforts.

Systems thinking is an essential skill set for today's health care clinicians. Mastery and development of systems thinking require attention to distinctions (D), systems rules (S), relationship rules (R), and perspective rules (P). Derek and Laura Cabrera (2015) believe that systems-thinking skills can be mastered with attention to the DSRP model of systems thinking. Care coordination systems thinking requires that the advanced practice clinician be able to make distinctions among ideas or things, recognizes that any idea or thing can be split into parts or lumped into a whole, and any idea can relate to other ideas or things. Finally, any thing or idea can be the point or view of a perspective. Distinguishing standardized terminology becomes important in clinical reasoning. How clinicians split terms or lump them together becomes important in regard to relating issues to each other from disciplinary points of view or perspectives.

The Waters Foundation (2015) suggests that there are 14 habits that systems thinkers employ. Systems thinkers:

1. Seek to understand the big picture
2. Observe how elements within systems change over time, generating patterns and trends
3. Recognize that a system's structure generates its behavior
4. Identify the circular nature of complex cause-and-effect relationships
5. Make meaningful connections within and between systems
6. Change perspectives to increase understanding
7. Surface and test assumptions

8. Consider issues fully and resist the urge to come to quick conclusions
9. Consider how mental models affect current reality and the future
10. Use understanding of system structures to identify possible leverage actions
11. Consider short-term, long-term, and unintended consequences of actions
12. Pay attention to accumulations and their rates of change
13. Recognize the impact of time delays when exploring cause-and-effect relationships
14. Check results and change actions if needed: "successive approximation"

As you consider the systems in which you will find yourself using the clinical reasoning mind-set, ask yourself some of these basic questions about the skills and attitudes that are essential to fulfill the competencies to become a care coordinator (Table 1.3).

Think of a recent interaction with a patient. Stop and think about how to answer the following questions.

1. Did the patient have a story to tell?
2. What did I learn from listening to the patient's story?
3. How do patient stories influence me?
4. What were the moral or ethical dimensions to the patient's story?
5. How did I respond to the story?
6. What emotional responses did the patient's story invoke?
7. As I listened to the patient story, did it remind me of any patients in my past?
8. Did the story have a recognizable pattern or meaning?
9. How might I use patient stories as a guide for developing clinical reasoning skills?
10. How did I communicate and interact with the other members of the health care team?
11. To what degree did I consider the systems of care in which care was taking place?
12. How did I process and evaluate the services delivered to patients that were contributed from several clinics, providers, or other health care contexts?
13. How will the data and information I input on selected patients be used by the organization in the future to develop descriptive, comparative, prescriptive, or predictive health analytics that might inform population health care plans?

A LOOK AHEAD

This book describes ways to think and reason about patient stories and to be open to multiple perspectives in the service of care coordination. In the next few chapters, we emphasize the value and importance of standard terminologies to the clinical reasoning process. We trace the development of the concept and practice of care coordination clinical reasoning, and the essential types of thinking skills that support clinical reasoning. We discuss the importance and need to consider care coordination and multiple levels of perspective: the patients' needs and perspective, the perspective of the health care provider, the perspective of the team, and the perspective of the health care system or organizations in which care occurs. Obviously,

TABLE 1.3 Prompts for a Clinical Reasoning Mind-Set

Knowledge Work and Clinical Reasoning

1. Do I know basic nursing facts, parameters, norms, and possible deviations from the norm?
2. Am I familiar with current knowledge classifications and up to date on your understanding of nursing informatics? Unified medical languages? Advancements in the use of electronic health records? Different types of health analytic techniques? (Chapter 2 describes and discusses the knowledge complexity archetype and contemporary issues related to the application and use of a unified medical language system that supports universal standards in regard to health care informatics work.)

Intention

1. Do I reason with purpose and intention?
2. Do I start with the end result in mind?
3. How do I organize my thinking to get to the end result?

Reflection

1. Am I able to see or describe myself in action?

Curiosity

1. Do I eagerly search out new knowledge about the situation?
2. Am I comfortable asking questions?

Tolerance for Ambiguity

1. How do I feel about the situation?
2. Am I aware of my reasoning and how I organize my thinking?
3. How can ambiguity be useful?

Perspective Taking and Systems Thinking

1. How do I manage my perspective taking and concurrently process information about the patient, the team and the system or organization in which services are provided?
2. As I review the habits of a systems thinker, which one best describes me?
3. Which of the systems-thinking skills do I need to spend more time developing?

Self-Confidence

1. What do I believe about my skills in this situation?
2. What professional motivates me?
3. How will I know I am the best nurse I can be?

there are systems nested within other systems. These systems sometimes interact in synergistic or complicated ways that represent and illustrate both the art and science of clinical reasoning in nursing.

Albert Einstein (1927) wrote:

> If what is seen and experienced is portrayed in the language of logic, we are engaged in science. If it is communicated through forms whose connections are not accessible to the conscious mind, but are recognized intuitively as meaningful, then we are engaged in art. (p. 30)

Nursing is both art and science. The science of nursing helps nurses analyze and evaluate data and make sound decisions concerning patient care. The science of nursing is about logic. The art of nursing enables nurses to use intuition and experience to build meaningful relationships with patients and colleagues. The art of clinical reasoning involves connections that are recognized intuitively as meaningful. Nurses use knowledge from science as they work with and understand people's health care needs. This book is devoted to helping you understand how to reason more effectively about nursing care needs of individuals while paying attention to the interprofessional health care team dynamics given the context of organizations and services where care is provided.

We believe the knowledge work in nursing requires both differentiation and integration in order to think and reason about complex patient stories. The next chapter discusses the importance of contemporary developments in the area of standardized languages, nursing informatics, and unified medical language systems to support clinical reasoning. In subsequent chapters, we build on the OPT model of clinical reasoning and step up the reasoning process from the perspective of the individual patient and provider to filter, frame, and focus on the interaction and negotiation of competing values of the team and then focus on the care coordination process across health care contexts. Our goal is to provide you with the building blocks of care coordination clinical reasoning so that you can master its art, science, and complexity.

SUMMARY

In this chapter, we discussed the social forces that are shaping nursing. Specifically, the ANA *Social Policy Statement*, AACN Essentials Series, CNL directives, and work of the NONPF to set the standards and expectations for nursing education and to outline the skills nurses need to practice in today's health care delivery contexts.

The concept of interprofessionality was introduced and defined and the interprofessional competencies required of a 21st-century health care worker have been identified. These national policy and competency expectations set the expectations for teamwork and the need for care coordination clinical reasoning. On a personal level, one needs to engage in reflection and value clarification regarding the characteristics essential for professional nursing practice. On a professional level, one needs to be up to date in regard to contemporary standards of practice, developments in unified medical languages, nursing informatics, and the knowledge work required to support the development of clinical reasoning skill sets. Teamwork requires people to negotiate competing values and play different leadership roles at different times. In terms of collaborating, members of the team may be facilitators or mentors. In regard to creating members of the team, they may be brokers and/or innovators. In terms of competing members of the team, they may take on the role of director or producer. With respect to control, members of the team may take on the role of coordinator and/or monitor.

Clinical reasoning skills are supported and enhanced through intention, reflective capacity, curiosity, tolerance for ambiguity, perspective taking and systems thinking, and self-confidence, which are inspired and supported by professional purpose and motivation. The degree to which nurses value these dimensions will determine the ratio of science, art, and practical intelligence in their clinical reasoning efforts. One of the keys to success in developing clinical reasoning skills is the conscious development of an action self and a reflective self. In the next chapter, we discuss the importance of standardized terminologies and the unified medical language systems and knowledge complexity.

The rest of this book outlines changes and transformations of the nursing process and proposes a new model of care coordination clinical reasoning. Once the foundation is established, we believe that nurses will be able to build on this foundation and become more adept in their thinking and reasoning. We also explain how the intentional application and use of self-regulation thinking strategies support the development and mastery of the complex thinking skills required of advanced practice clinicians, teams, and organizations of today. The later parts of the book illustrate application of the model, methods, and tools with specific patient cases so that you will be able to practice and master the art and science of care coordination clinical reasoning.

KEY CONCEPTS

1. National standards and competencies establish ways to measure and evaluate the essential knowledge, skills, and abilities nurses need to practice. The AACN and the NONPF have defined and developed core curriculum and competency expectations for advanced practice.
2. Nursing as an art involves establishing meaningful connections with patients; listening and learning from patient stories; and developing a rational, moral, and skillful mode of practice.
3. In addition to knowledge work, clinical reasoning is influenced by intention and mind-set. The prerequisite attitudes that you need for clinical reasoning are (a) intention, (b) reflection, (c) curiosity, (d) tolerance for ambiguity, (e) perspective taking and systems thinking, (f) self-confidence, and (g) professional motivation.
4. Development of clinical reasoning skills involves responsibility, reflection and the ability to shift perspectives, as well as thinking in terms of systems at the patient, team, and organizational levels. Reflection is becoming aware and actively using differences in an "action self" and "reflective self."

STUDY QUESTIONS AND ACTIVITIES

1. Read the current ANA (2015) *Social Policy Statement*: http://nursingworld.org/MainMenuCategories/ThePracticeofProfessionalNursing
2. Review the current AACN essential documents, which outline the expected competencies that graduates from baccalaureate and higher degrees are expected to have—to what degree has your educational program prepared you to meet these essentials? www.aacn.nche.edu/education-resources/essential-series
3. Explore the 2008 Advanced Practice Registered Nurse (APRN) Consensus model developed by the AACN. What is the current policy in your state about the APRN Consensus model? How do you believe the APRN Consensus model supports or hinders practice? www.aacn.nche.edu/education-resources/aprn-consensus-process

4. Explore the resource center of the National Center for Interprofessional Practice and Education: https://nexusipe.org/resource-exchange
5. Read the final report of the Interprofessional Education Collaborative Expert Panel. (2011). *Core Competencies for Interprofessional Collaborative Practice: Report of an Expert Panel*: www.aacn.nche.edu/education-resources/ipecreport.pdf
6. How do you explain the differences between an "action self" and a "reflective self"?
7. Explore Kolb's Model of Experiential Learning. Discover your learning style and reflect on how it supports or inhibits the development of your clinical reasoning skills: www.haygroup.com/leadershipandtalentondemand/enhancing/kolb.aspx
8. Create a personal plan of action for the development of these two parts of the self. What do you need to develop the reflective self part of your professional self?

REFERENCES

American Association of Colleges of Nursing (AACN). (2011). *The essentials of master's education in nursing*. Washington, DC. Author. Retrieved from http://www.aacn.nche.edu/education-resources/MastersEssentials11.pdf

American Association of Colleges of Nursing (AACN). (2015a). Washington, DC: Author. Retrieved from http://www.aacn.nche.edu

American Association of Colleges of Nursing (AACN). (2015b). *Core competencies for interprofessional practice*. Washington, DC: Author. Retrieved from http://www.aacn.nche.edu/education-resources/ipecreport.pdf

American Heritage Dictionary. (1985). *The American Heritage college dictionary* (2nd ed.). Boston, MA: Houghton Mifflin.

American Nurses Association (ANA). (1980). *Nursing: A social policy statement*. Washington, DC: Author.

American Nurses Association (ANA). (1995 edition). *Nursing: A social policy statement*. Washington, DC: Author.

American Nurses Association (ANA). (2010). *Nursing: A social policy statement*. Washington, DC: Author.

American Nurses Association (ANA). (2015). *Nursing: A social policy statement*. Washington, DC: Author.

Cabrera, D., & Cabrera, L. (2015). *Systems thinking made simple: New hope for solving wicked problems*. New York, NY: Odyssean Press.

D'Amour, D., & Oandasan, I. (2005). Interprofessionality as the field of interprofessional practice and interprofessional education: An emerging concept. *Journal of Interprofessional Care, 19*(Suppl. 1), 8–20.

Einstein, A. (1995). Letter to an editor of a German magazine. In A. Eddington (Ed.), *Essential Einstein* (p. 30, 1995). Rohnert Park, CA: Pomegranate Art Books. (Original letter written 1927)

Hawkins, D. R., Paul, R., & Elder, L. (2010). *The thinker's guide to clinical reasoning*. Tomales, CA: Foundation for Critical Thinking.

Henderson, V. (1961). *Basic principles of nursing care*. London, UK: International Council of Nurses. Retrieved from http://www.aacn.nche.edu/education-resources/ipecreport.pdf

Institute of Medicine (IOM). (2010). *The future of nursing: Leading change, advancing health*. Leading Change, Advancing Health Committee on the Robert Wood Johnson Foundation Initiative on the Future of Nursing, at the Institute of Medicine; National Academy of

Sciences. Retrieved from http://www.nap.edu/catalog/12956.html; http://www.thefutureofnursing.org/sites/default/files/4%20Transforming%20Education%20%28139-184%29.pdf

Interprofessional Education Collaborative Expert Panel. (2011). *Core competencies for interprofessional collaborative practice: Report of an expert panel.* Washington, DC: Interprofessional Education Collaborative. Retrieved from https://ipecollaborative.org/uploads/IPEC-Core-Competencies.pdf

Johnson, J. L. (1991). Nursing science: Basic, applied, or practical? Implications for the art of nursing. *Advances in Nursing Science, 14*(1), 7–16.

Johnson, J. L. (1994). A dialectical examination of nursing art. *Advances in Nursing Science, 17*(1), 1–14.

Kolb, A. Y., & Kolb, D. A. (2012). Experiential learning theory. In N. Seel (Ed.), *Encyclopedia of the sciences of learning* (pp. 1215–1219). New York, NY: Springer Publishing.

Kuiper, R. A. (2008). PDA use in clinical practice: A resource to support undergraduate baccalaureate nursing student clinical reasoning. *Computers Informatics Nursing, 26*(2), 80–89. Retrieved from http://journals.lww.com/cinjournal/toc/2008/03000

Kuiper, R. A., Heinrich, C., Matthias, A., Graham, M., & Bell-Kotwall, L. (2008). Evaluating situated cognition during simulation: Debriefing with the opt model of clinical reasoning. *International Journal of Nursing Education Scholarship, 5*(1), 1–14. Retrieved from http://www.bepress.com/ijnes/vol5/iss1/art17

Kuiper, R. A., Pesut, D., & Kautz, D. (2009). Promoting the self-regulation of clinical reasoning skills in nursing students. *Open Nursing Journal, 3*, 76–85. Retrieved from http://www.ncbi.nlm.nih.gov/pmc/articles/PMC2771264

Lamb, G. (2013). *Care coordination: The game changer.* American Nurses Association. Silver Spring, MD: Nurse Books.

National Council of State Boards of Nursing. (2008). Advanced Practice Registered Nurse (APRN) Consensus model. Retrieved from https://ncsbn.org/aprn.htm

National Council of State Boards of Nursing. (2012). Article XI of the 2012 Model Act for APRN Title and Scope of Practice document. Retrieved from https://ncsbn.org/2012_APRN_Model_and_Rules.pdf

National Organization of Nurse Practitioner Faculty (NONPF). (2015). Retrieved from http://www.nonpf.org/general/custom.asp?page=14

National Transitions of Care Coalition (NTOCC). (2008). *Improving transitions of care.* Washington, DC: Hogan & Hartson L.L.P. Retrieved from http://www.ntocc.org/Portals/0/PDF/Resources/TransitionsOfCare_Measures.pdf

Nightingale, F. (1946). *Notes on nursing: What it is and what it is not* (facsimile ed.). Philadelphia, PA: J. B. Lippincott. (Original work published 1859)

Pesut, D. J. (2001). Education: Clinical judgment: Foreground/background. *Journal of Professional Nursing: Official Journal of the American Association of Colleges of Nursing, 17*(5), 215.

Pesut, D. J. (2002). Nursing nomenclatures and eye-roll anxiety control. *Journal of Professional Nursing: Official Journal of the American Association of Colleges of Nursing, 18*(1), 3–4.

Pesut, D. J. (2004). Florence Nightingale: INTJ at work. *Reflections on nursing leadership/Sigma Theta Tau International, Honor Society of Nursing, 30*(3), 16–18, 44.

Pesut, D. J. (2006). 21st century nursing knowledge work: Reasoning into the future. In C. Weaver, C. W. Delaney, P. Weber, & R. Carr (Eds.), *Nursing and informatics for the 21st century: An international look at practice, trends and the future* (pp. 13–23). Chicago, IL: Health Care Information and Management Systems Society.

Pesut, D. J. (2008). Thoughts on thinking with complexity in mind. In C. Lindberg, S. Nash, & C. Lindberg (Eds.), *On the edge: Nursing in the age of complexity* (pp. 211–238). Bordentown, NJ: Plexus.

Pesut, D. J., & Herman, J. (1992). Metacognitive skills in diagnostic reasoning: Making the implicit explicit. *Nursing Diagnosis: ND: The Official Journal of the North American Nursing Diagnosis Association, 3*(4), 148–154.

Pesut, D. J., & Herman, J. (1998). OPT: Transformation of nursing process for contemporary practice. *Nursing Outlook, 46*(1), 29–36.

Pesut, D., & Herman, J. (1999). *Clinical reasoning: The art and science of critical and creative thinking.* New York, NY: Delmar.

Quinn, R. E., Bright, D., Faerman, S. R., Thompson, M. P., & McGrath, M. R. (2015). *Becoming a master manager: A competing values approach.* Hoboken, NJ: John Wiley & Sons.

Waters Foundation. (2015). *Habits of a systems thinker.* Pittsburgh, PA: Waters Foundation. Retrieved from http://watersfoundation.org/systems-thinking/habits-of-a-systems-thinker

CHAPTER 2

KNOWLEDGE COMPLEXITY AND CLINICAL REASONING: STANDARDIZED TERMINOLOGIES

In this chapter, the topics of knowledge complexity, nursing informatics, and standardized terminologies are discussed. Given the developments in nursing informatics over the years, nursing knowledge representation and knowledge complexity influence the way providers think and reason, as well as how they record and capture data with technology. Standardized terminologies provide clinicians with a clinical reasoning vocabulary. The value and importance of technology and developments in the field of nursing informatics are discussed. Levels of nursing practice data relevant to the clinical reasoning processes are described. Different levels of nursing practice data are used in making decisions, allocating resources, and contributing to development of professional nursing practice. With the advent of the electronic health record (EHR) and the accumulation of large databases, the opportunity to use evidence and data in a new and novel way is likely to influence thinking and reasoning into the future (Pesut, 2006).

The Health Care Information and Management Systems Society (HIMSS) and the American Medical Informatics Society provide leadership and background resources for understanding the role of technology and health information developments to support clinical care and reasoning. The Nursing Work Group of the American Medical Informatics Association (AMIA) has a long history of setting international and national standards that support the use of nursing knowledge in the world of health care. Health analytics (Burke, 2013) is likely to transform health care and the way that interprofessional teams reason about individual, family, community, and population health. Topol (2012) notes that the superconvergence of human data capture is likely to lead to the creative destruction of medicine as humans become digitalized. Ritt (2014) observes that advancements in analytics will improve patient outcomes, promote health and safety, and foster data-driven decision making, which will positively impact practice. Knowledge work is an essential element in advancing nursing science and practice. Advanced practice nurses need awareness and insight into the role that standardized terminologies play in building future nursing knowledge. Health analytics will alter the future of health care and the life sciences (McNeill, 2014).

LEARNING OUTCOMES

After completing this chapter, the reader should be able to:

1. Explain why knowledge work and the clinical vocabulary contained in unified medical language systems are important for clinical reasoning and evidence-based practice
2. Describe the knowledge complexity archetype and its consequences for nursing practice
3. Explain how nursing knowledge and other unified medical language systems support knowledge building and modeling into the future
4. Define nursing informatics
5. Explain why nursing informatics and health care information and management systems are important for organized nursing knowledge and for future work in health analytics
6. Discover resources and organizations like NANDA International, the Center for Nursing Classification, the Nursing Informatics Working Group of the AMIA, and the International Institute for Analytics

KNOWLEDGE WORK: FILTERS, FRAMES, AND FOCUS

Clinical reasoning presupposes knowledge work. Understanding how knowledge is represented and how knowledge language systems evolve and develop supports insight into the world of knowledge management. Such insight and understanding are essential for a full appreciation of types of knowledge that support performance, action, and learning. Knowledge is complex.

Knowledge is represented in resources like the International Classification of Diseases (ICD; World Health Organization, 2015) and the Unified Medical Language System (UMLS) of the U.S. National Library of Medicine (2015). These nationally recognized resources are important because many EHRs are organized to capture the data in these knowledge-representation systems to support the identification and tracking of essential health information. Nursing terms are embedded in these systems and provide nurses with ways to capture essential nursing data and knowledge. Capturing this knowledge supports ongoing data mining and pattern recognition in regard to the epidemiology of nursing diagnoses, interventions, and outcomes and supports the evolution and development of health analytics (McNeill, 2014). A useful classification system has a specific purpose, well-defined criteria for inclusion of items in categories, criteria that consistently and reliably assign items to categories, and makes sense to informed users. When classification systems meet these criteria, they provide the clinical vocabulary for clinical reasoning and assist the nurse to name patient problems, communicate with peers concerning the patient, and communicate with other disciplines concerning the nature of nursing's contribution to care (American Nurses Association [ANA], 2012).

The knowledge classification or standardized terminology that the advanced practice clinician uses in practice often serves as a filter for recording and ultimately thinking and reasoning about the management of problems, outcomes, and interventions. Filters help support framing and give specific meanings to a set of facts. Framing and "meaning making" then enable the advanced practice clinician to focus on a specific problem, which, in turn, can be transformed into a desired outcome and influenced by the choice of an intervention in service of a clinical judgment about the degree of outcome achievement.

Often the EHR is the vehicle through which nursing data and information are captured and stored. Sometimes medical framing of problems, outcomes, and interventions is necessary and these medical problems and issues have nursing care consequences. Medical framing and nursing framing of problems are complementary in nature. Framing from a nursing perspective is valuable in the care coordination process. What is important in terms of filtering, framing, and focus is that clinicians be conscious and intentional about the way they frame the facts associated with a client or a patient's story. Nursing informatics scholars have spent many years representing and coding nursing languages to capture the nursing framing of client conditions. Such nursing knowledge work has helped nursing define its unique contribution to health care and also has built a foundation on which nursing research and data science can evolve. The distinctions, system rules, relationships, and perspectives are important to be able to fully appreciate the contributions of disciplines to care coordination efforts and to support a systems-thinking mind-set.

NURSING INFORMATICS: EVOLVING NURSING KNOWLEDGE WORK

In 2016, the American Medical Informatics Association (AMIA), the nursing special interest group, defines nursing informatics as the "science and practice [that] integrates nursing, its information and knowledge, with management of information and communication technologies to promote the health of people, families, and communities worldwide" (American Medical Informatics Association, 2016). The application of nursing informatics knowledge is empowering for all health care practitioners in achieving patient-centered care. Nurse informaticians work to advance health care as developers of communication and information technologies, educators, researchers, chief nursing officers, chief information officers, software engineers, implementation consultants, policy developers, and business owners. Core areas of work include:

1. Concept representation and standards to support evidence-based practice, research, and education
2. Data and communication standards to build an interoperable national data infrastructure
3. Research methodologies to disseminate new knowledge into practice
4. Information presentation and retrieval approaches to support safe patient-centered care
5. Information and communication technologies to address interprofessional workflow needs across all care venues
6. Vision and management for the development, design, and implementation of communication and information technology
7. Definition of health care policy to advance the public's health

The work of nurse informaticians and much of nursing informatics efforts have become a part of the U.S. National Library of Medicine Unified Medical Language System (UMLS), which categorizes many health and biomedical vocabularies to enable interoperability among computer systems. To learn more about UMLS visit the National Library of Medicine or review the quick start guide to UMLS (https://www.nlm.nih.gov/research/umls/quickstart.html; U.S. National Library of Medicine, 2015) about the mapping and tracking of nursing terminologies in the meta-thesaurus of unified medical language. Do you know what the seven standard nursing terminologies are that are included in the UMLS? If not, explore the explanation and description about the representation of nursing terminologies in the UMLS (www.ncbi.nlm.nih.gov/pmc/articles/PMC3243214).

In addition, there are other models for care coordination. Haas, Swan, and Haynes (2014) have identified essential competencies and the basics of a care coordination curriculum stemming from an ambulatory care model. The Care Coordination and Transition Model (CCTM) curriculum educates professional nurses in the areas of advocacy, education and the engagement of patients and families, coaching and counseling of patients and families, patient-centered care planning, support for self-management, nursing process as a proxy for monitoring and evaluation, teamwork and collaboration, cross-setting communications and care transitions, population health management, care coordination and transition management between acute care and ambulatory care, informatics nursing practice, and telehealth nursing practice (Haas et al., 2014). These competencies all require attention to knowledge archetypes and knowledge work.

THE KNOWLEDGE-COMPLEXITY ARCHETYPE

In the world of informatics there is the notion that data lead to information, information leads to knowledge, and knowledge evolves into wisdom. Allee (1997, 2003) suggests that there is more to the process and has proposed an archetype that makes explicit the complexity of knowledge. Table 2.1 illustrates the levels and categories of what Allee defines as the Knowledge Complexity Archetype (1997, 2003). Reflect on the dimensions of the Knowledge Complexity Archetype table and consider how each aspect or facet of knowledge and learning informs action and performance and clinical reasoning activities. Also give attention to the span of time and perspective that is required to appreciate and value how the knowledge elements fit together. How do you think this Knowledge Complexity Archetype relates to the development of clinical reasoning for care coordination?

In Allee's model, knowledge gained through instinctual learning supports sensing and feedback for here-and-now moments. Gathered data lead to the development of information, which can be used to support learning and help define the most efficient way to accomplish a goal or a task. As people gain experience and reflect on the information they have acquired, knowledge grows and develops. Through self-conscious reflection the advanced practice clinician can discern how best to use knowledge in the most effective ways. The meaning that the advanced practice clinician attributes to knowledge gained supports understanding and productivity, and the effective use of resources. This type of meaning making requires sensitivity to time and communal learning. Communal learning coupled with a sense of past

TABLE 2.1 Knowledge-Complexity Archetype

KNOWLEDGE AND LEARNING MODE	ACTION AND PERFORMANCE FOCUS	TIME PERSPECTIVE AND CONSCIOUSNESS
DATA (instinctual learning) *Sensing.* The data mode of learning is at the sensory or input level. Little actual learning takes place.	DATA (feedback) *Gathering information.* Receiving input, registering data without reflection.	Time perspective: immediate moment Consciousness: awareness
INFORMATION (single-loop learning) *Action without reflection.* Procedural learning entails redirecting a course of action to follow a predetermined course. Learning occurs mostly through trial and error.	PROCEDURAL (efficiency) *Doing something the most efficient way.* Conforming to standards or making simple adjustments and modifications. Focus is on developing and following procedures.	Time perspective: Very short (present—now) Consciousness: physical sentience
KNOWLEDGE (double-loop learning) *Self-conscious reflection.* This requires a broad perspective that involves evaluation and modification of the goal or objective, as well as design of the path or procedures used to get there. Learning requires self-conscious reflection.	FUNCTIONAL (effectiveness) *Doing it the best way.* Evaluating and choosing between two or more alternative paths. Goals are effective action and resolution of inconsistencies. Focus is on effective work design and engineering aspects such as process redesign.	Time perspective: short (immediate past and present) Consciousness: self-reflective
MEANING (communal learning) *Understanding context, relationships, and trends.* Learning requires the making of meaning, which includes understanding context, seeing trends, and generating alternatives. From this perspective, it is possible to detect relationships among components as well as to comprehend roles and relationships among people.	MANAGING (productivity) *Understanding what promotes or impedes effectiveness.* This involves effective management and allocation of resources and tasks, using conceptual frameworks to analyze and tack multiple variables. It encompasses planning and measuring results. Also attends to working roles, relationships, and culture.	Time perspective: medium to long (historic past, present, very near future) Consciousness: communal

(continued)

TABLE 2.1 Knowledge Complexity Archetype *(continued)*

KNOWLEDGE AND LEARNING MODE	ACTION AND PERFORMANCE FOCUS	TIME PERSPECTIVE AND CONSCIOUSNESS
PHILOSOPHY (secondary learning) *Self-organizing.* Integrative or systemic learning seeks to understand dynamic relationships and nonlinear processes, discerning the patterns that connect, including archetypes and metaphors. Requires recognition of the embeddedness and interdependence of systems.	INTEGRATING (optimization) *Seeing where an activity fits within the whole picture.* This involves understanding and managing sociocultural system dynamics. Focus is on long-term planning and the ability to adapt to a changing environment. Comprises long-range forecasting, development of multilevel strategies, and evaluating investments and policies with regard to long-term success.	Time perspective: long term (past, present, and future) Consciousness: pattern
WISDOM (generative learning) *Value driven.* This is learning for the joy of learning, in open interaction with the environment. It involves creative processes, heuristic, open-ended explorations, and profound self-questioning. Allows one to discover his or her highest capabilities and talents, purpose, and intentions.	RENEWING (integrity) *Finding or reconnecting with one's purpose.* This refers to defining or reconnecting with values, vision, and mission. Understanding purpose. Very long-term time frame leads to deep awareness of ecology, community, and ethical action.	Time perspective: very long term (very distant past to far distant future) Consciousness: ethical
UNION (synergistic) *Connection.* Learning integrates direct experience and appreciation of oneness or deep connection with the greater cosmos. Requires processes that connect purpose to the health and well-being of the larger community and the environment.	UNION (sustainability) *Understanding values in greater context.* An intergenerational time perspective evokes commitment to the greater good of society, the environment, and the planet. Performance is demonstrated in actions consistent with these deeper values.	Time perspective: inter-generational, timeless Consciousness: universal

Source: Allee (2003).

history and present circumstance lays the foundation for self-organization and the development of a philosophy of how things fit together in a system. Throughout time, the knowledge, learning, and action of communal learning leads to the development of wisdom about the importance of the ecology of communities and the world. Wisdom gained supports insight into the connections and dynamic relationships between and among people and things in the greater whole. In the end, the advanced practice clinician realizes that there is a unity of insight that is necessary if sustainability is to be achieved through actions, learning, and performance.

A wise and effective health care provider is a knowledge worker who is conscious of his or her filtering, framing, and focusing in terms of knowledge representations. Such a person understands and appreciates the work that has gone into the development of nursing knowledge classification systems, standardized terminologies, as well as the creation of the UMLS and how they are related to each other. And although nursing terms may be embedded in these systems, future health analytic work (Burke, 2013; McNeill, 2014) will depend on the ways and means that the nursing terminology can be cross referenced and mapped to contribute to the creation of comparative, descriptive, prescriptive, and predictive analytics (Ritt, 2014). There are different levels of data that can be aggregated and used to develop nursing analytics. Understanding the role that data play at different levels of perspective in regard to care coordination clinical reasoning is an important value-clarification exercise. Organizing nursing knowledge for purposes of practice, education, and research is a professional responsibility that supports the optimization, integrity, and sustainability of the Knowledge-Complexity Archetype model.

LEVELS OF NURSING PRACTICE DATA

The Center for Clinical Effectiveness at the University of Iowa developed the model shown in Figure 2.1 to illustrate three levels of nursing practice data: the individual level, the unit/organization level, and the network/state/country level (Center for Nursing Classification and Clinical Effectiveness, 2016). It is essential that advanced nurses understand and value the importance and the interdependence of each level of practice data from a systems-thinking perspective. Students and clinicians are likely to resolve the individual level of practice data for clinical reasoning. Knowledge in these systems contributes to the filters, frames, and focus that nurses employ to reason about patient-care needs and clinical decision making. Represented knowledge is also then used for documentation of care delivered. Managers and administrators are most likely to value the unit-level data. Administrators and researchers are most interested in the network-, state-, and country-level data. All nurses need to be informed about these levels of practice data because these data, taken together, help describe and define nursing's contribution to the health care enterprise. Such contributions are the foundation for future health-analytic work (McNeill, 2014). Clinical testing and evaluation of classification systems for practice is an ongoing professional responsibility and contributes to the analytics needed to monitor care, quality, and the effective use of resources to advance nursing science and knowledge work.

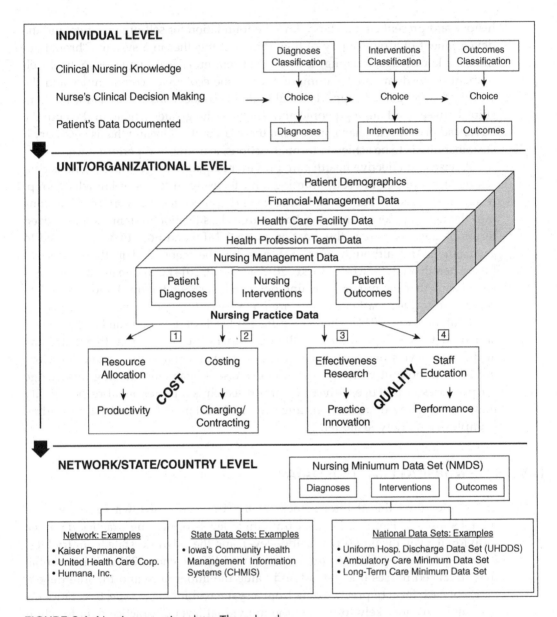

FIGURE 2.1 Nursing practice data: Three levels.

Reprinted with permission from Center for Nursing Classification and Clinical Effectiveness (2016).

Individual-Level Data

The level of immediate interest to most practicing nurses is the individual level. At this level, practice data are organized so that data are relevant and useful in explaining patient problems, nursing interventions, outcomes, and clinical choices and decisions that nurses can make. Information about the patient and the context is explained through the use of clinical knowledge that has been standardized in the form of classification systems or standardized terminology (ANA, 2012). If this information is collected and used according to a standardized system, it can be aggregated and used in a broader context at the unit or organizational level. Developments at this level are expanding, as groups and organizations continue to focus on development of nursing diagnoses, interventions, and outcomes.

Unit/Organization-Level Data

At the unit or organizational level, data about individual patients are combined into one system. This system can be linked to other information systems such as the medical care information system. At this level, analyses about common kinds of treatment can be performed according to four possible parameters: resources, costs, effectiveness, and education. Using data for resource allocation results in measures of productivity. Data related to costs provide information about charging and contracting. Using data used to support effectiveness research has consequences for practice innovations. Data about staff performance can be used for evaluation and planning. Each institution defines and specifies the type of information most useful for documenting patterns and trends for nursing service in the organization. If you have aspirations to become a nurse manager, unit/organizational-level data will be important.

Network/State/Country-Level Data

The network/state/country level represents the broadest scope of data about nursing activities. At this level, the Nursing Minimum Data Set (NMDS) provides an important contribution to the data-management needs of many systems. What do you think are essential pieces of nursing information? A group of nurse researchers believes the NMDS is a good place to start. The NMDS is a set of variables with uniform definitions and categories concerning the specific dimensions of nursing, which meets the information needs of multiple data users in the macro health care system (American Medical Informatics Association, 2016; Werley, Ryan, & Zorn, 1995). The purpose of the NMDS is to standardize information associated with nursing care that patients received in a variety of service settings. There are three elements in the data set: nursing care data, patient data, and service data. Nursing care data elements consist of (a) nursing diagnosis, (b) nursing intervention, (c) nursing outcome, and (d) intensity of nursing care. Patient data elements consist of (a) personal identification and (b) demographic characteristic such as date of birth, sex, ethnicity, and residence. Service data elements include (a) unique facility or service agency number, (b) unique health record of patient, (c) unique number of principal registered nurse providers, (d) episode admission or encounter date, (e) discharge date, (f) disposition of patient, and (g) expected payer.

Benefits of this kind of data set include uniform collection of data that can be compared across a variety of parameters, identification of trends related to patient problems and nursing care provided, and reliable data for quality-assurance evaluation and costing of nursing service. In addition, such a database promotes comparative research on nursing care, including research on nursing diagnoses, interventions, outcomes, and other clinical nursing research-based questions. Many efforts are being channeled to develop the NMDS. Many organizations and projects are devoted to developing the elements for the minimum data set. Consequences of this development include creation of a data bank to research projects about nursing care.

Most clinicians are most involved with the individual level of practice-relevant data. It is at this level that they make choices and decisions about the kind of patient problems or diagnoses identified, outcomes established, and the interventions chosen. Working in a team requires that the members of the team respect and value the filtering, framing, and perspective taking of the different disciplines. Nurses may collect data and cluster signs and symptoms inductively to build diagnoses using a nursing filter. However, the system in which the advanced practice clinician works may expect a different kind of filter or framing and require clinicians to use ICD-10 codes. Care coordination clinical reasoning challenges the advanced practice clinician to manage the competing values associated with both filters and frames to arrive at a focus. How does the advanced practice clinician negotiate and reconcile ICD-10 codes to gain insight into the nursing care issues and consequences associated with those medical diagnoses? As an advanced practice clinician, do you always filter and frame from a nursing perspective? Or perhaps you were taught to filter and frame information from a medical condition perspective? Filtering and framing are important aspects of the clinical reasoning process. Appreciating and valuing the long-term use and consequences of standardized data collection informs and influences one' motivation and understanding of how data can be used to generate knowledge that leads to insights and health analytic discoveries at different levels of perspective: patients, systems, populations.

Table 2.2 represents an attempt to illustrate nursing domains of practice from the filtering and framing perspective. In this conceptualization, one sees the four domains of nursing practice and interest: functional, physiological, psychosocial, and environmental. Under these major domains are classes of diagnoses, outcomes, and interventions. Many of the major nursing diagnoses, interventions, and outcomes are mapped in the UMLS and meta-thesaurus of the National Library of Medicine and thus are embedded in a number of EHRs in order to capture nursing-sensitive data for analysis, evaluation, and use in health analytic computations and projections.

Expanding the standardized language issue further, Table 2.3 represents a crosswalk from nursing domains to ICD-10 codes and medical diagnoses used by advanced practice nurses for reimbursement categorization. Harmonizing nursing domains with reimbursement codes captures the professional language of nursing, medicine, and other health professionals from the UMLS and meta-thesaurus of the National Library of Medicine. When the languages are united in the EHRs, the different interprofessional disciplines are united in focus and are in the best position to communicate and move toward the same patient outcomes. The harmonization of language can only bridge the gaps that currently exist between providers and offer the best data for health analytic computations and projections. Care coordination clinical reasoning presents a challenge because of the need to integrate and combine all of the health care team providers' disciplinary filters and frames to create and specify the focus of care and treatment. How the advanced practice clinician uses the knowledge stored in EHRs depends on the context of practice, knowledge, beliefs, values, and professional identity. As nursing continues to evolve, and data, information, and knowledge stored in EHRs become an important filter, frame, and

TABLE 2.2 Harmonizing Nursing Language and Domains Taxonomy of Nursing Practice: A Common Unified Structure for Nursing Language

	DOMAINS		
I. Functional Domain Includes diagnoses, outcomes, and interventions to promote basic needs	**II. Physiological Domain** Includes diagnoses, outcomes, and interventions to promote optimal biophysical health	**III. Psychosocial Domain** Includes diagnoses, outcomes, and interventions to promote optimal mental and emotional health and social functioning	**IV. Environmental Domain** Includes diagnoses, outcomes, and interventions to promote basic needs

CLASSES

Includes diagnoses, class outcomes, and interventions that pertain to:

I. Functional Domain	II. Physiological Domain	III. Psychosocial Domain	IV. Environmental Domain
Activity/Exercise—Physical activity, including energy conservation and expenditure	**Cardiac Function**—Cardiac mechanisms used to maintain tissue profusion	**Behavior**—Actions that promote, maintain, or restore health	**Health Care System**—Social, political, and economic structures and processes for the delivery of health care services.
Comfort—A sense of emotional, physical, and spiritual well-being and relative freedom from distress	**Elimination**—Processes related to secretion and excretion of body wastes	**Communication**—Receiving, interpreting, and expressing spoken, written, and nonverbal messages	**Populations**—Aggregates of individuals or communities with common characteristics
Growth and Development—Physical, emotional, and social growth and development milestones	**Fluid and Electrolyte**—Regulation of fluid/electrolytes and acid base balance	**Coping**—Adjusting or adapting to stressful events	**Risk Management**—Avoidance or control of identifiable health threats
Nutrition—Processes related to taking in, assimilating, and using nutrients	**Neurocognition**—Mechanisms related to the nervous system and neurocognitive functioning, including memory, thinking, and judgment	**Emotion**—A mental state or feeling that may influence perceptions of the world	

(continued)

43

TABLE 2.2 Harmonizing Nursing Language and Domains Taxonomy of Nursing Practice: A Common Unified Structure for Nursing Language (continued)

CLASSES		
Self-Care—Ability to accomplish basic and instrumental activities of daily living	**Pharmacological Function**—Effects (therapeutic and adverse) of medications or drugs and other pharmacologically active products	**Knowledge**—Information and skills applied to promote, maintain, and restore health
Sexuality—Maintenance or modification of sexual identity and patterns	**Physical Regulation**—Includes body temperature, endocrine and immune system responses to regulate cellular processes	**Roles/Relationships**—Maintenance and/or modification of expected social behaviors and emotional connectedness with others
Sleep/Rest—The quantity and quality of sleep, rest, and relaxation patterns	**Reproduction**—Processes related to human procreation and birth	**Self-Perception**—Awareness of one's body and personal identity
Values/Beliefs—Ideas, goals, perceptions, convictions that influence choices or decisions	**Respiratory Function**—Ventilation adequate to maintain arterial blood gases within normal limits	
	Sensation/Perception—Intake and interception of information through the senses, including seeing, hearing, touching, tasting, and smelling.	
	Tissue Integrity—Skin and mucous membrane protection to support secretion, excretion, and healing	

Source: Dochterman and Jones (2003).

TABLE 2.3 Harmonizing Nursing Domains and Medical Diagnoses

NURSING DOMAINS	ICD-10 CODES
Health Promotion • Deficient dimensional activity • Sedentary lifestyle • Deficient community health • Risk-prone health behavior • Ineffective health maintenance • Readiness for enhanced immunization status • Ineffective protection • Ineffective self-health management • Readiness for enhanced self-health management • Ineffective family therapeutic regimen management	C00–D49: Neoplasms E00–E89: Endocrine, nutritional, and metabolic diseases R00–R99: Symptoms, signs, and abnormal clinical and laboratory findings, not elsewhere classified
Nutrition • Insufficient breast milk • Ineffective infant feeding pattern • Imbalanced nutrition: less than bodily requirements • Imbalanced nutrition: more than bodily requirements • Readiness for enhanced nutrition • Impaired swallowing • Risk for unstable blood glucose level • Neonatal jaundice • Risk for neonatal jaundice • Risk for impaired liver function • Risk for electrolyte imbalance • Readiness for enhanced fluid balance • Deficient fluid volume • Excess fluid volume • Risk for deficient fluid volume • Risk for imbalanced fluid volume	C00–D49: Neoplasms E00–E89: Endocrine, nutritional, and metabolic diseases K00–K95: Diseases of the digestive system O00–O9A: Pregnancy, childbirth, and the puerperium
Elimination and Exchange • Functional urinary incontinence • Overflow urinary incontinence • Reflex urinary incontinence • Stress urinary incontinence • Urge urinary incontinence • Risk for urge urinary incontinence • Impaired urinary elimination • Readiness for enhanced urinary elimination • Urinary retention • Constipation • Perceived constipation • Risk for constipation	C00–D49: Neoplasms K00–K95: Diseases of the digestive system N00–N99: Diseases of the genitourinary system

(continued)

TABLE 2.3 Harmonizing Nursing Domains and Medical Diagnoses   *(continued)*

NURSING DOMAINS	ICD-10 CODES
<ul><li>Diarrhea</li><li>Dysfunctional gastrointestinal motility</li><li>Risk for dysfunctional gastrointestinal motility</li><li>Bowel incontinence</li><li>Impaired gas exchange</li></ul>	
Sexuality<ul><li>Sexual dysfunction</li><li>Ineffective sexuality pattern</li><li>Ineffective childbearing process</li><li>Readiness for enhanced childbearing process</li><li>Risk for ineffective childbearing process</li><li>Risk for disturbed maternal–fetal dyad</li></ul>	C00–D49: Neoplasms F01–F99: Mental, behavioral, and neurodevelopmental disorders N00–N99: Diseases of the genitourinary system O00–O9A: Pregnancy, childbirth, and the puerperium P00–P96: Certain conditions originating in the perinatal period Q00–Q99: Congenital malformations, deformations, and chromosomal abnormalities
Activity/Rest<ul><li>Insomnia</li><li>Sleep deprivation</li><li>Readiness for enhanced sleep</li><li>Disturbed sleep pattern</li><li>Risk for disuse syndrome</li><li>Impaired bed mobility</li><li>Impaired physical mobility</li><li>Impaired wheelchair mobility</li><li>Impaired transfer ability</li><li>Impaired walking</li><li>Disturbed energy field</li><li>Fatigue</li><li>Wandering</li><li>Activity intolerance</li><li>Risk for activity intolerance</li><li>Ineffective breathing pattern</li><li>Decreased cardiac output</li><li>Risk for ineffective gastrointestinal perfusion</li><li>Risk for ineffective renal perfusion</li><li>Impaired spontaneous ventilation</li><li>Ineffective peripheral tissue perfusion</li><li>Risk for decreased cardiac tissue perfusion</li></ul>	C00–D49: Neoplasms I00–I99: Diseases of the circulatory system J00–J99: Diseases of the respiratory system L00–L99: Diseases of the skin and subcutaneous tissue M00–M99: Diseases of the musculoskeletal system and connective tissue R00–R99: Symptoms, signs, and abnormal clinical and laboratory findings, not elsewhere classified V00–Y99: External causes of morbidity Z00–Z99: Factors influencing health status and contact with health services

(continued)

TABLE 2.3 Harmonizing Nursing Domains and Medical Diagnoses *(continued)*

NURSING DOMAINS	ICD-10 CODES
• Risk for ineffective cerebral tissue perfusion • Dysfunctional ventilatory-weaning response • Impaired home maintenance • Readiness for enhanced self-care • Bathing self-care deficit • Dressing self-care deficit • Feeding self-care deficit • Toileting self-care deficit • Self-neglect	
Perception/Cognition • Unilateral neglect • Impaired environmental interpretation syndrome • Acute confusion • Chronic confusion • Risk for acute confusion • Ineffective impulse control • Deficient knowledge • Readiness for enhanced knowledge • Impaired memory • Readiness for enhanced communication • Impaired verbal communication	C00–D49: Neoplasms F01–F99: Mental, behavioral, and neurodevelopmental disorders G00–G99: Diseases of the nervous system H00–H59: Diseases of the eye and adnexa H60–H95: Diseases of the ear and mastoid process R00–R99: Symptoms, signs, and abnormal clinical and laboratory findings, not elsewhere classified
Self-Perception • Hopelessness • Risk for compromised human dignity • Risk for loneliness • Disturbed personal identity • Risk for disturbed personal identity • Readiness for enhanced self-control • Chronic low self-esteem • Risk for chronic low self-esteem • Risk for situational low self-esteem • Situational low self-esteem • Disturbed body image	F01–F99: Mental, behavioral, and neurodevelopmental disorders
Role Relationships • Ineffective breastfeeding • Interrupted breastfeeding • Readiness for enhanced breastfeeding • Caregiver role strain • Risk for caregiver role strain • Impaired parenting • Readiness for enhanced parenting • Risk for impaired parenting	F01–F99: Mental, behavioral, and neurodevelopmental disorders O00–O9A: Pregnancy, childbirth, and the puerperium Q00–Q99: Congenital malformations, deformations, and chromosomal abnormalities Z00–Z99: Factors influencing health status and contact with health services

(continued)

TABLE 2.3 Harmonizing Nursing Domains and Medical Diagnoses *(continued)*

NURSING DOMAINS	ICD-10 CODES
• Risk for impaired attachment • Dysfunctional family processes • Interrupted family processes • Readiness for enhanced family processes • Ineffective relationship • Readiness for enhanced relationship • Risk for ineffective relationship • Parental role conflict • Ineffective role performance • Impaired social interaction **Coping/Stress Tolerance** • Posttraumatic stress disorder • Risk for posttrauma syndrome • Rape-trauma syndrome • Relocation stress syndrome • Risk for relocation stress syndrome • Ineffective activity planning • Risk for ineffective activity planning • Anxiety • Compromised family coping • Defensive coping • Disabled family coping • Ineffective coping • Ineffective community coping • Readiness for enhanced coping • Readiness for enhanced family coping • Death anxiety • Ineffective denial • Adult failure to thrive • Fear • Grieving • Complicated grieving • Risk for complicated grieving • Readiness for enhanced power • Powerlessness • Risk for powerlessness • Impaired individual resilience • Readiness for enhanced resilience • Risk for compromised resilience • Chronic sorrow • Stress overload	C00–D49: Neoplasms F01–F99: Mental, behavioral, and neurodevelopmental disorders G00–G99: Diseases of the nervous system R00–R99: Symptoms, signs, and abnormal clinical and laboratory findings, not elsewhere classified Z00–Z99: Factors influencing health status and contact with health services

(continued)

TABLE 2.3 Harmonizing Nursing Domains and Medical Diagnoses *(continued)*

NURSING DOMAINS	ICD-10 CODES
• Risk for disorganized infant behavior • Autonomic dysreflexia • Disorganized infant behavior • Readiness for enhanced organized infant behavior • Decreased intracranial capacity	
Growth/Development • Risk for disproportionate growth • Delayed growth and development • Risk for delayed development	C00–D49: Neoplasms E00–E89: Endocrine, nutritional, and metabolic diseases F01–F99: Mental, behavioral, and neurodevelopmental disorders Z00–Z99: Factors influencing health status and contact with health services
Life Principles • Readiness for enhanced hope • Readiness for enhanced spiritual well-being • Readiness for enhanced decision making • Decisional conflict • Moral distress • Noncompliance • Impaired religiosity • Readiness for enhanced religiosity • Risk for impaired religiosity • Spiritual distress • Risk for spiritual distress	C00–D49: Neoplasms F01–F99: Mental, behavioral, and neurodevelopmental disorders R00–R99: Symptoms, signs, and abnormal clinical and laboratory findings, not elsewhere classified Z00–Z99: Factors influencing health status and contact with health services
Safety/Protection • Risk for infection • Ineffective airway clearance • Risk for aspiration • Risk for bleeding • Impaired dentition • Risk for dry eye • Risk for falls • Risk for injury • Impaired oral mucous membrane • Risk for perioperative positioning injury • Risk for peripheral neurovascular dysfunction • Risk for shock • Impaired skin integrity • Risk for impaired skin integrity • Risk for sudden infant death syndrome	A00–B99: Certain infectious and parasitic diseases E00–E89: Endocrine, nutritional, and metabolic diseases D50–D89: Diseases of the blood and blood-forming organs and certain disorders involving the immune mechanism F01–F99: Mental, behavioral, and neurodevelopmental disorders H00–H59: Diseases of the eye and adnexa

(continued)

TABLE 2.3 Harmonizing Nursing Domains and Medical Diagnoses (*continued*)

NURSING DOMAINS	ICD-10 CODES
• Risk for suffocation • Risk for thermal injury • Risk for trauma • Risk for vascular trauma • Risk for other directed violence • Risk for self-directed violence • Self-mutilation • Risk for suicide • Contamination • Risk for contamination • Risk for poisoning • Risk for adverse reaction to iodinated contrast media • Latex allergy response • Risk for imbalanced body temperature • Hyperthermia • Hypothermia • Ineffective thermoregulation	I00–I99: Diseases of the circulatory system J00–J99: Diseases of the respiratory system L00–L99: Diseases of the skin and subcutaneous tissues P00–P96: Certain conditions originating in the perinatal period S00–T88: Injury, poisoning, and certain other consequences of external causes Z00–Z99: Factors influencing health status and contact with health services
Comfort • Impaired comfort • Readiness for enhanced comfort • Nausea • Acute pain • Chronic pain • Readiness for enhanced comfort • Social isolation	F01–F99: Mental, behavioral, and neurodevelopmental disorders R00–R99: Symptoms, signs, and abnormal clinical and laboratory findings, not elsewhere classified

ICD-10, International Classification of Diseases, 10th edition.
Source: World Health Organization (2015).

focus, clinical scholarship will evolve to produce comparative, descriptive, prescriptive, and predictive health analytics (Burke, 2013, McNeill, 2014; Ritt, 2014).

Members of the profession have an obligation and responsibility to stay informed, use, and refine the knowledge contained in these systems. Such responsibility requires communal learning and the development of a philosophy that supports the integration and optimization of the Knowledge-Complexity Archetype for the profession (Allee, 2003). The knowledge captured in these systems is the vocabulary that is used for clinical reasoning. Imagine what the next 10 to 20 years will be like, as hospitals and health care agencies begin to incorporate standardized nursing language into the information systems and electronic records. Pesut (2006) suggests that over the next 10 years, the fourth generation of nursing process (2020–2040) might be devoted to and organized around knowledge building and predictive analytics. As databases and systems are linked together with a common nursing language system it then becomes possible to discover and data mine these repositories so that we can learn from analysis of the patterns and relationships between and among nursing diagnoses, interventions, and outcomes.

As data accrue, it is likely that we will begin to develop predictive analytics from nursing data that is empirically based and can inform best practices and provide new treatment options based on experience and clinical insights (Burke, 2013; McNeill, 2014). As we refine these archetypes of care, we can learn about the occurrence and epidemiology of nursing diagnoses, interventions, and outcomes for specific patient populations. We might also sort the data by type of institution or level of primary, secondary, or tertiary care needs. As we gain more experience and understanding of what patterns are occurring, nurses can plan the care patients need more effectively and efficiently. Simulations of patient care scenarios may in fact aid us in clinical reasoning, clinical decision making, and better clinical judgments. Evolution of these developments will focus nurses on the knowledge development and management strategies that support nursing care practices.

The fact is that nursing process has changed and evolved over and through time (Pesut, 2006). In the next chapter, we discuss the evolution and transformation of nursing process and describe how the traditional conceptions of nursing process have changed in response to developments in nursing knowledge work, the adoption of standardized terminology, the press and push for use of EHRs and evidence regarding how humans process information and reason about complex and uncertain reasoning challenges.

As you will see in subsequent chapters, the Outcome-Present State-Test (OPT) model provides a structure that uses standardized terminology in a logical and artful way. Key to the success of this knowledge-complexity work is appreciating and valuing the importance and use of standardized terminology, the use of the EHR, and the evolving developments in nursing knowledge work supported by informatics and health analytic techniques and discoveries.

SUMMARY

Four trends supporting continued change and transformations of the clinical reasoning and nursing knowledge work are (a) developments in nursing informatics, (b) use of standardized nursing knowledge classification systems and the UMLS, (c) use of EHRs, and (d) use of more sophisticated data-analysis techniques. As data and experience with nursing care practices are captured, health services researchers are able to analyze and evaluate nurse-sensitive patient-care data and information that support 21st-century nursing knowledge work.

KEY CONCEPTS

1. The development of classification systems is important in order to standardize language about nursing diagnoses, interventions, and outcomes as well as other unified medical language terminologies and systems.
2. Each discipline uses knowledge representation and terminology to filter, frame, and focus on problem identification, outcome specification, and interventions.

3. In addition to classification systems, there are three levels of nursing practice data relevant to nurses. The individual level; the unit or organization level; and the state, national, or local level.
4. NANDA International has a rich history and many resources that trace the development and evolution of nursing diagnoses and nursing knowledge classification systems.
5. The Center for Nursing Classification and Clinical effectiveness (CNCC) provides references and resources for understanding the development of nursing diagnoses, interventions, and outcomes.
6. Health analytics is an emerging field of health study that is likely to accelerate knowledge work and life science insights through the use of data science.

STUDY QUESTIONS AND ACTIVITIES

1. Discover the latest information about the ICD at the World Health Organization website: www.who.int/classifications/icd/en
2. Explore the AMIA: www.amia.org/about-amia/mission-and-history
3. Review the history and development of NANDA International: www.nanda .org/nanda-international-history.html
4. Visit the Nursing Working Group of the American Medical Informatics Association: www.amia.org/programs/working-groups/nursing-informatics
5. Explore representation of nursing terminologies in the UMLS of the National Library of Medicine: www.ncbi.nlm.nih.gov/pmc/articles/PMC3243214
6. Listen to this tutorial regarding searching for nursing terms in the UMLS of the National Library of Medicine: www.nlm.nih.gov/research/umls/user_ education/quick_tours/Nursing_tutorial.html
7. Visit the Center for Nursing Classification and Clinical Effectiveness website at the University of Iowa to learn more about nursing intervention and nursing outcome classifications systems: www.nursing.uiowa.edu/ center-for-nursing-classification-and-clinical-effectiveness

REFERENCES

Allee, V. (1997). *The knowledge evolution: Expanding organizational intelligence.* Boston, MA: Butterworth Heinemann.

Allee, V. (2003). *The future of knowledge: Increasing prosperity through value networks.* Burlington, MA: Elsevier.

American Medical Informatics Association (AMIA). (2016). *Nursing Informatics Working Group.* Retrieved from https://www.amia.org/programs/working-groups/nursing-informatics

American Nurses Association (ANA). (2012). *ANA recognized terminologies that support nursing practice.* Silver Spring, MD: American Nurses Association. Retrieved from http:// www.nursingworld.org/MainMenuCategories/ThePracticeofProfessionalNursing/ NursingStandards/Recognized-Nursing-Practice-Terminologies.pdf

Burke, J. (2013). *Health analytics: Gaining insight to transform health care.* Hoboken, NJ: John Wiley & Sons.

Center for Nursing Classification and Clinical Effectiveness. (2016). Iowa City, IA: College of Nursing, The University of Iowa. Retrieved from http://www.nursing.uiowa.edu/center-for-nursing-classification-and-clinical-effectiveness

Dochterman, J. M., & Jones, D. A. (Eds.). (2003). *Unifying nursing language: The harmonization of NANDA, NIC and NOC*. Washington, DC: Nursebooks.org

Haas, S. A., Swan, B. A., & Haynes, T. S. (2014). *Care coordination and transition management core curriculum*. Pitman, NJ: American Academy of Ambulatory Care Nursing.

McNeill, D. (2014). *Analytics in healthcare and the life sciences: Strategies, implementation and best practices*. International Institute for Analytics. Upper Saddle River, NJ: Pearson.

NANDA International. (n.d.). *History, Philadelphia: North American Nursing Diagnosis Association*. Retrieved from http://www.nanda.org/nanda-international-history.html

Pesut, D. J. (2006). Twenty-first century nursing knowledge work: Reasoning into the future. In C. Weaver, C. Delany, P. Weber, & R. Carr (Eds.), *Nursing informatics for the 21st century: An international look at practice, trends and the future* (pp. 13–23). Chicago, IL: Health Care Information and Management Systems Society. Retrieved from http://acquire.cqu.edu.au:8080/vital/access/manager/Repository/cqu:5046

Ritt, E. (2014). Essential analytics in nursing education: Building capacity to improve clinical practice. *Journal of Nursing Education and Practice, 4*(2), 9–12.

Topol, E. (2012). *The creative destruction of medicine*. New York, NY: Basic Books.

U. S. National Library of Medicine. (2015). *Unified medical language system*. Bethesda, MD: U. S. National Library of Medicine. Retrieved from https://www.nlm.nih.gov/research/umls

Werley, H. H., Ryan, P., & Zorn, C. R. (1995). The Nursing Minimum Data Set (NMDS): A framework for the organization of nursing language. In N. M. Lang (Ed.), *Nursing data system: The emerging framework* (pp. 19–30). Washington, DC: American Nurses Association.

World Health Organization (WHO). (2015). *Manual of the International Classification of Diseases and related health problems* (10th rev. ed.). Geneva, Switzerland: Author. Retrieved from http://www.icd10data.com

CHAPTER 3

THE EVOLVING NATURE OF NURSING PROCESS AND CLINICAL REASONING

The nursing process in its various forms has always been the foundation for patient problem management since Florence Nightingale (1859/1946) first described it. When considering the evolution of the nursing process over time, one has to appreciate the evolving nature of professional identity; developments in informatics; knowledge representation and classification systems; and concurrent insights and developments related to critical, creative, systems and complexity-thinking processes. The major phases in the nursing process and associated clinical-thinking strategies have been described in the literature, which spans six decades of change and can be classified into several generations.

LEARNING OUTCOMES

After completing this chapter, the reader should be able to:

1. Describe the evolution and development of nursing process models through time
2. Appreciate the role and development of nursing knowledge work through time and the impact and influence informatics and nursing knowledge representation have on clinical reasoning
3. Describe how to create and develop a clinical reasoning web to help visualize and represent the complexity and dynamic relationships between and among patient care problems and nursing care interventions, outcomes, and judgments
4. Master the self-regulatory thinking processes that support the Outcome-Present State-Test (OPT) model

DEVELOPMENTAL GENERATIONS OF NURSING PROCESS

Before the 1950s, there was not much attention paid to the thinking skills nurses needed to practice. Once nursing education moved from hospitals into university settings, the need developed for an academic discipline to discern the unique thinking strategies and skills nurses used to reason about patient care challenges. The first-generation (1950–1970) nursing process proposed was based on a problem-solving model and consisted of the following steps: assess, plan, implement, and evaluate (APIE). This structured, stepwise logic model was taught and learned as a linear process that focused on problems and pieces of a patient story, medical conditions, and associated nursing care responses. Evaluation was linked with problem identification and goal achievement. Over time, nurses realized that the problem–solutions they identified in practice were redundant and could be classified and categorized according to the evolving nature and scope of nursing practice.

Nursing informatics as a specialty influenced the development of and quest for ways to represent nursing knowledge. Nursing diagnoses were developed and assimilated into the traditional APIE nursing process model. Nursing process evolved from a four-step process (APIE) to a five-step model: assess, diagnose, plan, implement, and evaluate (ADPIE). This development had profound implications on how nurses began to teach, learn, think, and reason about nursing care situations. With the advent of nursing knowledge representation systems and the beginning use of standardized nursing language, it was clear that nursing knowledge could be captured, analyzed, and evaluated and could yield insights into nursing patterns of care. Data could be transformed into information. Information could be transformed into knowledge. Knowledge could influence the way nurses think and reason and establish a repository of nursing knowledge that could be tested, evaluated, and support the development of nursing science. As nurses gained experience with the process, nursing knowledge classification models emerged and were based on nurses creating and naming phenomena of concern. Grand nursing theories gave way to more middle-range challenges in terms of specifying human responses to actual or potential health problems, which became the purview and definition of nursing. The North American Nursing Diagnosis Association (NANDA, 1994, 1996) assumed a leadership role in the creation and vetting of nursing diagnoses. Given the nursing diagnosis development work, the second generation of nursing process focused on the nature of diagnostic reasoning using the evolving diagnostic labels.

The second generation of nursing process (1970–1990) focused on developing insights and understanding regarding the nature of diagnosis and reasoning in nursing. Research in the area of diagnostic reasoning led to discoveries and insights about the advantages and disadvantages of the nursing process as a model and a method. Diagnosis of nursing problems shifted the nursing process model from one of problem identification and solution finding to thinking and reasoning about hypotheses and diagnoses. Diagnostic reasoning involved the recognition and clustering of cues and analysis of data given specific clinical situations. The shift from problem identification and solving to diagnostic reasoning was a revolution in thinking that continues to have ripple effects in contemporary nursing practice.

Studies on diagnostic reasoning and the critical thinking involved in nursing practice emerged (Facione & Facione, 1996; Jones & Brown, 1993; Kintgen-Andrews, 1991; Miller & Malcolm, 1990). *Nursing Diagnosis: Process and Application* by Marjory Gordon (1994) and *Diagnostic Reasoning in Nursing* by Carnevali, Mitchell, Woods, and Tanner (1984) described a way of thinking that offered an enhancement of the nursing process and was proposed to help nurses manage information and make decisions. They defined diagnostic reasoning as a pattern of steps beginning with pre-encounter data; entry into the data search field; shaping direction of data gathering, cue clustering, determining diagnostic hypotheses, focused cue search, and testing hypotheses for "goodness of fit" in order to derive a diagnosis. The nature and type of terms linked at that time with thinking in nursing changed from problem identification to hypothesis formulation and testing. Critical and creative thinking skills were essential to the development of nursing diagnoses and nursing knowledge. Continued evolution and development of nursing knowledge classification systems as well as continued research into the dynamics of clinical reasoning set the stage for another transformation of the nursing process. Table 3.1 outlines the American Nurses Association (ANA)-approved nursing languages and the classification systems or approved terminologies most often used by advanced practice providers (American Nurses Association [ANA], 2012).

The third generation of nursing process emerged (1990–2020) and highlighted a nursing process model that emphasized reflection, outcome specification, and testing given a patient's story. The OPT clinical reasoning model (Pesut & Herman, 1999), built on the heritage of the nursing process, was more responsive and relevant to contemporary nursing practice needs. Definitions and distinctions among the terms *clinical reasoning*, *clinical decision making*, and *clinical judgment* were made (Pesut & Herman, 1999).

Concurrently, Dr. Patricia Benner (1988) and her colleagues (Benner, Tanner, & Chesla, 1997) were studying nurses, thinking and discovered that novice nurses were not as sophisticated in their thinking skills as expert nurses. Based on her research, Benner (1988) reframed and renamed many of the daily activities in which nurses were involved. Her studies indicated that expert nurses did not necessarily use the nursing process, but relied on experience and intuition and a combination of practical and academic intelligence. Exemplars illustrated how nurses coupled thinking with caring and ethics. The role of intuition and the person as

TABLE 3.1 Standardized Nursing Languages

AMERICAN NURSES ASSOCIATION APPROVED LANGUAGES	ADVANCED PRACTICE LANGUAGES
1. NANDA International (NANDA-I)	1. International Classifications of Diseases (ICD-10) codes
2. Nursing Interventions Classifications (NIC)	2. The Omaha System
3. Nursing Outcomes Classification (NOC)	3. Systemized Nomenclature of Medicine—Clinical Terms (SNOMED CT)
4. Clinical Care Classification (CCC)	4. Clinical Care Classification (CCC)
5. The Omaha System	
6. Perioperative Nursing Data Set (PNDS)	
7. International Classification for Nursing Practice (ICNP)	
8. Systemized Nomenclature of Medicine—Clinical Terms (SNOMED CT)	
9. Logical Observation Identifiers Names and Codes (LOINC)	
10. Nursing Minimum Data Set (NMDS)	
11. Nursing Management Minimum Data Set (NMMDS)	
12. ABC Codes	

ABC, Alternative Billing Concepts.

Source: American Nurses Association (2012).

the focus in reasoning about care needs was highlighted. Rather than retrofit new knowledge into an old, linear, problem-solving process model, there was a need for an expanded model of reasoning. It was becoming clear that clinical reasoning included more than critical thinking and involved elements of creative thinking, systems thinking, ethical reasoning, and outcome specification. The development of the OPT clinical reasoning model accommodated the changes in nursing process over time. In this model, clinical reasoning is defined as the critical, reflective, concurrent, and creative thinking embedded in nursing practice that results in the juxtaposition of problems and outcomes that are subject to interventions and clinical judgments (Kuiper, 2002; Pesut & Herman, 1999).

The OPT clinical reasoning model provides a structure, a process, and strategies for thinking about multiple competing patient care needs in the context of the patient's story. As the nurse or clinicians reflect on and analyze how each of these needs or issues impacts and influences all the other needs, patterns emerge that reveal leverage points of intervention that can accelerate the specification of outcomes and provide foci for effective and efficient interventions. The OPT model supports contemporary definitions of the nursing process, which include assessment, diagnosis, outcome identification, planning, implementation, coordination of care, health teaching and promotion, and evaluation (ANA, 2015). The OPT clinical reasoning model differs considerably from the earlier generations of the nursing process. Its strengths include the following: the model builds on a foundation of reflective judgment and is derived from empirical data, the model honors the holistic nature of nursing, the model approaches patient situations in terms of outcomes, the model identifies the thinking skills and strategies involved in making clinical decisions and judgments, and the model can be used with interprofessional taxonomies that provide the content for clinical reasoning.

The OPT clinical reasoning model (Figure 3.1) uses the patient's story, diagnostic cluster cue and web logic, keystone priority, present to outcome states to determine tests, and interventions for health and illness management, all of which support the development and acquisition of skills in clinical reasoning and judgment.

MASTERING THE OPT MODEL OF CLINICAL REASONING

Patient-centered clinical reasoning is the first phase of care coordination and is used to determine the priorities between and among comorbidities the patient is dealing with. The OPT model provides a structure, a process, and a method that support patient-centered clinical reasoning. The major difference between the OPT clinical reasoning model and previous models is the OPT's emphasis on filters, framing, and focusing a situation and the gaps that exist between the problems identified and the outcomes desired. The gaps are based on the story of the patient, which is determined by an examination and history. The explicit focus on the patient's story is a way to frame relationships among contexts, present states, and desired outcomes. The OPT clinical reasoning model underscores the fact that reasoning is concurrent and iterative as side-by-side comparisons of outcomes with present-state information from the patient story create gaps that can be analyzed and evaluated as test conditions about which judgments and conclusions are made given decisions

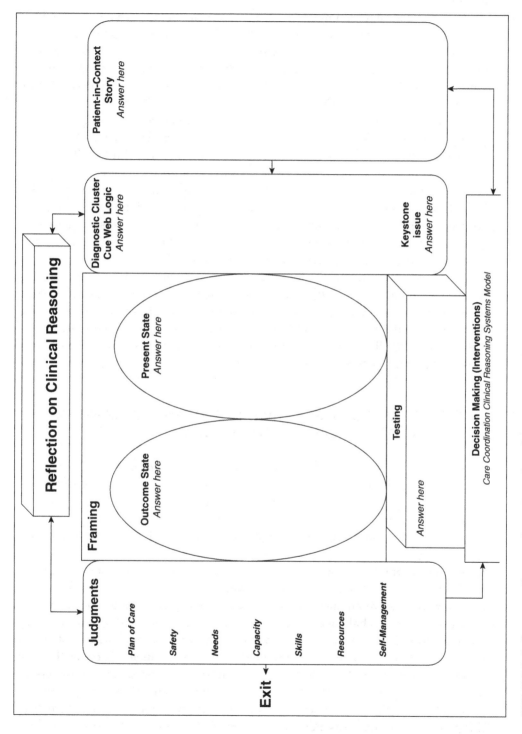

FIGURE 3.1 Outcome-Present State-Test clinical reasoning model.

and actions that fill the gaps. The OPT clinical reasoning model relies on higher order critical thinking skills, such as analysis, synthesis, evaluation, creativity, and judgment.

The OPT clinical reasoning model is a way to help identify what is important in a patient case and what outcomes you are trying to achieve for health and wellness. Based on the facts of the situation, providers make choices to get to the most acceptable outcomes from the patient-and-family story. The OPT clinical reasoning model is more likely than other models to be able to accommodate present and future knowledge development activities in nursing and other disciplines.

The first level of perspective challenge of patient-centered clinical reasoning is to represent all the issues and needs that patients' reveal. The second challenge is to consider how all these issues are related to one another. The third challenge is to find the keystone or priority issue that organizes the focus of care based on the story. Once the keystone issue is identified, other diagnostic concerns may resolve through activities surrounding the keystone issue. The OPT clinical reasoning web worksheet helps the advanced practice clinician define relationships among issues and highlights potential keystone issues. Developing a clinical reasoning web helps illustrate the art and science of clinical reasoning. The OPT clinical reasoning model is circular and fluid, and allows for visualization of several problems and the "big picture" at the same time. Delineating each problem and how it is related to all the others, and then developing a picture of the whole dynamic interaction, helps the nurse focus on the what, why, and how of a patient scenario once an outcome is specified to act to fill the gaps between problems and outcomes and promote transitions from present to desired states.

PATIENT-CENTERED REASONING: ACTIVATING SYSTEMS-THINKING SKILLS THROUGH THE USE OF CLINICAL REASONING WEBS

Patient stories are complex but with a little analysis and synthesis, complex stories can be simplified into key issues. An OPT clinical reasoning web is a useful method and tool used to illustrate the functional relationships between and among diagnoses, conditions, and diagnostic hypotheses derived from critical thinking that can result in divergent and convergent identification of central issues that necessitate nursing care.

Advanced practice clinicians could begin with a medical diagnosis or a nursing diagnosis in mind when they begin planning of care. Whichever is primarily in the forefront, there are medical and nursing consequences to be considered for each. The reasoning challenge begins with a description and understanding of the patient's story. Framing the story and discerning the issues that need attention are crucial. Thinking about one's thinking helps one evaluate, discover flaws in thinking, and adjust and develop one's clinical reasoning skills. One of the essential parts of the OPT clinical reasoning is reflection. Some of the components of self-regulatory reflection are self-monitoring, self-evaluation, and self-correction. This process is referred to as metacognition. For example, one way to begin patient-centered reasoning is to spin and weave a web of relationships among identified nursing diagnoses associated with medical conditions.

Spinning and weaving a web is the process of using thinking strategies to analyze and synthesize functional relationships between and among diagnostic hypotheses associated with a patient's health status. The steps to the creation of an OPT clinical reasoning web using the worksheet are as follows:

1. Place a general description of the patient in the respective middle circle.
2. Place the major medical diagnoses in the respective middle circle.
3. Place the major nursing diagnoses in the respective middle circle.
4. Choose the nursing domain for which each medical nursing diagnosis is appropriate.
5. Generate all the International Classification of Diseases (ICD)-10 codes that would result from the particular patient-and-family story that coincide with the nursing domains (World Health Organization, 2015).
6. Reflect on the total picture on the worksheet and begin to draw lines of relationship, connection, or association among the diagnoses. As you draw the lines, try to justify and explain your reasons for connecting these diagnoses.
7. Determine which pattern has the highest priority for care coordination and most efficiently and effectively represents the keystone nursing care needs of the patient.
8. Look once again at the sets of relationships and determine the theme that summarizes the patient-in-context or the patient's story.

The OPT clinical reasoning web worksheet seen in Figure 3.2 shows a template with the patient health care situation, medical diagnoses, and nursing diagnoses in the center. Around the outer edges of the web are nursing domains with ICD-10 codes derived from history and physical assessment associated with the patient story. The multidirectional arrows that create the web effect are functional relationships between and among the diagnostic possibilities. Through the use of self-talk and if–then thinking, clinicians can challenge themselves to explain the explicit relationships between and among the competing issues. How does one condition affect the other? What are the relationships, consequences, and/or impact and outcome of the concurrent conditions? As one can see, the domains and ICD-10 codes with more arrows converging on one of the circles display the priority problem or keystone, in this case, activity and rest. Keystone issues are one or more central supporting elements of the patient's story that guide reasoning and care coordination based on an analysis and synthesis of diagnostic possibilities as represented in the web.

THE OPT CLINICAL REASONING MODEL

After considering the whole picture using the clinical reasoning web worksheet, the next step is to use the OPT clinical reasoning model worksheet to structure the provider's reasoning about relationships between and among problems, outcomes, interventions, decision making, and judgments. As the provider thinks about the patient, he or she will concurrently consider the frame, the outcome state, and the present state. Each aspect of the OPT clinical reasoning model contributes to the other. The OPT clinical reasoning model worksheet is a map of the structure, which is

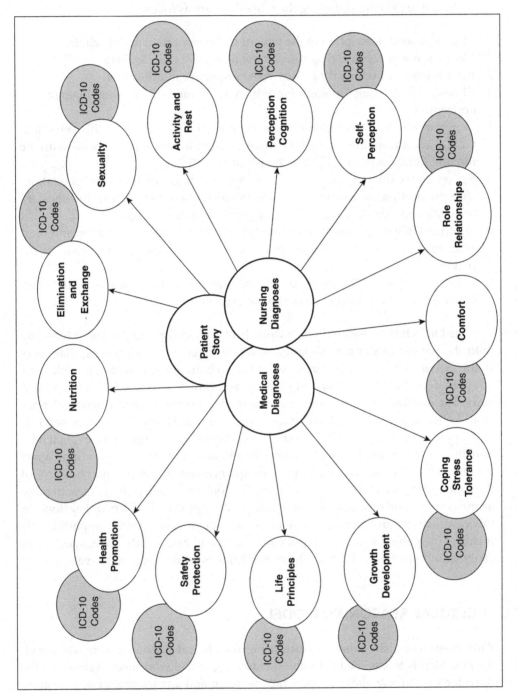

FIGURE 3.2 Outcome-Present State-Test clinical reasoning web worksheet.
ICD-10, International Classification of Diseases, 10th edition.

designed to provide a representation and guide thinking about relationships between and among competing issues, problems, outcomes, interventions, and judgments.

By writing each element on the worksheet, it is easy to see how parts of the model relate to each other. For example, as seen in Figure 3.1, on the far right-hand side, there is space to write the patient's story. This space is called the patient-in-context. It is a place for the provider to make notes and jot down relevant facts of the story. Moving to the left, there are places to write down inferences and conclusions that result from the provider's logic and analysis of the facts between and among the diagnoses and relationships. Remember diagnostic cluster cue web logic is supported by the use of inductive and deductive thinking.

At the center and background of the worksheet are places to indicate the frame or theme that best represents the background issues regarding thinking about the patient story. The frame is the theme that often emerges after the creation of an OPT clinical reasoning web. The frame helps organize the present state and the outcome state, and illustrates the gap and provides insights about what tests or interventions are needed to fill the gap. Frames depend on the advanced practice clinician's filters and on distinctions being made about salient features of the case and story. Decision making and reflection surround the framing as the advanced practice clinician thinks of all the patient-centered elements concurrently. Reflective thinking is used to monitor thinking and self-regulate thinking.

At the center of the worksheet are spaces to place the present state and outcome state side by side. Putting the two states together in this way creates a gap analysis that naturally shows where and what the goals are in terms of the patient's care. The gap between where the patient is and where you want the patient to be is one way to create a test. Tests are really gap analyses. Clinical decisions are choices made about interventions that will help the patient transition from present state to a desired outcome state. One is constantly updating and "testing" the degree to which outcomes are being achieved or are not based on the results of the interventions. Testing is concurrent and iterative as one gets closer and closer in successive increments toward goal achievement.

The "reflection on clinical reasoning" box at the top of Figure 3.1 is a reminder of the thinking strategies used for the patient situation. These strategies also help make explicit many of the relationships among ideas and issues associated with the patient's problems. Finally, the judgment space on the far left-hand side of the figure is the place to write in the results of the conclusions drawn from a test. Based on the degree of gap or comparison of where the patient is and where the provider wants the patient to be, there may or may not be an evidence gap. Once the provider gets evidence that fills that gap, he or she has to attribute meaning to the data. Making judgments about clinical issues is all about the meaning the provider attributes to the evidence derived from the test or gap analysis of the present to the desired state.

Once a provider has experience coordinating care for patients, the cases become part of a clinical reasoning learning history. These schema experiences inform future thinking with patients who are similar to those with whom the provider has had experiences. These schemata and experience build on each other over time and result in the development of pattern recognition for future clinical reasoning applications. If the scenario results in a negative judgment, or progress is not being made to transition patients from present to desired states, the provider may have to reframe the situation and reconsider the problem to be solved, the outcome to be achieved, or the framing of the situation.

CLINICAL REASONING: FRAMING AND PERSPECTIVES

A patient's story provides important information about the context and major issues for clinical reasoning. Listening to patients, connecting with them in meaningful ways, attributing meaning to their stories, and getting the facts of their situation constitute the art of nursing. Stories are a key element of clinical reasoning. How you "frame" a story has implications for how you reason. For example, consider the following case: George Appleton is a 99-year-old gentleman in a long-term care facility with a diagnosis of end-stage renal disease. If you "frame" this situation as the need to keep George comfortable and maintain a urinary output to excrete metabolic waste products, how does such a frame guide and direct your thinking and doing? Would your thinking and doing be different if the "frame" or lens you used to view this situation involved "promoting a peaceful death?" How would your thinking and actions be different given these two different perspectives?

We constantly frame situations. Frames are mental models or perceptual positions we have about issues, events, and meanings. Peter Senge (1990) discusses mental models in his book *The Fifth Discipline*. Mental models determine how we make sense of the world and take action. Senge writes:

> Mental models can be simple generalizations such as "people are untrustworthy" or they can be complex theories, such as assumptions about why members of my family interact as they do. But what is most important to grasp is that mental models are active—they shape how we act. If we believe people are untrustworthy, we act differently from the way we would if we believed they were trustworthy. If I believe that my son lacks self-confidence and my daughter is highly aggressive, I will continually intervene in their exchanges to prevent her from damaging his ego. (1990, p. 175)

Frames are mental models that influence and guide our perception and behavior. Becoming aware of mental models in regard to patient stories is an important aspect of clinical reasoning. In their book, *The Art of Framing*, Fairhurst and Sarr (1996) write, "to hold the frame of a subject is to choose one particular meaning or set of meanings over another" (p. 21). Here are some other observations they have about the importance of framing:

1. Framing is a way to manage meaning. It involves the selection and highlighting of one or more aspects of a subject while excluding others.
2. Framing involves use of language, thought, and forethought. Language helps to focus, classify, remember, and understand one thing in terms of another.
3. Framing increases our chances of implementing goals and getting people's agreement because once the right frames are in place the right behavior follows.
4. Framing requires initiative, which includes both a clarity of purpose and a thorough understanding of those for whom we are managing meaning.

5. Opportunities for framing occur with every communication.
6. Our values play an important role in the kind of framing that we do and in the way that we and our frames are perceived (p. 22).

Think of frames as different types of camera lenses. A wide-angle lens frames a scene much differently than a close-up zoom lens. Becoming aware of mental models and the frames we put on patient stories is crucial to successful clinical reasoning. We become aware of frames through stories patients share with us and the meanings we attribute to those stories. The meaning we attribute to patient stories is often translated into shorthand themes. For example, after listening to some one's story, we might conclude that it is an issue about frustration, anxiety, coping, or some other theme. Framing is understandable when we take time to reflect on what we see, hear, know, and feel in the clinical moment. Framing is like the headline or caption of a patient's situation or story. Critical thinking skills, reflective reasoning, and specific thinking strategies support framing and reasoning.

REFLECTION

When using the OPT clinical reasoning model worksheets, the provider engages in reflection as a component of executive-thinking processes; reflection consists of critical, creative, and concurrent systems and complexity thinking. Reflection is the process of observing one's thinking while simultaneously thinking about patient situations. The goal of reflection is to achieve the best possible thought processes. The greater the reflection, the higher the quality of care delivered. Reflection involves use of the skills of monitoring, analyzing, predicting, planning, evaluating, and revising. Critical thinking consists of developing the following skills of interpretation: analysis, inference, explanation, evaluation, and self-regulation (Facione & Facione, 1996). Some questions that guide the use of the OPT clinical reasoning model are shown in Table 3.2 (Pesut, 2008).

Working with the OPT clinical reasoning model worksheets involves critical, creative, complexity, and systems thinking as one considers multiple interactions of various elements in a situation (Pesut, 2008). The knowledge representation and framing of nursing phenomena involving patient care needs is complex and nurses have to adjust their thinking along with it. The specific critical, creative, and complexity-thinking activities that enable one to perform clinical reasoning are gained through practice, conscious reflection, and attention to issues associated with a patient's story and context of practice. The patient-centered systems thinking defined in the OPT clinical reasoning model is derived from critical thinking, creative thinking, and complexity thinking principles and practices that lead to framing, understanding system dynamics, and ultimately the juxtaposition of present states with desired outcome states. Keystone issues are the central supporting element of the patient story derived from analysis of system dynamics and the complexity of relationships among identified diagnoses. Combining all types of thinking with an understanding of the complexity of relationships embedded in a particular patient story gives rise to the challenge of complexity thinking about how the individual patient and family needs interact as a system of care, and are

TABLE 3.2 Questions That Guide the Use of the OPT Model

Patient-in-context	What is the patient story?
Diagnostic cue/web logic	What diagnoses have you generated?
	What outcomes do you have in mind given the diagnoses?
	What evidence supports those diagnoses?
	How does a reasoning web reveal relationships among the identified problems (diagnoses)?
	What keystone issue(s) emerge?
Framing	How are you framing the situation?
Present state	How is the present state defined?
Outcome state	What are the desired outcomes?
	What are the gaps or complementary pairs (~) of outcomes and present states?
Test	What are the clinical indicators of the desired outcomes?
	On what scales will the desired outcomes be rated?
	How will you know when the desired outcomes are achieved?
	How are you defining your testing in this particular case?
Decision making (interventions)	What clinical decisions or interventions help to achieve the outcomes?
	What specific intervention activities will you implement?
	Why are you considering these activities?
Judgment	Given your testing, what is your clinical judgment?
	Based on your judgment, have you achieved the outcome or do you need to reframe the situation?
	How, specifically, will you take this experience and learning with you into the future as you reason about similar cases?

OPT, Outcome-Present State-Test.

Adapted from Pesut (2008).

affected by relationships with care providers and the context in which they live and work. Providers seldom take time to compare and contrast the framing of patient issues and the complexity of relationships between and among those issues when considering a patient's needs.

It is important to reflect on the framing and complexity of patient issues to plan interventions to achieve outcomes. The prompts listed in Table 3.3 can be used to support reflection framing and patient-centered care planning. In the next section, thinking skills and strategies that support clinical reasoning are described, defined, and discussed.

STRATEGIES THAT SUPPORT THE DEVELOPMENT OF CLINICAL REASONING

There are some specific thinking strategies that support the development of clinical-reasoning skills. Many of these strategies are metacognitive in nature. Each of the

TABLE 3.3 Reflection Prompts to Support Self-Regulated Clinical Reasoning

1. The essence of this story is...
2. When I think about this situation, I think...
3. The particular diagnoses I would identify for this situation...
4. When I search for the evidence that supports these diagnoses, I think I...
5. When I look back on the themes that emerge...
6. When I prepare to frame the situation I...
7. In framing this situation I should have
   a. spent more time on...
   b. spent less time on...
8. I made sure I defined the present state by...
9. I made sure I defined the outcome state by...
10. When I think about the gap between the outcome and present situation...
11. When I need resources to determine evidence to fill this gap...
12. My impression of the desired outcomes...
13. As I look back, I know the outcome was achieved by...
14. The clinical decisions that help the patient to transition...
15. I think my ability to make clinical judgments for this situation...
16. When I am considering the choices and decisions...and if I need help...
17. The environment in which I must make clinical judgments...
18. My reaction to my clinical judgments...
19. The past experiences I have that influenced my thinking in this situation...
20. The consequence of the reasoning web for this situation shows...

Source: Kuiper, Pesut, and Kautz (2009). Used with permission.

following strategies is discussed: attention to knowledge work, self-talk, prototype identification or pattern recognition (schema searches), hypothesizing, activation of if–then thinking, comparative analysis, juxtaposing to ascertain gaps between present and desired states, activating reflexive comparisons, reframing, and reflection checks.

Clinical reasoning presupposes that you have done the *knowledge work* of reading, memorizing, drilling, writing, and practicing. This knowledge work is necessary to gain the clinical vocabulary of the classification systems in order to interpret data about the patient-in-context. Oftentimes the knowledge work that one needs is provided by the electronic health care record or the systems of care processes that are in place in an organization. It is very difficult to generate diagnostic hypotheses for a patient case if one does not know the definitions and classifications of disease states or domains of nursing care knowledge that provide the disciplinary knowledge base for the provider. Other fundamental knowledge areas needed to plan care for patients include knowledge about physiological, psychological, and sociological functioning. Fundamental knowledge in these areas includes such things as normal and abnormal laboratory values, and the psychodynamics of anxiety and fear. Fundamental knowledge in these areas helps one to interpret, analyze, explain, and infer what is going on in a case to support clinical reasoning. The thinking strategies of self-talk, schema search, prototype identification, hypothesizing, if–then/how-so thinking, comparative analysis, juxtaposing, and reflexive comparison are defined and described here.

Self-talk is the process of expressing one's thoughts to one's self. Self-talk answers the question: What are the nursing diagnostic possibilities associated with the medical conditions of disease states? The answer to this question results in the identification of the diagnostic hypotheses relevant to the case. For example, the human responses to emphysema include such things as ineffective breathing pattern, impaired gas exchange, fatigue, anxiety, and fear. Self-talk also is useful when spinning and weaving clinical reasoning webs. One has to think out loud and reason about the possible relationships and give voice to connections among diagnostic hypotheses and their relationships to one another.

Schema search is the process of accessing general and/or specific patterns of past experiences that might apply to the current situation. The reason that advanced practice students prefer to have a large number of clinical experiences is the fact that those experiences help them build schemata. Past clinical experiences are helpful in reasoning about a specific case. One way to develop expertise is to use self-talk as you build schemata. Each experience you have with a patient creates a web in your mind. The more experiences you have, the more complex the web, the greater the number of patterns developed, and the easier it is to access those patterns or neural networks. Novices are in the process of spinning and weaving memory webs with each clinical experience. Experts have multiple webs superimposed on one another. That is why they can reason about situations so effectively and quickly. The schema includes what a particular patient exhibited, what interventions were made, and what the outcomes were. These memories become the foundation for clinical reasoning expertise.

Prototype identification is using a model case as a reference point for comparative analysis. A patient with a disease condition represents one instance of a person with that disease. Knowing what the prototypical patient in an acute crisis is likely to exhibit serves as a standard. With prototype identification, one uses textbook cases as the standard and a reference point for comparative analysis. Prototypes or simulations enable one to create the neural network connections that lead to the formation and development of patterns that can be recognized. A major part of clinical reasoning is the pattern-recognition match between what one knows and has experienced and comparing that information with what one is observing and assessing. Through time, patterns of experience help with the development of schemata. Prototype identification activates and reinforces schema development.

Hypothesizing is determining an explanation that accounts for a set of facts that can be tested by further investigation. Hypothesizing presupposes use and understanding of clinical vocabulary. Explanations for circumstances in a case are called diagnostic hypotheses. They are guesses about what might explain a situation and high-risk sequelae. Testing the hypotheses we make about patient cases has to be supported by data or we have to keep searching for the reality in a situation.

The diagnostic hypotheses become the origins and insertion points for making associations when one develops a clinical reasoning web. Hypothesizing includes if–then/how-so thinking; however, it is a more formal statement or declaration about how specifically sets of facts are related. Hypothesis testing requires gathering evidence under controlled conditions to affirm or negate the proposed relationship. Spinning and weaving the webs for individual case care coordination result in a number of diagnostic hypotheses. Once diagnoses are identified, it is easier to see how these diagnoses might be related through hypothesizing.

If–then/how-so thinking involves linking ideas and consequences together in a logical sequence. This type of thinking is used to connect diagnoses and care coordination needs in the respective webs. The linking of ideas and consequences together in a logical sequence is at the heart of clinical reasoning. It is also the place to start developing the plan of care and determining what resources are required for care coordination.

Comparative analysis is a thinking strategy that involves considering the strengths and weaknesses of competing alternatives. Once diagnostic hypotheses and their relationships are made explicit using the webs, comparative analysis is used to determine which of these relationships is the keystone or the central supporting issues of a situation. Identifying the keystone issues enables the advanced practice nurse to focus on care. Once a keystone issue is identified, it has a domino effect in that it can influence other problems and needs.

Juxtaposing is another essential strategy. Think of juxtaposing as creation of a gap analysis. Juxtaposing involves putting the present-state condition next to the outcome state. The side-by-side contrast of one state with the other illustrates the differences or gaps between the two states. The differences or gaps evident from the present to the desired state help establish the conditions for the creation of a test in the OPT model. A test is satisfied if the gap is closed. As one determines the practice issues, interventions, and outcomes in the care coordination model, the successive achievement of the desired outcome helps to close the gap and successfully pass the test(s). Juxtaposing enables one to set up essential elements between two states. Decisions that one makes and interventions one initiates help bridge the gap between juxtaposed conditions.

Reflexive comparison is the strategy that involves constant comparison of the patient's state from one time period of observation to another period of observation. For example, each time a laboratory test value is reviewed, the advanced practice nurse or provider compares a patient's progress from one observation to the next. In this way, the advanced practice nurse or provider is using the patient as his or her own standard in terms of making progress toward the desired outcome state. This represents an ipsative versus a normative model of comparison.

Reframing is the strategy that attributes different meaning to the content or context of a situation given a set of cues, tests, decisions, or judgments. Remember, clinical reasoning combines reflective, concurrent, creative, critical, systems, and complexity thinking embedded in nursing practice that nurses use to frame, juxtapose, and test the match between a patient's present state and the desired outcome state. It may be that one needs to reframe the keystone issue. The challenge now becomes how one assists a patient transition from one state to another. Another way to reframe the situation is to consider how, through care coordination, the patient and family can more effectively manage their own therapeutic regimen. Reframing is the thinking strategy that enables one to attribute different meaning given the story and context and reflection on the situation.

A *reflection check* involves reflecting and analyzing the patient-centered, team-centered, and organization-centered thinking using critical, creative, complexity, and systems strategies that support clinical reasoning. Reflection check is the process

TABLE 3.4 Thinking Strategies and Definitions

THINKING STRATEGY	DEFINITION
Knowledge work	Active use of reading, memorizing, drilling, writing, reviewing, and practicing to learn clinical vocabulary
Self-talk	Expressing one's thoughts to one's self
Schema search	Accessing general and/or specific patterns of past experiences that might apply to the current situation
Prototype identification	Using a model case as a reference point for comparative analysis
Hypothesizing	Determining an explanation that accounts for a set of facts that can be tested by further investigation
If–then/how-so thinking	Linking ideas and consequences together in a logical sequence with an explanation of how they are related
Comparative analysis	Considering the strengths and weaknesses of competing alternatives
Juxtaposing	Putting the present-state condition next to the outcome state in a side-by-side comparison
Reflexive comparison	Constantly comparing the patient's state from one time of observation to another time of observation
Reframing	Attributing a different meaning to the content or context of a situation based on tests, decisions, or judgments
Reflection check	Self-examination and self-correction of critical thinking skills and thinking strategies that support clinical reasoning

of intentionally using self-regulation strategies of self-monitoring, self-correcting, self-reinforcing, and self-evaluating one's own thinking about a specific task or situation (Herman, Pesut, & Conard, 1994; Kuiper & Pesut, 2004; Pesut & Herman, 1992; Worrell, 1990). A reflection check pinpoints all that you have done correctly, identifies errors, and provides an opportunity to understand how to correct them. A reflection check involves understanding how the thinking skills and strategies described thus far support reflective clinical reasoning. Table 3.4 defines the thinking strategies described previously.

The strategies previously described and displayed in Table 3.5 come together during case analysis to make clinical decisions. Clinical decision making involves the selection of interventions, actions, and issues that move patients from a presenting state to a specified or desired outcome state. In other words, what interprofessional actions and interventions, as coordinated by the advanced practice nurse, are necessary to bring the present state and the outcome state closer together? Decision making is supported through the use and application of schema searches and prototype identification. Comparative analysis is the process of considering the strengths and weaknesses of competing alternatives. If–then/how-so thinking also supports decision making.

During testing, the advanced practice nurse determines how well the gap has been filled between the present and the outcome state. Testing is accomplished

TABLE 3.5 Comparison of Thinking Strategies, Critical Thinking Skills, and Reflective Clinical Reasoning

THINKING STRATEGIES	CRITICAL THINKING SKILLS	REFLECTIVE CLINICAL REASONING
Reading	Interpretation	Knowledge work
Memorizing	Categorize	Clinical vocabulary
Drilling	Decode sentences	Standardized terminologies
Writing	Clarify meaning	
Reviewing		
Practicing		
Self-talk	Analysis	Web logic
Schema search	Examine ideas	Cue connection
Prototype identification	Identify arguments	Induction
Hypothesizing	Analyze arguments	Deduction
		Retroduction
Schema search	Inference	Framing
Prototype identification	Query evidence	Cue connection
Hypothesizing	Conjecture alternatives	Scenario development
If–then/how-so thinking	Draw conclusions	Outcome specification
		Test creation
Schema search	Explanation	Decision making
Prototype identification	State results	Interventions
Comparative analysis	Justify procedures	Alternatives
If–then/how-so thinking	Present arguments	Consequences
Juxtaposing	Evaluation	Testing
Comparative analysis	Assess claims	Conduct test
Reflexive comparison	Assess arguments	Evaluate
Reframing	Self-regulation	Judgment
Reflection check	Self-examination	Attribute meaning to the test outcome
	Self-correction	Frame new situation
		Create new test

through the use and application of comparative analysis and reflexive comparison, which is the process of making a judgment about the state of a situation after gauging the presence or absence of some quality against a standard using the current case as a reference criterion (Fowler, 1994). For example, how does a wound look 1 week after treatment? Conclusions related to tests are the bases of clinical judgments.

Judgments are made by drawing conclusions based on the findings from the tests of comparing the present state to a specified outcome state, and the result of organizational systems thinking. Once judgments of the present state closely match the desired outcomes (a wound is healed), the advanced practice nurse can reason about other things. If a match or test is unsatisfactory (infection still present), reflection activates critical, creative, concurrent thinking and decision making. In terms of judgments, three conclusions are possible: (a) a perfect match between the outcome state and the present state (e.g., wound is healed), (b) a partial match of the outcome state with the present state (wound healing is progressing but not complete), and (c) no match between the outcome and the present state (wound is not healed and looks worse). Judgments result in reflection and clinical decision making about achieving a satisfactory match between patient's present state and the outcome state. Thinking strategies that support judgment are reframing or the process of attributing a different meaning to the facts or evidence at hand. Finally, a reflection about the entire process results in self-correction.

Clinically, focusing on the present state or presenting problems does not provide explicit direction for action. Once outcomes are specified, the path of action is clear and the tests of achievement are explicit. Transforming problems into outcomes involves thinking beyond the present to the end results of action. This must include care coordination activities and reflection on the provider, team, and organizational systems in order to achieve success. One can appreciate how thinking strategies and critical thinking skills are embedded in reflective clinical reasoning. Table 3.5 compares thinking strategies, critical thinking skills, and reflective clinical reasoning, all of which are used during the process of systems thinking at the provider, team, and organizational levels.

SUMMARY

The OPT clinical reasoning model provides the structure for clinical reasoning for the provider so that he or she can reason and think systemically about the individual patient-and-family case. The OPT model provides the foundational level for identification of the patients' essential needs and their related practice issues, interventions, outcomes, and values. The thinking strategies discussed in this chapter provide the tools to support and scaffold the strategies and skills required to achieve insights about the problems that need to be managed. The learning tools introduced in this chapter serve as the foundation for reasoning about patient-centered cases across various contexts. The next chapter introduces the care coordination clinical reasoning model. This model builds on the foundation of the OPT model and is enhanced with special attention to the team, care coordination, and health system perspectives that are essential to care coordination across health care contexts and services.

KEY CONCEPTS

1. Clinical reasoning for care coordination can be promoted in advanced practice nursing students with a framework that includes structure, content, and process.
2. A supporting framework for care coordination clinical reasoning begins with case management using provider systems thinking and the OPT clinical reasoning model.

3. Specific thinking strategies and tools that support the mastery of the OPT clinical reasoning model include intentional use of knowledge, self-talk, schema search, prototype identification and pattern recognition, hypothesizing, juxtaposing, if–then/how-so thinking, comparative analysis, reflexive comparison, reframing, and self-monitoring of reflection.

STUDY QUESTIONS AND ACTIVITIES

1. Describe in your own words the benefits and the process of using the OPT clinical reasoning model in identifying priority problems in a case with which you are familiar. What do you appreciate about the OPT model? How does it influence your thinking?
2. Identify all the possible standardized health care languages that were used or considered in a case in which you were recently involved. What were their similarities and differences? Did language have an impact on communication and the patient outcomes?
3. Identify the relationship among critical, creative, systems, and complexity thinking as these skills relate to critical reflection and thinking strategies as they are applied to the OPT model.

REFERENCES

American Nurses Association (ANA). (2012). *ANA recognized terminologies that support nursing practice.* Silver Spring, MD: Author. Retrieved from http://www.nursingworld.org/MainMenuCategories/ThePracticeofProfessionalNursing/NursingStandards/Recognized-Nursing-Practice-Terminologies.pdf

American Nurses Association (ANA). (2015). *Scope and standards of practice* (3rd ed.). Silver Spring, MD: Author.

Benner, P. (1988). *From novice to expert.* Menlo Park, CA: Addison Wesley.

Benner, P., Tanner, C., & Chesla, C. (1997). *Expertise in nursing practice.* New York, NY: Springer Publishing.

Carnevali, D., Mitchell, P., Woods, N., & Tanner, C. (1984). *Diagnostic reasoning in nursing.* Philadelphia, PA: Lippincott.

Facione, N. C., & Facione, P. A. (1996). Externalizing the critical thinking in knowledge development and clinical judgment. *Nursing Outlook, 44*(3), 129–136.

Fairhurst, G., & Sarr, R. (1996). *The art of framing.* San Francisco, CA: Jossey-Bass.

Fowler, L. (1994). *Clinical reasoning of home health nurses: A verbal protocol analysis.* Unpublished doctoral dissertation, University of South Carolina, College of Nursing, Columbia, South Carolina.

Gordon, M. (1994). *Nursing diagnosis: Process and application.* St. Louis, MI: Mosby.

Herman, J., Pesut, D., & Conard, L. (1994). Using metacognitive skills: The quality audit tool. *Nursing Diagnosis, 5*(2), 56–64.

Jones, S. A., & Brown, L. N. (1993). Alternative views on defining critical thinking through the nursing process. *Holistic Nursing Practice, 7*(3), 71–75.

Kintgen-Andrews, J. (1991). Critical thinking and nursing education: Perplexities and insights. *Journal of Nursing Education, 7*(4), 152–157.

Kuiper, R. A. (2002). Enhancing metacognition through the reflective use of self-regulated learning strategies. *Journal of Continuing Education in Nursing, 33*(2), 78–87.

Kuiper, R. A., & Pesut, D. J. (2004). Promoting cognitive and metacognitive reflective clinical reasoning skills in nursing practice: Self-regulated learning theory. *Journal of Advanced Nursing, 45*(4), 381–391.

Kuiper, R., Pesut, D., & Kautz, D. (2009). Promoting the self-regulation of clinical reasoning skills in nursing students. *Open Nursing Journal, 3*, 76–85. Retrieved from http://www.ncbi.nlm.nih.gov/pmc/articles/PMC2771264

Miller, M. A., & Malcolm, N. S. (1990). Critical thinking in the nursing curriculum. *Nursing Health Care, 11*(2), 67–73.

Nightingale, F. (1946). *Notes on nursing: What it is and what it is not* (facsimile ed.). Philadelphia, PA: J.B. Lippincott. (Original work published 1859)

North American Nursing Diagnosis Association (NANDA). (1994). *Nursing diagnoses: Definitions and classification 1994–1996.* Philadelphia, PA: Author.

North American Nursing Diagnosis Association (NANDA). (1996). *Nursing diagnoses: Definitions and classifications 1997–1998.* Philadelphia, PA: Author.

Pesut, D. J. (2008). Thoughts on thinking with complexity in mind. In C. Lindberg, S. Nash, & C. Lindberg (Eds.), *On the edge: Nursing in the age of complexity* (pp. 211–238). Bordentown, NJ: Plexus Press.

Pesut, D. J., & Herman, J. (1999). *Clinical reasoning: The art and science of critical and creative thinking.* Albany, NY: Delmar.

Pesut, D. J., & Herman, J. A. (1992). Reflection skills in diagnostic reasoning. *Nursing Diagnosis, 3*(4), 148–154.

Senge, P. (1990). *The fifth discipline.* New York, NY: Doubleday.

World Health Organization (WHO). (2015). *Manual of the International Classification of Diseases and related health problems* (10th rev. ed.). Geneva, Switzerland: Author. Retrieved from http://www.icd10data.com

Worrell, P. (1990). Metacognition: Implications for instruction in nursing education. *Journal of Nursing Education, 29*, 170–175.

CHAPTER 4

ESSENTIALS OF CARE COORDINATION CLINICAL REASONING

In the current health care arena, nursing practice requires critical, creative, systems, and complexity thinking. Articulating and managing competing values are also a necessary component of care coordination. In many health care settings, nursing care plans have been replaced by interprofessional checklists, care maps, and critical pathways. These critical paths are road maps that help determine the progress that a patient is or is not making along a predetermined treatment plan. Maps and pathways do not absolve nurses from clinical reasoning responsibilities or making clinical judgments about care patients receive. What happens, for instance, if a patient deviates from the path? How does one reason about deviations from the norm? Clinical reasoning is essential when there is no standard plan or when patients deviate from the expected trajectory. Under these circumstances, professional nurses draw on past experiences, use accumulated knowledge, analyze existing data, consult with colleagues across health care contexts, and jointly formulate a plan of care to remedy patient issues.

The major focus of current health care practice is achieving positive patient health outcomes. To function effectively in this arena, nurses need outcome-specification skills. Previous nursing process models and many nursing diagnoses were organized around problem lists. Clinical reasoning that focuses on outcomes is more valuable and cost-effective than clinical reasoning that focuses on problems. In fact, a well-formed outcome is the opposite of a defined problem. However, identification of outcomes is insufficient without attention to intervention and activities that support how outcomes will be achieved. So, in many instances, nurses and other health care providers must manage and negotiate competing values. Patients benefit from care coordination and case management (American Nurses Association [ANA], 2015) through management of competing values and making explicit the intangible value exchanges between and among providers on the team. The role of a case manager and a care coordinator is becoming essential for meeting patient health care outcomes. Advanced practice nurses, nurse practitioners, clinical nurse specialists, clinical nurse leaders, and other health care providers benefit from enhanced ways of thinking and reasoning that support successful care coordination on a day-to-day basis. Such care coordination is enhanced if advanced practice nurses are able to practice to the full extent of their education and license (Greiner & Kneber, 2003). Clinical reasoning for care coordination addresses the essentials of patient and family needs in dealing with health care problems and prioritizing activities.

LEARNING OUTCOMES

After completing this chapter, the reader should be able to:

1. Explain the levels of perspective of a care coordination framework that are needed to manage the problems, interventions, and outcomes of people across health care services
2. Describe the competing values and value impact framework and relate the models collaborating, creating, competing, and controlling to care coordination processes
3. Describe how the standardized terminologies and communication among inter-professional health care team members are essential for care coordination to address patient and family needs
4. Describe the processes that support clinical reasoning skills and thinking strategies for determining priorities in care coordination cases
5. Define the self-regulatory thinking and reflective practices that support provider reflection associated with levels and perspectives of care coordination
6. Describe team-centered systems thinking and reflection practices that support the effectiveness of care coordination activities in health care contexts

CARE COORDINATION AND COMPETING VALUES

The Competing Values Framework (CVF), developed by Quinn and Rohrbough (1983), provides guidance and insights into some of the essential areas of organizational life and care coordination, for example, collaborating, creating, competing, and controlling. The model suggests that all organizations and groups must manage tensions between external and internal demands or forces as well as the dynamics of flexibility versus control. The juxtaposition of these elements creates four different domains, as well as tensions and polarities to manage among the values of collaborating and competing, and creating and controlling (Quinn, Bright, Faerman, Thompson, & McGrath, 2014).

Each of the four quadrants in the CVF is necessary for an organization or activity to realize efficiency, effectiveness, and success (Figure 4.1). For example, in terms of *collaboration*, people must understand themselves and communicate honestly and effectively. Collaboratively, individuals mentor and develop others and know how to participate and lead teams. Often this knowledge requires encouraging and managing constructive conflict. *Competition* enhances productivity and profitability. In this domain, vision and goal setting are a path to motivating oneself and others so that the systems can be developed and organized to get results. *Creating* and promoting the adoption of new ideas or clinical innovations require attention to judicious use of power and ethics as well as championing new ideas and innovations through negotiating commitments and agreements for implementing and sustaining change. *Control* contributes to the development of stability and continuity as

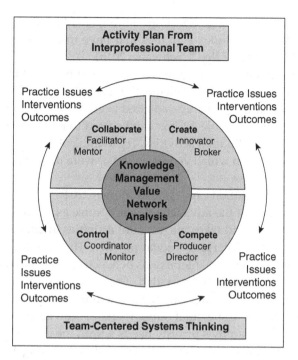

FIGURE 4.1 Competing Values Framework for care coordination clinical reasoning.

people work and manage across functions, organize information exchange, measure and monitor performance and quality, and enable compliance.

To what degree do health care providers explicitly consider the values exchanged in the context of a care coordination scenario? Making value exchanges explicit in the care coordination process is likely to result in new insights, knowledge, learning, performance, and expectations in future health care systems (Allee, 1997). Discussions about value exchanges between and among patients and caregivers and providers are likely to result in role clarity and contributions that support more high-quality performance (Allee, 2003). *Value network analysis* is a method that comes from the business world to help explain the value-added aspects of individual, group, and team contributions to a business transaction or enterprise. Inviting discussions about intangible value exchanges highlights and underscores important contributions and relational dynamics among health care providers in the context of care coordination (Allee, 2008).

When a group of people get together to make something happen, it does not evolve in a linear and/or hierarchical way. Value networks help make explicit the collaboration and values exchanged in human-to-human network interactions (Allee & Schwabe, 2015). As the center of attention for health care needs moves from management hubs to diffuse and distributed webs of relationships between and among providers, each interaction supports a specific value exchange as participants partner for success (Allee, 2003). The dynamic relationships among individuals are collaborative, trusting, dynamic, and interdependent. In addition, they are embedded in the competing values of creating, competing with markets, controlling, and collaborating. Digital connectivity also impacts value networking through greater access to knowledge and information, enabling one to provide quick and effective work with complex activities that have multiple variables and frequent exceptions (Allee, 2003; Allee & Schwabe, 2015).

For example, review the types of values defined in Table 4.1. Consider the degree to which these value exchanges impact and contribute to care coordination. The definitions of the values, adapted from Allee and Schwabe (2015), are also framed as questions in Table 4.1 and can be used to make explicit the value-added elements of care coordination activities. Try to think about a situation or transaction in your own practice in which you provided or were the recipient of one or more of these intangible values.

The Care Coordination Clinical Reasoning (CCCR) model proposed in this book emphasizes the role of the advanced practice nurse as a care coordinator, enhances the nursing process, and takes into account activities intended to navigate competing values related to interprofessional practice. The CCCR framework highlights the complexity and systems interactions between and among the patient issues, the care needed, and the services provided. The CCCR systems model web discussed in this chapter enables one to visually represent the complexities and essential care coordination practice issues that support the organized thinking that focuses on the patients and/or family's priority needs within the context of services provided within and between health care delivery systems. Taking the time to build the model and see connections between and among complementary and/or competing patient care needs and team values helps create desired outcomes and effective and efficient care coordination.

CLINICAL REASONING AND CARE COORDINATION: LEVELS AND PERSPECTIVES

The CCCR systems model provides a blueprint for consideration of the care coordination practice issues. The reality is that clinicians must think using multiple levels of perspective and transcend and transverse these different levels. Every patient has a story that is analyzed and evaluated by the disciplinary perspective and knowledge classification representations and systems unique to the discipline. As clinicians interpret and evaluate the patient's story they filter the story through their disciplinary knowledge base. Such filtering leads each clinician to frame the story and give meaning to the fact patterns associated with the patient's story. A specific patient frame results from filtering a patient's story through a disciplinary lens of nursing, medicine, culture, gender, race, family, and/or pharmacological perspectives. Disciplinary framing then leads to a focus for intervention and care planning. Sometimes filters and frames must be negotiated with competing values in mind.

For example, each discipline reasons with a patient-centered focus. One has to think about the patient's needs, problems, and outcomes. Once disciplines process patient-centered thinking, they move to the next level of reasoning, which is team centered, as the advanced practice clinician has to take into consideration the team deliberations and dynamics related to the care coordination process—collaborating, creating, competing, and controlling. Finally, team members must consider the

TABLE 4.1 Value-Added Reflection Questions

	VALUE DEFINITIONS AND REFLECTION QUESTIONS
Deliverable	The specific values or objects that are conveyed from one role or participant to another role or participant. What are the deliverables that you offer and expect of others?
Exchange	Two or more transactions between two or more roles or participants that evoke reciprocity. A process in which one role as agent receives resources from another role or agents and provides resources in return. What are the resource exchanges between roles or participants on your interprofessional health care team?
Explicit knowledge	The knowledge that is codified and conveyed to others through dialogue, demonstration, or media. What is the explicit knowledge shared among members of the team?
Feedback	Information returned about the impact of an activity. It can also mean the return of a portion of the output of a process as new input. What feedback is returned about activities or outputs in your care coordination activities? How does feedback influence team dynamics and goal attainment?
Human capital/ competence	The knowledge, skills, and competencies that reside in individuals who work in an organization or that are embedded in the organization's internal and external social networks. What human capital resources are needed in order for care coordination in your context to be successful?
Impact analysis	An assessment of how an input for a role is handled. What are the tangible/intangible costs, gains, or values from the input that generate a response or activity, or increase/decrease tangible assets?
Knowledge management	The degree to which the team facilitates and supports processes for creating, sustaining, sharing, and renewing organizational knowledge in order to generate social or economic gain or improve performance. Who is responsible and how is knowledge managed in the care coordination process?
Perceived value	The degree of value participants feel they receive from individual deliverables, which can come from roles, participants, or the network. What are the value-added dimensions of individual, collective, team, and organizational networks?
Resilience	The degree to which the network is able to reconfigure to respond to changing conditions and then return to original form. What is the resilience capacity of the team and organization in which you work?
Structural capital	The infrastructure, routines, concepts, models, information systems, work systems, and business processes that support productivity and sustainability. To what degree does the structural capital and infrastructure support interprofessional teamwork and care coordination processes?
Systems thinking	An analysis and synthesis of the forces and interrelationships that shape the behavior of systems. To what degree do members of the team think about the system dynamics at the individual, group, team, or organizational levels?
Value realization	The degree to which tangible or intangible values turn the input into gains, benefits, capabilities, or assets that contribute to the success of an individual, group, organization, or network (Allee, 2008). To what degree do members of the team intentionally negotiate and manage competing values related to collaborating, creating, competing, and/or controlling?

Adapted from Allee, Schwabe, and Babb (2015).

context and systems as well as organizational challenges that exist in supporting care coordination. All three of these levels must be taken into consideration to fully appreciate and efficiently manage the care coordination process. The following sections explain in detail the structure, the content, and the process of clinical reasoning at different levels of perspective that guide and support advanced practice nursing professionals (and other health care providers) in the development of a care coordination competency mind-set. The clinical reasoning framework proposed suggests structure that can be used as a scaffold to support clinical reasoning. Worksheets provide ways and means for people to create visual representations of issues and relationships between and among issues. The proposed model can be used to support teaching and learning and also to stimulate a pedagogical research agenda (Quinn, Heynoski, Thomas, & Spreitzer, 2014; Rahim & Goolamally, 2014).

The Outcome-Present State-Test (OPT) clinical reasoning model and the CCCR systems model provide the structure to organize the systems and complexity of reflective thinking needed to pinpoint the juxtaposition of present states with desired health outcome states. It is essential that disciplines and individual providers of care be alert and attentive to the philosophy, beliefs, and values, as well as the standardized health care language used to document problems, interventions, and outcomes for each of the health care disciplines involved in the care coordination process. The clinical vocabulary or knowledge content for clinical reasoning consists of the standardized languages or knowledge representations that are used to communicate between and among interprofessional health care providers. Knowledge regarding how domains of practice are influenced by standardized language is useful for interprofessional communication. As individual providers reflect on care coordination contributions and competing values, it influences and affects team reflection and leads to yet another level of reflection in the contexts of organizations and systems in which care is provided. These multiple levels of perspective provide insights and guidance related to the evaluation and effectiveness of care coordination efforts.

CLINICAL REASONING CARE COORDINATION ESSENTIALS

To reiterate from Chapter 1, the core competencies suggested by the Institute of Medicine (IOM) include providing patient-centered care, working in interprofessional teams, employing evidence-based practice, applying quality improvement, and using informatics (Greiner & Knebel, 2003). These competencies are embedded in a number of essential documents (American Association of Colleges of Nursing [AACN], 2011). The CVF described earlier in this chapter also is a useful lens through which to consider how teams best navigate issues of collaboration, creating, competing, and controlling in service of making intangible value exchanges explicit in the care coordination process.

When the advanced practice clinician surveys the various care coordination models and programs, there are care coordination essential needs included in each case management situation to help guide the plan of care toward successful outcomes. These responsibilities and foci are necessary for the individual care provider as well as the team who is responsible for patient-centered care coordination. In addition, Haas, Swan, and Haynes (2014) have identified the essential competencies and essentials of care coordination in a curriculum for ambulatory care nurses. Some of the essentials that all these models share are:

1. Conducting a needs assessment
2. Initiating medical care services
3. Testing, evaluation of capacity, resources, and skills
4. Developing an individualized plan of care
5. Engaging, coaching, and educating the patient and family
6. Monitoring and safety
7. Promoting self-management
8. Team collaboration

Cases are complex, but organizing, mapping, and analyzing needs with visual aids help simplify key issues. The functional relationships among care coordination essential needs derived from the perspective and level of the individual provider, and the level of the team-systems thinking, results in a convergence and identification of central issues that require health care team attention. Spinning and weaving a web of relationships with concurrent consideration of competing values and value exchange among identified common key areas associated with a patient and family situation simplifies and expedites the identification and achievement of care coordination across settings, and care transitions.

CREATING A CCCR SYSTEMS MODEL WEB

The CCCR systems model web worksheet builds on the foundation of the OPT model and helps the advanced practice clinician visually represent and determine relationships between and among essential patient care problems, needs, and issues. Concurrent consideration of all the needs and issues is essential in order for the health provider team to appreciate the complexity of the challenges and the interaction of system dynamics at play, and also manages the cross-setting communication and care transitions. A big-picture representation helps individual clinicians as well as the team to discern, evaluate, and communicate priority needs. For example, essential needs are placed in the CCCR systems model web worksheet (Figure 4.2) to visualize the case dynamics and assist the care coordinator in determining priorities for team interaction, communication, and systems thinking.

The steps to the creation of a CCCR systems model web using the worksheet are as follows:

1. Create and draw a CCCR systems model web and place a general description of the patient, medical diagnoses, and priority nursing domains/International Classification of Diseases (ICD)-10 codes into the center circles as depicted in Figure 4.2. Filtering information leads to framing and the ability to focus on the issue(s) which are are important first steps in clinical reasoning process.
2. Provide the evidence and defining characteristics under each essential care coordination need that will be of consequence in this particular patient and family story. This helps make implicit knowledge explicit and contributes to knowledge management, perceived value, and value realization. Care coordination needs relate to a needs assessment, an individualized plan of care, attention to safety

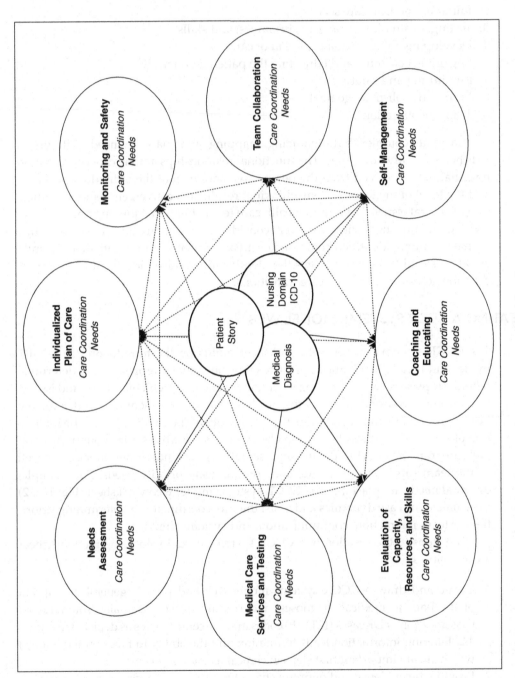

FIGURE 4.2 Care Coordination Clinical Reasoning systems model web.

ICD-10, International Classifications of Diseases, 10th edition.

and monitoring, team collaboration, patient self-management, coaching and education, medical care services and testing, evaluation of capacity resources and skills, and cross-setting communication. Each of these needs may be linked with a medical and/or nursing concern, given the client story.

3. As needs are identified, one can reflect on the total picture on the worksheet and begin to draw lines of relationship, connection, or association among the essential needs. This supports systems thinking, value analysis, feedback, and exchange. As you draw the lines, try to justify and explain reasons as you "think out loud" to explain the relationships and connections between and among the needs from the perspective of a clinician planning a patient-centered level of care.

4. Concurrent iterations will reveal patterns and associations. Determine which needs have the highest priority for care coordination and most efficiently and effectively represents the key needs of the patient.

5. Look once again at the patterns and connections among the needs and the lines of relationships and decide whether there is an emergent frame that summarizes the patient-in-context or the patient's story.

The CCCR systems model web worksheet shown in Figure 4.2 is an adaptation of the OPT clinical reasoning model worksheets. Around the outer edges of the web are care coordination essential needs associated with the patient's story. In this worksheet, under each need, are two to three cues or evidence to support care coordination needs. Directional arrows that create the web effect are functional relationships between and among the needs. As one can see, there are many more arrows converging on one of the priorities. Essential needs are central supporting elements in the patient's story that guide thinking, clinical reasoning, and care coordination based on an analysis and synthesis and impact of possible priorities as represented in the CCCR systems model web.

CREATING A CCCR SYSTEMS MODEL

The CCCR systems model web worksheet (Figure 4.3) is designed to provide a visual representation or map of the structure of the CCCR systems model and to be a guide used to help make explicit the value exchanges in teamwork and the perspectives that emerge when thinking at the level of the team. By writing each element on the worksheet, it is easy to see how parts of the model relate to each other. As seen in Figure 4.3, on the far left-hand side, there is space to write the description of the patient's health care situation. Then three essential needs are placed in the first boxes to the right; basic needs assessment, medical care services and testing, and coaching and education. From provider-systems thinking activities used to create the OPT clinical reasoning model worksheets, an individualized plan of care is considered along with monitoring of safety needs, assessment, and the ongoing plan of care. The interprofessional team then engages in communication to collaborate, create, compete, and control the dynamics derived from the CVF to realize the intangible value exchanges used to develop an activity plan. This activity plan includes considerations and interventions from the individualized plan of care, monitoring process, evaluation of patient and family capacity with regard to

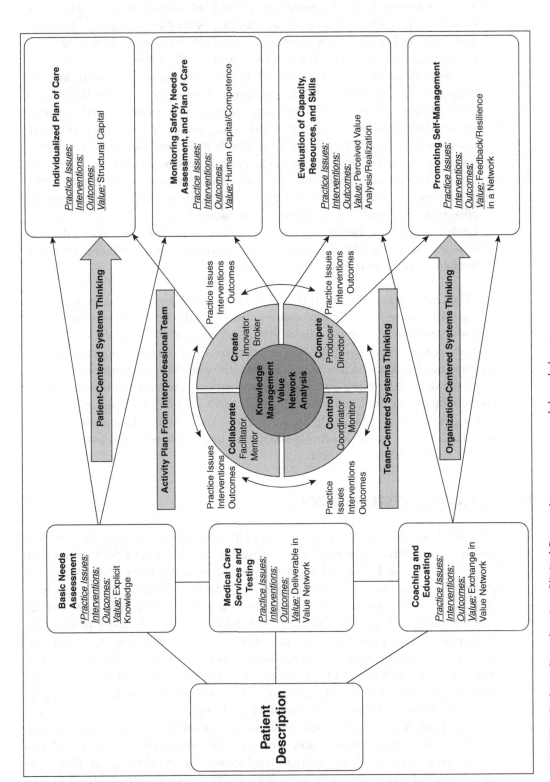

FIGURE 4.3 Care Coordination Clinical Reasoning systems model worksheet.

[a] Practice issues can be from any discipline: nursing, medicine, pharmacy, social work, and so on.

resources and skills, and promotion of self-management. Finally, consideration of the care coordination process at the level or perspective of organization, care coordination thinking, coaching, and education of the patient and family is activated as the team evaluates the capacity of the patient and/or family in regard to health promotion and self-management. With the use of the patient-centered, team-centered, and organization-centered systems thinking depicted in this model, an overlap and coverage of all the essential needs of care coordination are addressed by the entire interprofessional team. The model that is built from this activity serves as a resource to stimulate communication among the members of the team across settings.

Further consequences for health care providers within each of the care coordination essential needs include practice issues, interventions, outcomes, and values assigned to them by the team. In the book *Care Coordination: The Game Changer*, Haas and Swan (2013) discuss the need for evaluation strategies to determine whether objectives of the plan of care are being met. Furthermore, providers must be prepared to address practice issues by developing evidence-based interventions, implementing measures of adherence, and evaluating processes and outcomes. The practice issues, interventions, and outcomes used for patient and family care coordination stem from the National Quality Forum (NQF, 2010) and Agency for Healthcare Research and Quality (AHRQ, 2014).

Mosser and Begun (2014) note that there are seven defining characteristics of a work team. Work teams have a common team goal and share responsibility for achieving that goal. Work teams have defined membership and authority for taking action to achieve shared team goals. Work teams are interdependent and there is an absence of independent subgroups. Finally, work teams are accountable to the larger organization in which they work.

In order for the interprofessional team to have a successful activity plan, it must be purpose centered, internally directed, other focused, and externally open; these are the key ingredients to team-centric systems thinking, the negotiation of competing values, and communication in the CCCR model (Quinn & Quinn, 2015), and the development of positive organizations (Quinn, 2015). As a team member, being externally open leads to openness to challenges, feedback, freedom from labels, higher performance, the cultivation and development of communities of practice based on the value and benefit people derive from shared joy in others' success. Challenges to this outcome are stereotypes of a team member's abilities are fixed and some people are more valued than others in the context of competitive versus collaborative goals. Team success is also influenced by being other focused, as this state cultivates empathy, rapport, energy, and calmness. Creating this state encourages a sense of safety and security, a willingness to take risks and to act with trust, integrity, and resilience. Creating such a culture supports a spirit of inquiry, learning, and experimentation, which results in higher performance. Being other focused is only possible when one is internally directed and intentional about activating one's highest values and operates with freedom, strength, and dignity. Such behavior requires the activation of a reflective self in contrast to automatic self-justification and reactive modes of being and communicating. In order to be a positive influence and bring a state of leadership to the team, each member of the team needs to be vigilant about being purpose centered, choosing goals that create focus, energy, and meaning for the team. Such purpose management requires more complex and creative thinking and results in high performance of self and others. A focused purpose-centered team is likely to attract and create resources related to the reasoning required to communicate across settings to achieve care coordination clinical reasoning goals. There are four key questions that advanced practice clinicians could ask of themselves to help them become purpose centered and to take the four dimensions of the CVF into consideration in the context of teamwork in the CCCR model (Quinn, 2015; Quinn & Quinn, 2015):

- What result do I want to create?
- What would my story be if I were living the values I expect from others?
- How do others feel about this situation?
- What are the three (or four or five) strategies I could use to accomplish my purpose for this situation?

THE VALUE DIMENSIONS OF CCCR

The final phase of clinical reasoning for overall system effectiveness in is to determine whether outcomes were met and whether care coordination activities were successful. The OPT model of clinical reasoning is revisited for the next level of perspective in care coordination, where judgments are made about achieving outcomes from the interprofessional team activity plan. Figure 4.3 is the OPT model clinical reasoning worksheet used for provider systems thinking and case management care planning. Taking it a level further, judgments are made about the care coordination essentials (needs; individualized plan of care; safety; capacity, resources, skills, self-management). Shifting to the next level of perspective, using team-centered systems-thinking activities, collaboration and coordination of the plan of care leads to evaluation of services provided. Shifting to the next level of perspective requires application of critical team reflection using systems thinking to arrive at judgments as to whether outcomes were reached as the team monitors safety, needs, and the plan of care; evaluates capacity, resources, and skills; and promotes patient and family self-management. In the end, the care coordinator should be able to determine success toward goals and/or need for further adjustments in the plan of care, taking into consideration the provider, team, and organizational levels of perspective. Taking into account the organizational perspectives, several issues and questions emerge to prompt reflection and evaluation.

Did the organization or services provide resources and achieve care coordination outcomes for the case? The care coordinator must review the processes to determine whether there were any changes to the interconnections of the systems that affected the outcomes. Did the organizational dynamics support behaviors for the purposes of fulfilling the needs for this case? Did the feedback loop promote communication among and between the health care providers, and patient and family? Did the complexity of the system hinder or enhance the achievement of outcomes? As care coordinator the advanced practice nurse considers each level of perspective individually and then collectively and is the key integrator and systems thinker who communicates with the team regarding the efficiency and effectiveness of the processes for care outcomes.

Chapter 5 emphasizes that a sense of agency is the desire to control events that affect people so they perceive that they work on their own behalf (Bandura, 1997). Success for the provider is promoted through metacognitive strategies to pursue and sustain behaviors, cognitions, and emotions for goal attainment (Zimmerman & Schunk, 2001). As advanced practice nurses use clinical reasoning for care coordination, they choose courses of action for case management. Self-reflection is the phase in which judgments are made about the behaviors and actions taken (Zimmerman, 1998, 2000). The self-regulation activities during care coordination clinical reasoning result in individual-level self-reflections, where there will be evidence of strategic thinking for care coordination and positive health care outcomes for patients. Self-regulatory reflective questions can also be used by the team to promote reflection and support clinical reasoning judgments about the achievement of patient and family outcomes. For examples, see some of the reflection prompts listed in Table 4.2.

The particular systems-thinking skills and strategies used at the patient-centered level can also be applied to the team-centered level of reflection (Figure 4.4) and build on and coincide with the critical, creative systems, and complexity thinking employed during the work with the OPT clinical reasoning and CCCR systems model worksheets. Richmond (1993) notes that key concepts of systems thinking are:

1. All systems are composed of interconnected parts and a change to any part or connection affects the entire system.
2. Structure or pattern of connections between and among parts is how the system is organized and determines its behavior.
3. System behavior is an emergent phenomenon, as its parts and structure are constantly changing through feedback loops.
4. Feedback loops control a system's major dynamic behavior, as each part influences the others in a circular pattern creating a great deal of complexity.

Solving difficult complex social system problems requires the use of systems thinking with a process that uniquely fits the problem at hand within the system dynamics. Advanced practice nurses must understand the whole system of human activity in the environment in which it exists. Vygotsky (1978) suggests that environments mediate learning, including the collaborative social environment of language, symbols, and cultural artifacts. Self-regulatory critical, reflective questions that can be used to promote clinical reasoning to make judgments about the achievement of team outcomes and organizational systems success are shown in Table 4.3.

The self-regulation-, critical-, creative-, systems-, and complexity-thinking processes that are used for care coordination stream across levels from the patient-centered level to the team-centered level to the organization-centered level. The systems thinking used to organize data at the patient-centered level informs the team-centered systems thinking and reflective practices that support analysis and agreement about care coordination needs. Finally, the care coordinator and the team at the organization-centered level adopts the data and thinking used to organize information at the team-centered level to evaluate the case management outcomes with organization-centered systems thinking and reflective practices that use complexity thinking. Judgments are made about whether the case management

TABLE 4.2 Patient-Centered Systems-Thinking Reflection Questions

SELF-REGULATION ACTIVITIES	REFLECTION QUESTIONS

Monitoring thinking	I. **Reflect on the thinking processes you used with the care coordination of this case.**
	1. The baseline needs I identify in this case are…I think I can identify future adjustments in the plan of care by…if I have difficulty I…
	2. When I think about my feelings during the care coordination of this case, I describe them as…and I handle them by…
	3. When I try to remember or understand important facts to develop the plan of care, coach, and educate the patient/family I…
	4. As I look back on meaningful activities, the resources I could have spent:
	   a. More time on…
	   b. Less time on…

Monitoring the environment	II. **Reflect on the environmental circumstances you encountered in the care coordination of this case.** 5. When I prepare to carry out coaching and education activities for care coordination, I… 6. When I think about particular distractions to facilitating medical care services and supports for care coordination, I… 7. When I work and communicate with interprofessional partners for care coordination of this case, I… 8. If I had the chance to redo the care coordination activities, I would do…instead of…because…

Monitoring behavior	III. **Reflect on your behaviors and reactions to the care coordination of this case.**
	9. My impression of my performance in evaluating capacity, energy, support, readiness, and skills to organize and manage the plan of care is…
	10. I make sure I will update the needs assessment and individualized plan of care by… and if I need to make changes, I….
	11. I make sure I empower the patient/family for self-management of health care needs by…and if I need to make changes, I…
	12. Reaction to care coordination of this case…
	   a. My reaction to what I like about the care coordination of this case…
	   b. My reaction to what I do not like about the care coordination of this case…
	Optional prompt: Other comments I have about the care coordination of this case…

Adapted from Kuiper, Pesut, and Kautz (2009).

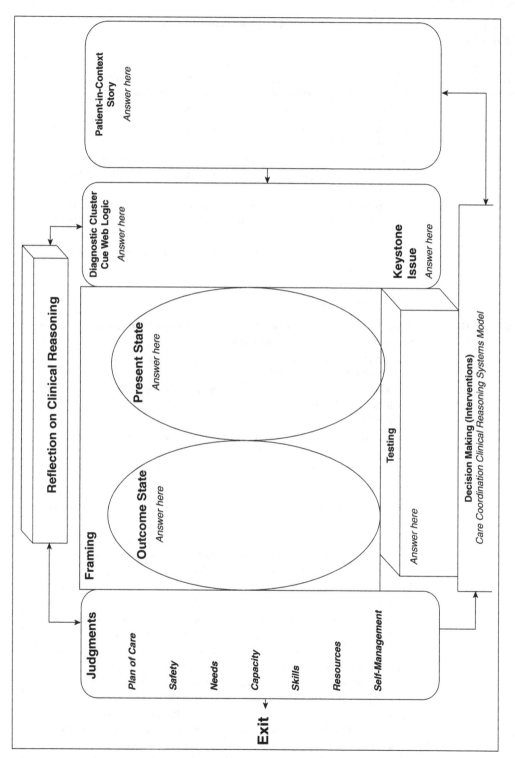

FIGURE 4.4 Outcome-Present State-Test clinical reasoning model.

Source: © Pesut and Herman (1999).

TABLE 4.3 Team-Centered and Organization-Centered Systems-Thinking Reflection Questions

SELF-REGULATION ACTIVITIES	REFLECTION QUESTIONS

Monitoring thinking	I. **Reflect on the thinking processes the team used to navigate organizational systems for care coordination of this case.**
	1. The baseline needs identified by the team in this case are…
	2. Adjustments in the plan of care for future successes include…and difficulties were resolved by…
	3. Team reactions during the care coordination of this case in regard to organizational systems could be described as…and it was handled by…
	4. When the team was dealing with important facts to develop the plan of care, coach, and educate the patient/family about organizational systems, it…
	5. Looking back on meaningful activities, the resources the team could have spent:
	   a. More time on…
	   b. Less time on…

Monitoring the environment	II. **Reflect on the environmental circumstances the team encountered in the care coordination of this case.** 6. When the team prepares to carry out coaching and education activities for care coordination, it… 7. When the team considers particular distractions in the organizations that impede medical care services and supports for care coordination, it… 8. When the team works and communicates with organizational partners for care coordination of this case, it… 9. If the team had the chance to redo the care coordination activities, it would do…instead of…because….

Monitoring behavior	III. **Reflect on team behaviors and reactions to the care coordination of this case.**
	10. Impressions of the team performance in evaluating capacity, energy, support, readiness, and skills to organize and manage the plan of care within organizational systems are…
	11. The team assures it updates the needs assessment and individualized plan of care by…and if it needs to make changes, it….
	12. The team makes sure it empowers the patient/family to navigate through organizational systems for management of health care needs by…and if it needs to make changes, it…
	13. The team reaction to care coordination of this case…
	   a. Reaction to what it likes about the navigation of organizational systems to facilitate the care coordination of this case…
	   b. Reaction to what it does not like about the navigation of organizational systems to facilitate the care coordination of this case…
	Optional prompt: Other comments about the care coordination of this case…

Adapted from Kuiper, Pesut, and Kautz (2009).

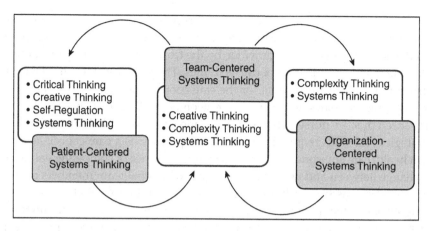

FIGURE 4.5 Flow of thinking.

outcomes have been achieved, and the information is iteratively shared to revise or enhance the plan of care.

Researchers from the business discipline have shown that the use of multiple levels of systems thinking are associated with better overall performance in decision making because there is a better understanding of problems and careful assessment of decision outcomes (Maani & Mahara, 2004). In contrast with the linear thinking inherent in historical versions of the nursing process, a cycle of problem identification, planning, and action from a systems perspective using the various thinking skills we have identified in Figure 4.5 leads to a reiterative analytic process that builds understanding and better health care decisions. We have applied these principles to the systems-thinking model for advanced practice care coordination clinical reasoning. Analytical decisions based on systems thinking promote the integration of patient-centered, team-centered, and organization-centered contributions to patient outcomes, leading to the promotion of safety, reduced risks, reduced costs, disease prevention, and health equity (Ritt, 2014).

SUMMARY

Becoming aware of the specific thinking strategies used to support reflective clinical reasoning by the use of the CCCR systems model helps one develop "purposeful self-regulatory judgment which results in interpretation, analysis, evaluation, and inference as well as the explanation of the evidential, conceptual, methodological, criteriological or contextual considerations upon which that judgment was based" (Facione & Facione, 1996, p. 36).

The reasoning challenge begins with a description and an understanding of the patient's story. Disciplines filter and organize information differently. Such filtering leads to framing. Framing a problem or situation helps pinpoint a focus for reasoning and care coordination planning. Thinking about thinking helps one to evaluate successful strategies, discover flaws in thinking, and correct clinical reasoning skills. Thinking strategies are specific reflection techniques and strategies that nurses use when engaged in reflective clinical reasoning. The CCCR model provides the structure for clinical reasoning at multiple levels of perspective. Each level uses different types of thinking to support clinical reasoning effectiveness. The CCCR structure and process is used at several levels by the provider, by the team, and by the organization to discern alignment and coordination of care activities. The CCCR systems model provides the structure for clinical reasoning for the care coordination of essential needs and their related practice issues, interventions, outcomes, and values. These tools provide the advanced practice nurse with the support and scaffold needed to exercise the thinking strategies and skills required to achieve competency as a care coordinator in the current health care environment. Attention to the presence of competing values and value exchange between and among health care professional team members makes explicit the contributions that each makes to the team and the CCCR challenge. Developing insights about the advanced practice clinician's professional contributions supports professional role clarification and enables the health care team to explicitly explain the value-added benefits of care coordination efforts.

The learning tools introduced in this chapter serve as the foundation for reasoning about particular patient cases across levels of perspective and contexts. Part II of the book introduces care coordination cases across the health care continuum for the advanced practice nurse clinician in the contexts of primary community health, acute care, rehabilitative care, and long-term care within multiple contexts and systems.

KEY CONCEPTS

1. Clinical reasoning for care coordination can be promoted in advanced practice nursing students with a framework that includes structure, content, and process.
2. A supporting framework for care coordination clinical reasoning extends case management using the OPT clinical reasoning model across levels of perspective to align care coordination activities.
3. The process of care coordination clinical reasoning involves critical reflection on all phases of case management through the use of patient-centered, team-centered, and organization-centered systems thinking.
4. Attention to issues of competing values and value analysis helps to define and describe the unique contributions that individual providers make to care coordination clinical reasoning efforts.
5. Effective team dynamics include being purpose centered, internally directed, other focused, and externally open.
6. A supporting framework for care coordination clinical reasoning includes attention to the organizational systems thinking to make judgments about care coordination essentials and uses the CCCR model to communicate across care settings and contexts.

STUDY QUESTIONS AND ACTIVITIES

1. Describe in your own words the benefits and processes of using the CCCR systems model in identifying priority of essential needs in a case with which you are familiar. Were you able to identify system issues in order to proceed with care coordination and interconnect with the interprofessional team?

2. Using the CCCR systems model, identify the care coordination essential needs of a case you are familiar with and identify the primary values operating in the case.
3. Learn more about the CVF and relate the concepts, ideas, and principles to your interprofessional practice challenges. See the octogram: http://www.octogram .net
4. To what degree do you explicitly identify and describe the value exchange associated with your interprofessional work?
5. Using the CCCR systems model, give some examples of monitoring safety, evaluation of capacity and self-management promotion that would require interprofessional health care team input.
6. Identify all the possible standardized health care languages that were used/considered in a case in which you were recently involved. What were their similarities and differences? Did language impact on communication and the patient outcomes? How does a discipline-specific framework influence the use and understanding of standardized health care languages?
7. Identify the relationship between critical reflection and thinking strategies as they are applied to the three levels of system-thinking perspectives required—patient, team, and organizations. What does it take to shift from a focus on the provider and patient to a focus on the team and organization?

REFERENCES

Agency for Healthcare Research and Quality (AHRQ). (2014). *Care coordination measures atlas–June 2014 update.* Rockville, MD: Author. Retrieved from http://www.ahrq. gov/sites/default/files/wysiwyg/professionals/prevention-chronic-care/improve/ coordination/atlas2014/appendix4a.pdf

Allee, V. (1997). *The knowledge evolution: Expanding organizational intelligence.* Burlington, MA: Butterworth-Heinemann.

Allee, V. (2003). *The future of knowledge: Increasing prosperity through value networks.* Burlington, MA: Elsevier.

Allee, V. (2008). Value network analysis and value conversion of tangible and intangible assets. *Journal of Intellectual Capital, 9*(1), 5–24.

Allee, V., Schwabe, O., & Babb, M. K. (Eds.). (2015). *Value networks and the true nature of collaboration.* Tampa, FL: Megher–Kifer Press, ValueNet Works and Verna Allee Associates. Retrieved from http://valuenetworksandcollaboration.com/downloads/glossaryof-terms.html

American Association of Colleges of Nursing (AACN). (2011). *The essentials of master's education in nursing.* Washington, DC: Author. Retrieved from http://www.aacn.nche.edu/ education-resources/MastersEssentials11.pdf

American Nurses Association. (2015). *Scope and standards of practice* (3rd ed.). Silver Spring, MD: Author.

Bandura, A. (1997). *Self-efficacy: The exercise of control.* New York, NY: W. H. Freeman and Company.

Facione, N. C., & Facione, P. A. (1996). Externalizing the critical thinking in knowledge development and clinical judgment. *Nursing Outlook, 44*(3), 129–136.

Greiner, A., & Knebel, E. (Eds.). (2003). *Health professions education: A bridge to quality.* Washington, DC: The National Academies Press.

Haas, S., & Swan, B. A. (2013). Quality and safety outcomes for patients and families. In G. Lamb (Ed.), *Care coordination: The game changer: How nursing is revolutionizing quality care* (pp. 1–9). Silver Spring, MD: American Nurses Association, Nursesbooks. org. Retrieved from www.nursingworld.org

Haas, S. A., Swan, B. A., & Haynes, T. S. (Eds.). (2014). *Care coordination and transition management core curriculum.* Pittman, NJ: American Academy of Ambulatory Care Nursing.

Kuiper, R., Pesut, D., & Kautz, D. (2009). Promoting the self-regulation of clinical reasoning skills in nursing students. *Open Nursing Journal, 3,* 76–85. Retrieved from http://www .ncbi.nlm.nih.gov/pmc/articles/PMC2771264

Maani, K. E., & Maharaj, V. (2004). Links between systems thinking and complex decision making. *System Dynamics Review, 20*(1), 21–48.

Mosser, G., & Begun, J. (2014). *Understanding teamwork in health care.* New York, NY: McGraw-Hill.

National Quality Forum. (2010). *Quality connections: Care coordination.* Retrieved from http://www.qualityforum.org/Publications/2010/10/Quality_Connections__Care_ Coordination.aspx

Quinn, R. (2015). *The positive organization: Breaking free from conventional cultures, constraints, and beliefs.* Oakland: CA: Berrett-Koehler.

Quinn, R., & Quinn, R. E. (2015). *Lift: Becoming a positive force in any situation.* San Francisco, CA: Berrett-Koehler.

Quinn, R. E., Bright, D., Faerman, S. R., Thompson, M. P., & McGrath, M. R. (2014). *Becoming a master manager: A competing values approach.* Hoboken, NJ: John Wiley & Sons.

Quinn, R. E., Heynoski, K., Thomas, M., & Spreitzer, G. M. (2014). *The best teacher in you: How to accelerate learning and change lives.* San Francisco, CA: Berrett-Koehler.

Quinn, R. E., & Rohrbough, J. (1983). A spatial model of effectiveness criteria: Towards a competing values approach to organizational analysis. *Management Science, 29,* 363–377.

Rahim, R. A., & Goolamally, N. (2014). Pedagogical model to inculcate clinical reasoning skills among nursing students in the open distance learning institution. In *Seminar Kebangsaan Pembelajaran Sepanjang Hayat.* Seminar conducted at the Open University Malaysia, Kuala Lampur, Malaysia.

Richmond, B. (1993). Systems thinking: Critical thinking skills for the 1990s and beyond. *System Dynamics Review, 9*(2), 13–133.

Ritt, E. (2014). Essential analytics in nursing education: Building capacity to improve clinical practice. *Journal of Nursing Education and Practice, 4*(12), 9–16.

Vygotsky, L. S. (1978). *Mind in society: The development of higher psychological processes.* Cambridge, MA: Harvard University Press.

Zimmerman, B. (1998). Developing self-fulfilling cycles of academic regulation: An analysis of examplary instructional models. In D. H. Schunk & B. J. Zimmerman (Eds.), *Self-regulated learning: From teaching to self-reflective practice* (pp. 1–19). New York, NY: Guilford Press.

Zimmerman, B. (2000). Attaining self-regulation: A social cognitive perspective. In M. Boekaerts, P. R. Pintrich, & M. Zeidner (Eds.), *Handbook of self-regulation* (pp. 13–39). San Diego, CA: Academic Press.

Zimmerman, B., & Schunk, D. S. (2001). *Self-regulated learning and academic thought.* Mahwah, NJ: Lawrence Erlbaum.

CHAPTER 5

THINKING SKILLS THAT SUPPORT CARE COORDINATION CLINICAL REASONING

This chapter offers an introduction and overview of the thinking skills that support care coordination clinical reasoning (CCCR). Although not a new concept, care coordination is an evolving model of care that supports the desired achievement of triple aim, with goals for improved patient experiences of high-quality care, reduced costs, improving the health of populations. The information presented explores differences between case management and care coordination, and develops the argument that nurses, especially advanced practice nurses, by virtue of their knowledge, skills, and experiences, are in the best position to coordinate care. The discussion highlights the importance and value of advanced practice preparation and development of a CCCR skill set as the means to influence and lead care coordination at the provider, interprofessional team, and organizational levels.

Advanced practice registered nurses (APRNs) add value to care coordination because the education and training they receive promote the development of clinical reasoning skills that are necessary to manage all facets of the health care landscape and because they value and include the patient as a key member of the health care team (Yang & Meiners, 2014). Care coordination combines evidence-based practice with patient preferences (Goeree & Levin, 2006; Haas, Swan, & Haynes, 2014). CCCR skills can be enhanced with didactic and clinical learning experiences that employ different types of thinking skills.

The complexity of CCCR involves several types of thinking providers use to reason about individual patient problems while concurrently considering the care coordination issues of working with a multiprofessional team within organizational and system contexts. The quality of care provided through these synchronized efforts can be evaluated by looking at value exchange and the impact of structure (facilities and organizational health care systems that manage care), processes (behavior of the provider when diagnosing and treating), and outcomes (resulting change in health status and satisfaction of the patient; Mullnix & Bucholtz, 2009).

LEARNING OUTCOMES

After completing this chapter, the reader should be able to:

1. Describe different types of care coordination concepts and models proposed for advanced practice nursing roles

2. Explain why care coordination is a solution to the health care system problems of cost, uneven quality, and poor patient outcomes
3. Compare and contrast the concept of case management with care coordination
4. Define care coordination clinical reasoning (CCCR) and explain how this skill supports safe, effective, efficient, high-quality advanced practice nursing care
5. Define the different types of thinking that support CCCR
6. Describe the interface of cognitive strategies (critical thinking) with metacognitive strategies (creative thinking) as well as systems and complexity thinking for clinical reasoning skill development

THE NEED FOR CARE COORDINATION

Given health care complexity, reforms are being put in place to include the proper use of resources and best practices that involve models and interventions that improve the quality of patient care. The misalignment of resources and incentives prevents effective allocation and coordination of care that supports good patient outcomes. The Institute of Medicine reported an analysis of a large group of Medicaid and Medicare/Medicaid patient claims for five large states to determine the cost of uncoordinated care (Owens, 2010). The uncoordinated care analysis in this report revealed costs that were 75% higher than matched patients whose care was coordinated.

The health professional who historically has coordinated patient and family care has been the nurse. In fact, advanced practice nurses are highly qualified health care practitioners who provide cost-effective, accessible, patient-centered care and have the education to provide care coordination and case management services sought in the context of health care reform (Stanley, Werner, & Apple, 2009). Thus, care coordination is evolving as a key focus for accountable care organizations (ACOs) because of the emphasis and need to promote shared plans of care and improve costs across health care services and settings (Patient Protection and Affordable Care Act, 2010). Care coordination is an essential skill that is familiar to nurses at all levels. Care coordination is an expected standard and core competency of professional nursing practice (American Nurses Association [ANA], 2015). The current attention to inter-professional education and practice is giving rise to new opportunities for nurses to educate colleagues about the care coordination they have been providing to patients and families for many years.

The difference in scope of practice between RNs and advanced practice nurses is significant for future care coordination models because advanced practice nurses can directly, autonomously, and, with great flexibility, manage care activities and be compensated for their coordination activities (Laughlin & Beisel, 2010; Naylor et al., 2004). When RNs are to be used for care coordination efforts, educational strategies to prepare them and additional costs in practice overhead are incurred in order for their work to be sustained (Moore & Coddington, 2011).

Persons aged 85 years and older are growing at four times the rate of the U.S. population and, by 2030, one in every five people will be 65 years and older (Tabloski, 2014). American's average life expectancy has increased; at the same time, death rates for the 65- to 84-year-old age group have decreased (Touhy & Jett, 2012).

The growth in this population is only one reason our nation is already experiencing a shortage of primary care physicians; this shortage is expected to increase dramatically at the same time nurse practitioner (NP) programs are "educating three primary care NPs to every one primary care physician" (Sustaita, Zeigler, & Brogan, 2013, p. 42). It has been projected that NPs and physician assistants will fill this gap and be able to competently provide primary care medical homes. The American Association of Nurse Practitioners (AANP, 2013) recognizes that 90% of credentialed NPs are actively practicing, with enrollment and graduation rates of NP programs steadily increasing. With decreasing reimbursement rates from the Centers for Medicare & Medicaid Services (CMS), the vast majority of NPs continue to see Medicare and Medicaid recipients. Primary care providers often need to coordinate care and perform the role of a care coordinator because they are the central point of care for the patient. Not only are NPs educated and fully competent to provide primary care medical homes, their efforts are also cost-effective.

APRNs, specifically NPs, are being touted as the future of primary care by the following organizations: American Academy of Nurse Practitioners, American Association of Nurse Practitioners, Gerontological Advanced Practice Nurse Association, National Association of Pediatric Nurse Practitioners, National Association of Nurse Practitioners in Women's Health, and National Organization of Nurse Practitioner Faculties. To date, many of the advanced practice nurse–led models of care have demonstrated better coordinated care at lower costs for patients with multiple social and health care needs (Craig, Eby, & Whittington, 2011). Advanced practice nurses have the knowledge, skills, and abilities to be the key care coordinating agents in a system. The care coordination of the future is likely to be different from the case management of the past.

CONTRASTING CASE MANAGEMENT WITH EVOLVING DEFINITIONS OF CARE COORDINATION

Past notions of case management often referred to intense and extensive care coordination of individuals with complex physical, emotional, and social health care needs who are at risk of complications from comorbidities and high costs (Schraeder & Shelton, 2013). In these case management instances, individuals, with all of their complexities, were managed with cost-effectiveness in mind. APRNs in the role of clinical nurse specialists (CNSs) have had a positive impact on care organization through case management (Foss & Koerner, 1997). However, the emergence of new technologies and standardized documentation have impacted the nursing care coordination practice to include more intense management for at-risk and vulnerable populations across all settings. A holistic approach to care coordination provided by nurses includes physical health and social, mental, and spiritual needs. Nurses bring a unique perspective to care coordination through their roles and scope of practice (Institute of Medicine [IOM], 2001).

The relationship of case management and care coordination for APRNs is determined by their scope of practice. *Scope of practice* is defined as the activities an individual health care practitioner is allowed to perform within a profession as determined by the law and standards of care (Safriet, 2002). Other boundaries of the scope of practice include clinical competence, skill, knowledge, and training that evolves over time as needs and operations (technology) of the health care milieu are redesigned (Milstead, 2008). Although the debate between scope-of-practice laws and reimbursement for NP services continues across the country, it has been noticed that nurses are the health care providers who take initiative in patient care and are key facilitators for communication between patients and all providers (Yang & Meiners, 2014).

Nurses have historically worked collaboratively with other health care providers for many years to provide care management. And when they are in positions of managing models of interprofessional teams, results show the best clinical outcomes and reduced costs (Schraeder & Shelton, 2013). In the advanced practice role, the APRN is in a key position to provide horizontal or lateral leadership to manage and coordinate care to improve primary care availability, provide care of the underserved, redesign the role of public health, and restructure hospitals (Aiken & Salmon, 1994; American Association of Colleges of Nursing [AACN], 2004; Lancaster, Lancaster, & Onega, 2000; Radzyminski, 2005). As evidence-based practice is used by advanced practice nurses to inform clinical decisions, theory and values inform case management and the coordination of team efforts to provide quality care (IOM, 2001). New definitions are evolving regarding the elements, dimensions, and values of care coordination across health care contexts.

The National Quality Forum (NQF) defines care coordination as a "function that helps ensure that the patient's needs and preferences for health services and information sharing across people, functions, and sites that are met over time" (NQF, 2014, p. 5). The framework for examining and understanding care coordination identified five key domains: health care "home," proactive plan of care and follow-up, communication, information systems, and transitions or handoffs (NQF, 2014). When care coordination is successful, it is associated with higher quality, improved efficiency, better patient experiences, and reduced costs. When it is not successful, inaccurate transmission of information, inadequate communication, inappropriate follow-up care, medical error, and overall lower quality outcomes are obvious. The care coordination focus for nursing is helping the patient/family navigate health care systems and transitions between and among providers and services. Therefore, a definition of care coordination seen from a nursing perspective provides a foundation on which educational methods and strategies support the development of clinical reasoning skills that provide the foundation for care coordination.

The Agency for Healthcare Research and Quality (AHRQ) considered several definitions of care coordination when developing the following:

> Care coordination is the deliberate organization of patient care activities
> between two or more participants (including the patient) involved
> in a patient's care to facilitate the appropriate delivery of health
> care services. Organizing care involves the marshaling of personnel
> and other resources needed to carry out all required patient care
> activities and is often managed by the exchange of information among
> participants responsible for different aspects of care. (AHRQ, 2015, p. 1).

The ANA (2015) supports and advances the core elements of care coordination (AHRQ, 2015; NQF, 2010) and espouses the following. Care coordination is the deliberate organization of patient care activities between two or more partici-pants (including the patient) involved in a patient's care to facilitate the appropriate delivery of health care services. RNs have demonstrated leadership and innova-tion in the design, implementation, and evaluation of successful care coordination processes and models using a team approach. These methods help ensure that the patient's needs and preferences are met over time with respect to health services and information sharing across people, functions, and sites. As a core professional standard and competency for all registered nursing practice, partnerships guided by the health care consumer's and family's needs and preferences are essential to the outcomes of quality care, satisfaction, and the effective and efficient use of health care resources. Qualified and educated RNs are positioned to provide care coordination services, particularly with high-risk and vulnerable populations.

What is common across all definitions of care coordination is the emphasis on attending to the needs and preferences of patients and families through the integra-tive activities of communication and mobilization of resources (Lamb, 2013). The advanced practice nurse is poised to facilitate the relay of information between pro-viders and across settings for effective implementation of services. The model that the ANA proposes is evident in primary care, where the patient receives care from an integrated, multidisciplinary team with a staff care coordinator (ANA, 2012). The models vary however, in which case managers, care transition programs, disease management, and health information technologies are used to manage services. Although not all care coordination activities show benefit (Ayanian, 2009; Peikes et al., 2009), many of the models show that the nurse is the most appropriate care coordinator.

EXAMPLES OF CARE COORDINATION MODELS

The American Academy of Nursing (AAN) has highlighted more than 50 nurse-driven programs in various settings with a variety of populations to reflect new thinking for the current reforms in health care systems (AAN, 2012). For example, models for acute care coordination use advanced practice nurses, patient naviga-tors, and social workers. Results in one study showed greater telephone contact, increased use of home health RNs, rehabilitation services, and reduced emergency department visits that resulted in readmission after the placement of a care coordi-nation program for care coordination (Robles et al., 2011). Care coordination with complementary therapies in a program managed by specially educated nurses and patient navigators showed a decrease in medical costs and an increase in hospital savings (Kligler et al., 2011). RNs and social workers were shown to impact inpatient health care costs by assessing and managing financial, social, and emotional needs of patients to obtain resources to manage care at home. The results are reduced inpatient-related costs as a result of decreased numbers of visits and the visits were less critical and shorter (Gundersen Lutheran Health System, 2013).

Care coordination involving transitions into the home was addressed by a study with NPs who specifically targeted frail elderly patients with multiple comorbidities (Naylor et al., 2004). Interventions included home visits for 3 months postdischarge and resulted in cost savings, increased survival time, and fewer readmissions.

The significant impact of this model was shown by the NP flexibility to individualize the evidence-based plan of care with interventions appropriate to on-site and real-time patient needs.

Community-based care coordination has shown cost reductions while ensuring safety with chronically ill elderly patients by using interprofessional teams that include RNs, NPs, and recommended social worker interventions to educate and empower patients to manage their own home care (Atherly & Thorpe, 2011; Coleman, Parry, Chalmers, & Min, 2006; Laughlin & Biesel, 2010). Patients are in need of medication knowledge, financial access to medications, caregiver support, and other services for chronic illness and cognitive decline that could promote aging in place.

Another population in need of care coordination is children with special health care needs. Models that use interprofessional teams with RNs and NPs as care coordinators have shown to decrease unnecessary resource use, decreased emergency department visits, decreased hospital admissions, decreased medical office visits, and improved functional status of the children (Antonelli, Stille, & Antonelli, 2008; Farmer, Clark, Drewel, Swenson, & Ge, 2011; Gordon et al., 2007). The value-model project used certified pediatric NPs as care coordinators, which resulted in improved patient satisfaction and reduced navigation of barriers to care resulting from the practitioner's autonomy to manage all aspects of care (Looman et al., 2012). Care coordination models in mental health care have shown reduced barriers to management of mental health conditions (Oxman et al., 2002) and greater response to treatment as compared with usual care (Dietrich et al., 2004). Depression outcome measures were met in many instances in a review of 55 randomized controlled trials with case management and monitoring by RNs (Christensen et al., 2008).

The benefit of team-based care with specially educated nurses as care coordinators, interfacing with physicians, pharmacists, social workers, nutritionists, and rehabilitation services, promotes the health care model of the future. As part of ACOs, nurses function as team members working alongside other providers to coordinate care across settings, including transitions into the community (Nursing Alliance for Quality Care [NAQC], 2014). In a cross-case analysis of six NP-led clinics, Shiu, Lee, and Chau (2012) discovered that physicians identified advanced practice nurses as the providers who promoted the integrated teamwork spirit and fostered collaboration of the multidisciplinary team.

Education, practice, and research initiatives are needed to promote and test the models and methods that achieve the best patient outcomes and most efficient use of resources. The core competencies that should be included in educational preparation to bridge the quality chasm in health care, as suggested by the Institute of Medicine, include providing patient-centered care, working in interprofessional teams, employing evidence-based practice, applying quality improvement, and using informatics (Greiner & Knebel, 2003). These competencies are embedded in the AACN (2011) essentials for advanced practice nurse education, so graduates are positioned for key roles to manage and coordinate care.

A review of the literature regarding disease-management program models across the globe reveals that successful programs have five characteristics in common: (a) larger programs yield better economic value, provide more reliable measurement results, allow ease for provider compliance, and use data to refine protocols and programs; (b) simplicity of care paths and single provider care coordination; (c) focus on patient needs and abilities for regular visits and preventative services; (d) information technology transparency to communicate goals, methods, outcomes, and data analysis; and (e) provide incentives for the patient and provider compliance (Brandt, Hartmann, & Hehner, 2010; Looman et al., 2012).

Synthesis of the literature in which reports and studies document nurse involvement in care coordination shows the following outcomes: (a) reductions in emergency department visits, (b) decreased medication costs, (c) reduced inpatient charges, (d) reduced overall charges for care, (e) average savings per patient, (f) increases in survival with fewer readmissions, (g) lower total annual Medicare costs for beneficiaries in pilot projects compared with control groups, (h) increased patient self-confidence in managing their own care, (i) improved quality of care, (j) increased safety of older adults during transition from acute care settings to home, (k) improved clinical outcomes and reduced costs, and (l) improved overall patient satisfaction (ANA, 2012). Nurses also play effective roles in relational coordination by developing relationships with patients and other types of care providers through the use of interpersonal communication skills (Yang & Meiners, 2014).

CCCR: LEVELS OF PERSPECTIVES AND TYPES OF THINKING

There is a complexity to CCCR, as nurses must reason about the individual client or patient while simultaneously considering the care coordination issues as they also grapple with the complexities of working in an interprofessional team that must struggle with organizational and/or system issues. So CCCR requires the concurrent consideration of several levels of perspective: patient-centered, team-centered, and system-centered reasoning.

If advanced practice nurses are to have a unique contribution to make for the future of care coordination models, it will require educational preparation and training to promote the clinical reasoning skills necessary to manage all the facets of the ever-changing health care landscape, and by including the patient as a key member of his or her own health team (Yang & Meiners, 2014).

Good practices in care coordination are clinical reasoning activities that examine the structure (facilities and management of the health care system), process (behavior of the provider when diagnosing and treating), and outcome (resulting change in health status and satisfaction of the patient) of clinical situations (Mullnix & Bucholtz, 2009).

The authors propose that CCCR skills are necessary to support the future development of care coordination skills of advanced practice nurses. The authors define CCCR as the application of critical, creative, systems, and complexity thinking to determine the practice issues, interdependencies, and interconnections of role relationships for collaborative work in service of caring for people to address problems, interventions and outcomes through time and across health care contexts and services.

CCCR skills require attention to several levels of perspectives and the development of various types of thinking to manage and self-regulate reasoning efforts.

Levels of perspective include the patient-centered dynamics of providers working with the patients and team-centered dynamics essential to the provider working with other professions to coordinate care. Finally, context or organization dynamics influence both team-centered and patient-centered dynamics. Based on the authors' experiences of helping people master the critical-, creative-, systems-, and complexity-thinking skills associated with clinical reasoning at the individual patient level, there are unique teaching and learning strategies that can be applied at the level of team and organization that support insights about the dynamics of care coordination for enhancing safe, effective, high-quality, and cost-effective care. The rest of this book provides a model, as well as methods, tools, and resources nurses can use as they master the thinking and reasoning skills needed at each level of perspective required for care coordination. The following discussion highlights types of thinking that support CCCR efforts at different levels of perspective.

SELF-REGULATION IN ACTION: THINKING PROCESSES THAT SUPPORT CLINICAL REASONING

Social cognitive theory states that people desire to control events that affect them and perceive themselves as agents working on their own behalf (Bandura, 1997). Key to this sense of agency is self-regulation, whereby individuals actively pursue and sustain behaviors, cognitions, and emotions that are geared toward goal attainment (Zimmerman & Schunk, 2001). Deliberate clinical reasoning presupposes skills in self-regulation, self-monitoring, self-evaluation, and self-reinforcement (Kuiper & Pesut, 2014; Pesut & Herman, 1999).

As health care providers interact with patients, families, and other providers within organizations and systems, their cognitive and metacognitive strategies are influenced by the environment and the people within it. As advanced practice nurses learn clinical reasoning for care coordination, they are faced with choices. For example, if the advanced practice nurse is working with an elderly patient who is to go home from an inpatient setting after a hip replacement, the self-regulation of behaviors, thinking activities, emotions, and environmental influences will determine the choices that are made for care coordination. The self-regulation processes that coincide with clinical reasoning are described by Zimmerman (1998, 2000) as forethought, performance control, and self-reflection. Applied to care coordination, the forethought phase precedes action and sets the stage for clinical reasoning. Performance control is the phase that coincides with clinical reasoning and affects the attention given to a situation and resulting actions. Self-reflection is the phase whereby people respond behaviorally and mentally to their actions. Social cognitive theory proposes that the interaction of the personal, behavioral, and environmental processes, during self-regulated thinking, is cyclic because the phases change as they are monitored during the process (Zimmerman 1998, 2000). Self-monitoring, a thinking activity used during self-regulation, leads to a change in an individual's strategies, cognitions, affects, and behaviors. When these thinking activities become habitual, as one repeats the processes in subsequent situations, learners develop self-efficacy to attain goals and employ self-evaluation during reflection to make attributions for performance (Kuiper & Pesut, 2004; Schunk, 2012). When effective clinical reasoning is employed, there is evidence of strategic thinking for care coordination and enhanced positive health care outcomes for patients. Such strategic thinking builds on the foundations of critical thinking.

Critical Thinking

According to Brookfield (2012), critical thinking happens when individuals try to discover assumptions that influence the way they think and act, check or appraise whether those assumptions are valid and reliable guides for action, look at these assumptions from multiple viewpoints or as others see them, and then take informed action.

The three different types of assumptions Brookfield proposes as one thinks critically are paradigmatic assumptions (ordering the world into fundamental categories), prescriptive assumptions (what we think ought to happen in a particular circumstance), and causal assumptions (how the world works and the conditions under which these can be changed). A similar description of critical thinking put forth by Watson and Glaser (1964) suggested that critical thinking is a composite of attitudes that enable a person to recognize problems, search for evidence to support truths, and accurately weigh logically determined evidence. Facione (1990) conducted an international Delphi study to determine a consensus statement on the essence of critical thinking and defined critical thinking as purposeful self-regulatory judgment. Scheffer and Rubenfeld (2000) surveyed expert nurse educators and developed a definition of critical thinking that includes the cognitive processes of information seeking, discriminating, analyzing, transforming knowledge, predicating, applying standards, and logical reasoning along with the characteristics of motivation, perseverance, fair-mindedness, and deliberate and careful attention to thinking. Brookfield (2012) points out that when critical thinking is linked to actions the issue of "values" is raised, because the next step in the process is to determine which actions are desirable and supported. Therefore, critical thinking is not just a mental process, but is done for a greater purpose and informed by the values of the situation and the context in which they occur. For example, an advanced practice nurse using critical-thinking skills will examine the assumptions and knowledge held by all parties concerned when decisions are made to vaccinate children. Knowing how to educate and present best evidence to parents will impact the values parents place on preventative health care measures for their child. Therefore, the critical thinking activities advanced practice nurses use for clinical reasoning in the context of care coordination are unique and driven by the values inherent in each situation.

The AACN makes the following statement about critical thinking in the *Essentials of Baccalaureate Nursing Education for Professional Nursing Practice*: "Critical thinking underlies independent and interdependent decision making. Critical thinking includes questioning, analysis, synthesis, interpretation, inference, inductive and deductive reasoning, intuition, application, and creativity" (AACN, 1998, p. 9).

Creative Thinking

Creative thinking is a metacognitive process that supports clinical reasoning by generating associations, attributes, elements, images, and operations to solve problems (Pesut, 2008). Creative thinking involves grappling with complementary pairs, tensions, and opposites. Creative problem solving, described in a model by Treffinger (1985) and Treffinger and Isaksen (2005), is comprised of three components: understanding a challenge, generating ideas, and preparing for action. It involves metacognitive processes such as planning, monitoring, and modifying behavior (Schunk, 2012). First, as a problem is considered, general strategies are implemented, which could be used across domains such as breaking down a problem into its components. Then domain-specific strategies would be used; for example, choosing which laboratory tests to conduct in order to diagnose particular diseases and health-related problems. These strategies are used early in creative thinking activities in order to understand the challenges in a problem.

Second, generating ideas would be accomplished by strategies such as generate-and-test, means–ends analysis, analogical reasoning, and brainstorming using domain-specific knowledge and experience (Schunk, 2012). The generate-and-test strategy uses knowledge to create a hierarchy of possible solutions and subsequent solution choice. Fundamental to creative thinking is the means–ends analysis activity, which compares the situation at hand with the desired goal and compares and contrasts the differences between them. By identifying subgoals and attaining each of them, one can move closer to a solution. Analogical reasoning is comparing a problem situation with one from experience, which requires good domain knowledge and previous exposure. Brainstorming requires defining a problem, generating solutions, determining criteria to judge solutions, and then selecting the best solution for the outcome. Brainstorming success is also determined by domain knowledge in order to be able to recognize the problem, generate workable solutions, and evaluate the outcome.

An example of the application and use of creative thinking is an advanced practice nurse who sees an adolescent with an eating disorder. After evaluating diagnostic studies to determine the extent of health-related problems resulting from the eating disorder, the APRN considers all the possible solutions based on the frame of the situation, and previous experience with these cases. The APRN determines that referral to a local support group is the best solution for this adolescent because the provider has seen significant success achieved with similar adolescent cases in the past. Providers develop schemas, models, and memories of past cases that support future reasoning efforts.

Third, preparing for action requires the use of production systems that are networks of condition–action sequences (Anderson, 1990, 1993, 2000). The conditions are the circumstances of the problem that activate the system, and the actions are the activities that occur. Proceeding through this stage of preparing for action requires the use of if–then comparisons synonymous with creative thinking. The "if" is the goal to be achieved and the "then" is the action. Problem solving in care coordination situations that are not clearly defined and difficult requires specific strategies, such as critical thinking and creative thinking, to maneuver through the health care systems of our day. Dealing with these systems will require additional strategies, such as complexity thinking, to manage the multiple factors influencing the health and uniqueness of patients.

Systems Thinking

Systems thinking was coined and described in 1993 by Barry Richmond (1993) as the art and science of making reliable inferences about behavior by developing an increasingly deep understanding of the world's underlying structures and that the world is a complex system whose behavior is controlled by its dynamic structure and interactive feedback loops. Peter Senge (1990) defined systems thinking as a way of thinking about, and a language for describing and understanding, the forces and interrelationships that shape the behavior of systems. Systems thinking revolves around four key concepts: (a) all systems are composed of interconnected parts and a change to any part or connection affects the entire system, (b) structure or pattern of part connections is how the system is organized and determines its behavior, (c) system behavior is an emergent phenomenon as its parts and structure are constantly changing through feedback loops, and (d) feedback loops control a system's major dynamic behavior as each part influences the others in a circular pattern, creating a great deal of complexity. Systems thinking defined more recently by Derek and Laura Cabrera (2015) is the mastery and development of thinking that requires attention to distinctions (D), systems rules (S), relationship rules (R), and perspective rules (P). Systems thinking requires one be able to make distinctions between and among ideas or things. And any idea or thing can be split into parts or lumped into a whole. And any idea can relate to other ideas or things. Finally, any thing or idea can be the point or view of a perspective. Distinguishing standardized terminology becomes important in clinical reasoning. How clinicians split terms or lump them together becomes important in regard to relating issues to each other from disciplinary points of view or perspectives.

The key to solving difficult complex social system problems is to use systems thinking with a process that uniquely fits the problem at hand within the system dynamics. For example, thinking and reasoning about balancing and reinforcing causal loops in a system dynamic are done by taking in the whole picture. Systems thinking is a framework that assists one to focus on relationships and patterns versus objects (Senge, 1990). Relationships, whether they be visible or invisible, become obvious with systems thinking as well as linkages and interactions among all the elements that comprise the whole situation (Senge, 1990). Understanding the whole system of human activity in the environment in which it exists is one of the challenges for the advanced practice nurse in care coordination. Instead of the traditional linear cause-and-effect relationship among patient comorbidities, treatments, and outcomes, the whole complex and bidirectional interrelationships are considered at the same time to expose interconnectedness (Pesut, 2008). Jennifer Mensik (2014) describes the importance of a systems-thinking mind-set for systems-based leadership in health care, and discusses the challenges of systems thinking from an individual organization up, and systems thinking from the corporate office down.

The final feature of systems thinking is consideration of the filter or frames one uses to interpret the facts in a situation. Frames or schemata, as defined by Lakoff (2010), are unconscious structures that include semantic roles, relations among roles, and relations to other frames. Furthermore, the frames that are established in cognitive and metacognitive processes in the brain belong to the system the frame is coming from (Lakoff, 2010). Frames are strengthened and maintained by language, evoke emotion, and inform unconscious reasoning (thinking). So developing a frame in terms of the system in which one is working assists with interpreting and considering facts that must be communicated to others. The various frames brought to a care coordination situation by each individual health care provider may prohibit providers from becoming involved in the system and understanding the real situation. For example, frames for care coordination that all providers and patients understand equally well require practice with systems thinking. Lakoff (2010) asserts that a lack of frames results in hypocognition. Some strategies to help with new frame development are (a) frame issues in terms of moral values; (b) provide stories that emphasize values and evoke emotion; (c) find general themes or narrative that incorporates important points; and (d) be aware of context and use words, visuals, and body language people can understand.

Complexity Thinking

Complexity thinking transcends and includes systems thinking. Complexity-thinking strategies emerged from complexity theory, which is based on mathematics and quantum physics, where "relationship is the key determiner of everything" (Wheatley, 1999, p. 11). The relationship of components in a situation reveals a pattern or configuration map of relationships (Capra, 1996). Complexity theory studies the interrelationship of multiple components, a weaving of forces, and interconnecting of parts that unite to create complex forms in motion (Gleick, 1987). Complexity theory applied to nursing and health care proposes that a multitude of factors influence health while acknowledging the uniqueness of each interaction with a patient. Complexity thinking then involves attention to the recursive nonlinear pattern recognition associated with the identification and creation of clinical reasoning webs, patient care needs, and nursing care responses. This nonlinearity is a difficult idea to accept in a society that is constantly seeking specific causes and solutions for problems. The individual, whether he or she is the patient or health care provider, is in relationships embedded in larger patterns such as families and health care communities. Some broader patterns that affect people are the environment, the economy, and the political system.

With complexity thinking, one considers multiple interactions of various elements in a situation (Pesut, 2008). The knowledge representation and framing of nursing phenomena involving patient care needs are complex and nurses have to adjust their thinking to accommodate them. The specific complex-thinking activities that enable one to perform clinical reasoning are gained through practice, conscious reflection, and attention to issues of complexity associated with a patient's story and context of practice. Complexity thinking defined in the clinical reasoning model for care coordination is derived from complexity principles and practices that lead to filtering, framing, and focus with concurrent understanding of system dynamics and, ultimately, the determination and juxtaposition of present states with desired outcome states.

In the Outcome-Present State-Test model of reflective clinical reasoning, keystone issues are derived from the application of systems and complexity thinking and help determine the central supporting element of the client story derived from analysis of system dynamics and complexity of relationships among identified diagnoses. Combining systems thinking with an understanding of the complexity of relationships embedded in a particular patient story gives rise to the challenge of care coordination and how the patient, at several levels of perspective, is affected by relationships with care providers and the context in which he or she lives and works. CCCR suggests that it is important to take into account the complexity of relationship/issues associated with thinking about a patient's needs, given the cast of providers and the health care delivery systems in which they practice.

Over time, nursing practice has changed in response to technological advances and expanded scope of practice, whereas the medical profession has adjusted as nurses assume responsibilities that once belonged to the medical profession. The exact nature of the specific interventions for patients varies depending on the patient needs; the history, filtering, framing, and focus of the practitioner; and the feedback related to the health care issues. In one situation, the pull of medical care may dominate, such as when the client has a physical illness requiring surgery. At another time, the patient may be more in need of treatments within the advanced practice nurses scope of practice, but the care from an advanced practice nurse is responsive to both nursing and medical sciences. Knowledge management informs nursing practice and other members of the health care team. The multiple skills and highly varied activities of nurses reflect the complex nature of the practice and health care arena. Complexity theory and thinking enable the nurse to consider many interrelated components with sensitivity to the filtering, framing, and focus that is required from each discipline, and with the health care team as a whole. Nursing as a holistic practice is always responsive to the unique and dynamic situations involving patient care as multiple interacting systems evolve and adapt (Waldrop, 1992). CCCR challenges nurses and all the members of the interprofessional team to think about their thinking and combine both cognitive and metacognitive skills in determining the practice issues, interventions, and outcomes that support activity plans of the interprofessional team.

METACOGNITION: THINKING ABOUT THE THINKING FOR CARE COORDINATION

Cognitive scientists have observed that people reason by using personal filters, frames, and foci, rather than careful assessment of facts, because they look for consistency with existing beliefs and preconceptions (Mariotto, 2010). The development and use of appropriate cognitive and metacognitive (thinking about thinking) processes used in thinking activities for clinical reasoning in a given situation transcend the limitations of the evidence and personal frames alone. Cognitive and metacognitive processes using specific thinking activities involve the application of knowledge and experience to identify patient problems and direct clinical judgments and actions, which results in positive patient outcomes (Benner, Hughes, & Sutphen, 2008; Kuiper & Pesut, 2004). If patient needs and wishes are not considered, and our thinking to choose appropriate interventions within a care coordination system is faulty, our practice interventions fail and they may turn to unscientific alternatives and contribute to hypocognition (Mariotto, 2010). Three strategies to solve issues of hypocognition are (a) relocate and integrate basic science into clinical reasoning skills, (b) practice translating evidence into practice from a pragmatic standpoint using the type of thinking that promotes this, and (c) be cautious about algorithms (that are created out of an attempt to synthesize overwhelming amounts of clinical research data) that deny individuality of clinical decision making (Mariotto, 2010).

CCCR skills are displayed in Table 5.1. Cognitive (critical thinking) and metacognitive (reflective self-regulation, creative thinking, systems thinking, and complexity thinking) thinking strategies are listed in categories to show how they are particular to types of thinking; yet, in practice, they are used simultaneously and recursively during the care coordination process.

Clinical expertise, clinical reasoning skills, and cognitive and metacognitive processes are needed to know when it is appropriate to deviate from evidence-based guidelines while also considering the values and preferences of individual patients, to deliver quality patient-centered, safe care (Cronenwett et al., 2007).

Understanding the nature of a whole situation from different levels of perspective is embedded in a sense of salience and reasoning in the situation or one's understanding (frame) of the situation (Benner, Hooper-Kyriakidis, & Stannard, 2011; Bordieu, 1990). This brings to the forefront the importance of advanced practice nurse abilities to self-regulate and manage different cognitive loads using the appropriate thinking activities for the context and health care problem at hand. As nurses filter, frame, and focus on different aspects of patient care needs, standardized terminology and knowledge representation systems provide ways to help them filter, frame, and focus disciplinary contributions to care.

SUMMARY

The CCCR model described in subsequent chapters of this book, and shown in Figure 5.1, includes and assumes the skills and thinking strategies described in Table 5.1. The CCCR model can be used as a pedagogical tool to help advanced practice nursing students hone their clinical reasoning abilities during field experiences.

The model illustrated previously integrates the elements of care coordination and highlights the importance of practice issues, interventions, outcomes, and values with attention to different levels of perspective. The levels of perspective are organized around patient-centered, team-centered, and organization-centered systems thinking. Knowledge management among team members is crucial and is accomplished through negotiation of the competing values of collaborating, creating, competing, and controlling. Team members act as facilitators, mentors, innovators, and brokers as they produce, direct and coordinate, and monitor practice issues, interventions, and outcomes in service of identified needs, individualized care planning, safety monitoring, evaluation, and use of resources that enable coaching and education to foster patient self-management.

TABLE 5.1 Care Coordination Clinical Reasoning Skills

COGNITIVE PROCESSES		METACOGNITIVE PROCESSES		
CRITICAL THINKING	REFLECTIVE SELF-REGULATION	CREATIVE THINKING	SYSTEMS THINKING	COMPLEXITY THINKING
A. Skills Information seeking Discriminating Interpreting Analyzing Explaining Transforming knowledge Predicating Applying standards Logical reasoning Inferring **B. Habits of Mind** Motivation Perseverance Fair-mindedness Deliberate and careful attention to thinking	**A. Forethought** Schema search Prototype identification **B. Performance Control** Attention to situation **C. Self-Regulation** 1. Self-reflection on behavior Self-monitoring Self-observation Self-judgment Self-reaction 2. Self-reflection on environment Skills/activities Context People 3. Self-evaluation/correction of thinking Self-efficacy Knowledge use Goals	**A. General Domain-Specific Strategies** Breaking down a problem Planning Monitoring Modifying behavior **B. Generating Ideas** Generate and test means–ends analysis Analogical reasoning Brainstorming **C. Preparing for Action** Indentifying complementary pairs Considering opposites Hypothesizing Recognizing tensions Using if–then thinking Comparative analysis	**A. Identify Interconnected Parts of the System Frame** Relationships Patterns **B. Identify the System Organization Frame** Bidirectional interrelationships **C. Identify the Frame of System Behaviors** Semantic roles Relations between roles Relations to other frames **D. Identify the Feedback Loops in the Frame** Circular and recursive communication General themes Language—words, visuals, body language	**A. Recursive Nonlinear Pattern Recognition** Families Health care communities Environment Economy Political system **B. Metacognitive Activities** Juxtaposition of present states with desired outcome states Practice conscious reflection on issues of complexity in patient's story and context Reframing

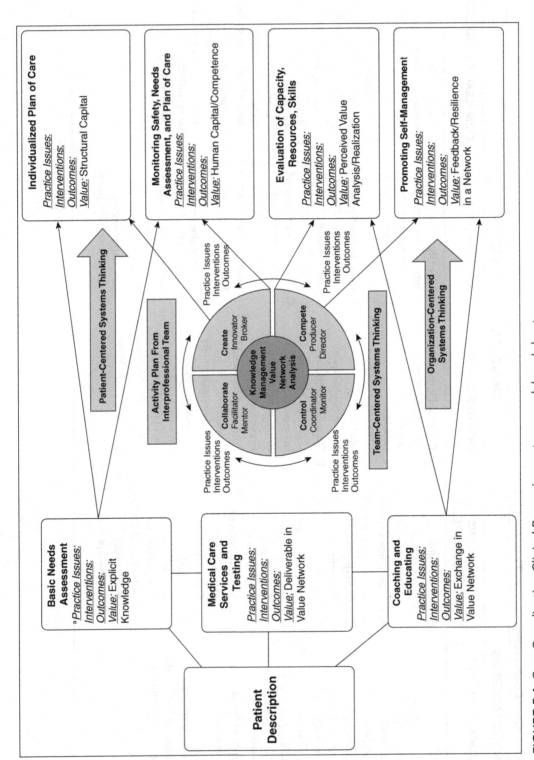

FIGURE 5.1 Care Coordination Clinical Reasoning systems model worksheet.

[a] Practice issues can be from any discipline: nursing, medicine, pharmacy, social work, and so on.

A significant point for the advanced practice nurse student to understand is that clinical reasoning in the context of care coordination requires practice so APRNs can develop competence and confidence with the thinking activities described in this chapter. Field experiences with preceptors who guide, mentor, and model clinical reasoning are essential; however, support by means of clinical reasoning models and worksheets is valuable to assist with training the mind to develop habits of good thinking.

KEY CONCEPTS

1. Health care in the United States is striving to meet the goals of the triple aim: positive patient experience, high quality, and cost-effectiveness.
2. Registered professional nurses have always had responsibilities for coordinating and advocating patient care experiences.
3. Case management evolved to help patients with comorbidities and complexities navigate health care systems.
4. Advanced practice nurses have the knowledge, skills, and abilities to evolve new models of care coordination that focus on patients, teams, and organizations.
5. The CCCR model builds on systems thinking, knowledge, skills, and abilities and attends to different levels of perspective in reasoning about clients, families, health care providers, and the systems in which they work.
6. Reflective self-regulation is an essential metacognitive process used to develop insight into thinking activities and changes needed for current and future care coordination models.
7. Clinical reasoning for care coordination involves the use of critical thinking, creative thinking, complexity thinking, and systems thinking.
8. Critical thinking and creative thinking are foundational for the advanced practice nurse to be able to apply knowledge and language when managing and communicating information in care coordination.
9. Advanced practice nurses must learn and use complexity- and systems-thinking activities in order to adapt to multiprofessional teams in dynamic health care systems.
10. The process of CCCR is influenced by the cognitive and metacognitive thinking activities that permit the advanced practice nurse to frame and consider the whole situation and associated relationships between and among problems, interventions, and outcomes in service of patient preferences for safe and effective care.

STUDY QUESTIONS AND ACTIVITIES

1. Develop a care coordination definition based on your practice experience. Does it match any of the definitions in the literature and would you change it based on the current health care environment?

2. Review the Institute of Medicine Report, *Crossing the Quality Chasm: A New Health System for the 21st Century* (2001) and determine whether the recommendations proposed therein have changed the scope of practice for contemporary advanced practice nurses as it relates to care coordination.

3. Compare and contrast the care coordination definitions presented in this chapter and determine which would be most appropriate for your practice setting. Explain why.

4. If you are practicing within a care coordination model, does it work and have positive outcomes/benefits been achieved for the patients in your practice?

5. Does the scope of practice and standards of care for advanced practice nurses in your state/country include the skills and activities required to coordinate care within multidisciplinary teams? If not, how would you begin to impact the necessary professional organizations and groups to promote the advanced practice nurse as the facilitator of care coordination teams?

REFERENCES

Agency for Healthcare Research and Quality (AHRQ). (2014). *What is care coordination? Care coordination measures atlas update*. Rockville, MD: Author. Retrieved from http://www.ahrq.gov/professionals/prevention-chronic-care/improve/coordination/index.html

Aiken, L. H., & Salmon, M. E. (1994). Health-care workforce priorities: What nursing should do now. *Inquiry, 31,* 318–329.

American Academy of Nursing (AAN). (2012). *Raise the voice: Transforming America's health care system through nursing solutions*. Retrieved from http://www.aannet.org/raisethevoice

American Association of Colleges of Nursing (AACN). (1998). *The essentials of baccalaureate education for professional nursing practice*. Washington, DC: Author.

American Association of Colleges of Nursing (AACN). (2004). *Working paper on the role of the clinical nurse leader*. Washington, DC: Author.

American Association of Colleges of Nursing (AACN). (2011). *The essentials of master's education in nursing*. Retrieved from http://www.aacn.nche.edu/education-resources/MastersEssentials11.pdf

American Association of Nurse Practitioners. (2013). *Nurse practitioners in primary care*. Retrieved from www.aanp.org

American Nurses Association (ANA). (2012). *Position statement: Care coordination and nurses' essential role*. Retrieved from http://www.nursingworld.org/MainMenuCategories/Policy-Advocacy/Positions-and-Resolutions/ANAPositionStatements/Position-Statements-Alphabetically/Care-Coordination-and-Registered-Nurses-Essential-Role.html

American Nurses Association (ANA). (2015). *Scope and standards of practice* (3rd ed.). Silver Spring, MD: Author.

Anderson, J. R. (1990). *Cognitive psychology and its implications* (3rd ed.). New York, NY: W. H. Freeman.

Anderson, J. R. (1993). Problem solving and learning. *American Psychologist, 48,* 35–44.

Anderson, J. R. (2000). *Learning and memory: An integrated approach* (2nd ed.). New York, NY: John Wiley & Sons.

Antonelli, R. C., Stille, C. J., & Antonelli, D. M. (2008). Care coordination for children and youth with special health care needs: A descriptive, multisite study of activities, personnel costs, and outcomes. *Pediatrics, 122*(1), e209–e216.

Atherly, A., & Thorpe, K. E. (2011). Analysis of the treatment effect of Healthway's Medicare health support phase 1 pilot on Medicare costs. *Population Health Management, 14*(1), 23–28.

Ayanian, J. (2009). The elusive quest for quality and cost savings in the Medicare program. *Journal of the American Medical Association, 301*(6), 668–670.

Bandura, A. (1997). *Self-efficacy: The exercise of control.* New York, NY: W. H. Freeman.

Benner, P., Hooper-Kyriakidis, P., & Stannard, D. (2011). *Clinical wisdom and intervention in acute and critical care: A thinking in action approach.* New York, NY: Springer Publishing.

Benner, P., Hughes, R. G., & Sutphen, M. (2008). Clinical reasoning, decision making, and action: Thinking critically and clinically. In R. G. Hughes (Ed.), *Patient safety and quality: An evidence-based handbook for nurses* (pp. 1–23). Washington, DC: Agency for Healthcare Research and Quality. Retrieved from http://www.ncbi.nlm.nih.bov/books/n/nursehb/ch6

Bordieu, P. (1990). *The logic of practice.* Stanford, CA: Stanford University Press.

Brandt, S., Hartmann, J., & Hehner, S. (2010). How to design a successful disease management program. *Health International, 101,* 68–79.

Brookfield, S. D. (2012). *Teaching for critical thinking: Tools and techniques to help students question their assumptions.* San Francisco, CA: Jossey-Bass.

Cabrera, D., & Cabrera, L. (2015). *Systems thinking made simple: New hope for solving wicked problems.* New York, NY: Odyssean Press.

Capra, F. (1996). *The web of life.* New York, NY: Doubleday.

Christensen, H., Griffiths, K. M., Gulliver, A., Clack, D., Kljakovic, M., & Wells, L. (2008). Models in the delivery of depression care: A systematic review of randomized and controlled intervention trials. *Family Practice, 9,* 25–35. Retrieved from http://www.biomedcentral.com/1471–2296/9/25

Coleman, E. A., Parry, C., Chalmers, S., & Min, S. J. (2006). The care transitions intervention: Results of a randomized controlled trial. *Archives of Internal Medicine, 166*(17), 1822–1828.

Craig, C., Eby, D., & Whittington, J. (2011). *Care coordination model: Better care at lower cost for people with multiple health and social needs.* Cambridge, MA: Institute for Healthcare Improvement.

Cronenwett, L., Sherwood, G., Barnsteiner, J., Disch, J., Johnson, J., Mitchell, P., . . . Warren, J. (2007). Quality and safety education for nurses. *Nursing Outlook, 55*(3), 122–131.

Dietrich, A. J., Oxman, T. E., Williams, J. W., Schulberg, H. C., Bruce, M. L, Lee, P. W., . . . Nuttting, P.A. (2004). Re-engineering systems for the treatment of depression in primary care: Cluster randomized controlled trial. *British Medical Journal, 329,* 602.

Facione, P. A. (1990). *The Delphi report: Executive summary;* critical thinking: A statement of expert consensus for purposes of educational assessment and instruction. Millbrae, CA: The California Academic Press.

Farmer, J. E., Clark, M. J., Drewel, E. H., Swenson, T. M., & Ge, B. (2011). Consultative care coordination through the medical home for CSHCN: A randomized controlled trial. *Maternal Child Health Journal, 15*(7), 1110–1118.

Foss, N., & Koerner, J. (1997). The advanced practice nurse's role in differentiated practice: Martha's story. *AACN Clinical Issues, 8,* 262–270.

Gleick, J. (1987). *Chaos: Making a new science.* New York, NY: Penguin Books.

Goeree, R., & Levin, L. (2006). Building bridges between academic research and policy formulation: The PRUFE framework—An integral part of Ontario's evidence-based HTPA process. *Pharmacoeconomics, 24,* 1143–1156.

Gordon, J. B., Colby, H. H., Bartelt, T., Jablonski, D., Krauthoefer M. L., & Havens, P. (2007). A tertiary care–primary care partnership model for medically complex and fragile children and youth with special health care needs. *Pediatric and Adolescent Medicine, 161*(10), 937–944. doi:10.1001/archpedi.161.10.937

Greiner, A., & Knebel, E. (Eds.). (2003). *Health professions education: A bridge to quality.* Washington, DC: The National Academies Press.

Gundersen Lutheran Health System. (2013). Care coordination cuts admissions, ED visits, LOS. *Hospital Case Management, 21*(5), 67–68. Retrieved from http://www.gundluth

.org/upload/docs/CareCoordination.pdf; http://www.refworks.com/refworks2/?site=025421125547200000%2fRWWS2A909793%2fPublications

Haas, S. A., Swan, B. A., & Haynes, T. S. (Eds.). (2014). *Care coordination and transition management core curriculum.* Pittman, NJ: American Academy of Ambulatory Care Nursing.

Institute of Medicine (IOM). (2001). *Crossing the quality chasm: A new health system for the 21st century.* Washington, DC: The National Academies Press.

Kligler, B., Homel, P., Harrison, L. B., Levenson, H. D., Kenney, J. B., & Merrell, W. (2011). Cost savings in inpatient oncology through an integrative medicine approach. *American Journal of Managed Care, 17*(12), 779–784.

Kuiper, R. A., & Pesut, D. J. (2004). Promoting cognitive and metacognitive reflective clinical reasoning skills in nursing practice: Self-regulated learning theory. *Journal of Advanced Nursing, 45*(4), 381–391.

Lakoff, G. (2010). Why it matters how we frame the environment. *Environmental Communication: A Journal of Nature and Culture, 4*(1), 70–81. doi:10.1080/17524030903529749

Lamb, G. (2013). Care coordination, quality, and nursing. In G. Lamb (Ed.), *Care coordination: The game changer how nursing is revolutionizing quality care* (pp. 1–9). Silver Spring, MD: American Nurses Association. Retrieved from Nursesbooks.org

Lancaster, J., Lancaster W., & Onega, L. L. (2000). New directions in health-care reform: The role of nurse practitioners. *Journal of Business Research, 48*, 207–212.

Laughlin, C. B., & Beisel, M. (2010). Evolution of the chronic care role of the registered nurse in primary care. *Nursing Economics, 28*(6), 409–414.

Looman, W. S., Presler, E., Erickson, M. M., Garwick, A. W., Cady, R. G., Kelly, A. M., & Finkelstein, S. M. (2013). Care coordination for children with complex special health care needs: The value of the advanced practice nurse's enhanced scope of knowledge and practice. *Journal of Pediatric Health Care, 27*(4), 293–303.

Mariotto, A. (2010). Hypocognition and evidence-based medicine. *Internal Medicine Journal, 40*, 80–82. doi:10.111?j.1445–5994.2009.02086.x

Mensik, J. (2014). *Lead, drive and thrive in the system.* Silver Spring, MD: American Nurses Association. Retrieved from Nursesbooks.org

Milstead, J. A. (2008). *Health policy and politics: A nurse's guide* (3rd Ed.). Sudbury, MA: Jones & Bartlett.

Moore, K. D., & Coddington, D. C. (2011). *ACO case study: Catholic medical partners.* Buffalo, NY: American Hospital Associating & McManis Consulting.

Mullnix, C., & Bucholtz, D. P. (2009). Role and quality of nurse practitioner practice: A policy issue. *Nursing Outlook, 57*, 93–96.

National Quality Forum (NQF). (2010). *Quality connections: Care coordination.* Retrieved from http://www.qualityforum.org/Publications/2010/10/Quality_Connections__Care_Coordination.aspx

National Quality Forum (NQF). (2014). *NQF endorses care coordination measures.* Retrieved from http://public.qualityforum.org/NQFDocuments/Phrasebook.pdf; http://www.qualityforum.org/News_And_Resources/Press_Releases/2012/NQF_Endorses_Care_Coordination_Measures.aspx

Naylor, M. D., Brooten, D. A., Campbell, R. L., Maislin, G., McCauley, K. M., & Schwartz, J. S. (2004). Transitional care of older adults hospitalized with heart failure: A randomized, controlled trial. *Journal of the American Geriatrics Society, 52*(5), 675–684.

Nursing Alliance for Quality Care [NAQC]. (2014). *The role of nurses in accountable care organizations.* Silver Spring, MD: Author. Retrieved from http://www.rwjf.org/files/research/Whatareaccountablecareorganizations.pdf

Owens, M. K. (2010). Costs of uncoordinated care. In P. L. Young, R. S. Saunders, & L. A. Olsen (Eds.), *The healthcare imperative: Lowering costs and improving outcomes: Workshop series summary* (pp. 109–140). Washington, DC: The National Academies Press.

Oxman, T. E, Dietrich, A. J., Williams, J. W., & Kroenke, K. (2002). A three-component model for re-engineering systems for the treatment of depression in primary care. *Psychosomatics, 43*, 441–450.

Patient Protection and Affordable Care Act, 42 U.S.C., § 18001 (2010). Pub Law No. 111–148.

Peikes, D., Chen, A., Schore, J., & Brown, R. (2009). Effects of care coordination on hospitalization, quality of care, and health care expenditures among Medicare beneficiaries. *Journal of the American Medical Association, 301*(6), 603–618.

Pesut, D. (2008). Thoughts on thinking with complexity in mind. In C. Lindberg, S. Nash, & C. Lindberg (Eds.), *On the edge: Nursing in the age of complexity* (pp. 211–238). CreateSpace Independent Publishing Platform, Plexus Press.

Pesut, D., & Herman, J. (1999). *Clinical reasoning: The art and science of critical and creative thinking*. New York, NY: Delmar.

Radzyminski, S. (2005). Advances in graduate nursing education: Beyond the advanced practice nurse. *Journal of Professional Nursing, 21*(2), 119–125.

Richmond, B. (1993) Systems thinking: Critical thinking skills for the 1990s and beyond. *System Dynamics Review, 9*(2), 13–133.

Robles, L., Slogoff, M., Ladwig-Scott, E., Zank, D., Larson, M. K., Aranha, G., & Shoup, M. (2011). The addition of a nurse practitioner to an inpatient surgical team results in improved use of resources. *Surgery, 150*(4), 711–717.

Safriet, B. J. (2002). Closing the gap between can and may in health-care providers' scopes of practice: A primer for policymakers. *Yale Journal of Regulation, 19*, 301–334.

Scheffer, B., & Rubenfeld, G. (2000). A consensus statement on critical thinking in nursing. *Journal of Nursing Education, 39*(8), 352–359, 356.

Schraeder, C., & Shelton, P. (2013). Effective care coordination models. In G. Lamb (Ed.), *Care coordination: The game changer how nursing is revolutionizing quality care* (pp. 57–79). Silver Spring, MD: American Nurses Association. Retrieved from Nursesbooks.org

Schunk, D. H. (2012). *Learning theories—An educational perspective* (6th ed.). Upper Saddle River, NJ: Pearson Prentice-Hall.

Senge, P. (1990). *The fifth discipline: The art and practice of the learning organization*. New York, NY: Doubleday Currency.

Shiu, A., Lee, D., & Chau, J. (2012). Exploring the scope of expanding advanced nursing practice in nurse-let clinics: A multiple-case study. *Journal of Advanced Nursing, 68*(8), 1780–1792.

Stanley, J. M., Werner, K. E., & Apple, K. (2009). Positioning advanced practice registered nurses for health care reform: Consensus on APRN regulation. *Journal of Professional Nursing, 25*(6), 340–348. doi:10.1016/j.profnurs.2009.10.001

Sustaita, A., Zeigler, V., & Brogan, M. (2013). Hiring a nurse practitioner: What's in it for the physician? *Nurse Practitioner, 11*(38) 41–45. doi:10.1097/01.NPR.0000435783.63014.1c.

Tabloski, P. (2014). *Gerontological nursing* (3rd ed.). Upper Saddle River, NJ: Pearson.

Touhy, T. A., & Jett, K. (2012). *Ebersole & Hess' toward healthy aging: Human needs & nursing response* (8th ed.). St. Louis, MI: Mosby Elsevier.

Treffinger, D. J. (1985). Review of the Torrance Tests of creative thinking. In J. Mitchell (Ed.), *Ninth mental measurements yearbook* (pp. 1633–1634). Lincoln, NE: Buros Institute of Mental Measurement.

Treffinger, D. J., & Isaksen, S. G. (2005). Creative problem solving: The history, development, and implications for gifted education and talent development. *Gifted Child Quarterly, 49*(4), 342–353. doi:10.1177/001698620504900407

Waldrop, M. (1992). *Complexity: The emerging science at the edge of chaos*. New York, NY: Simon and Schuster.

Watson, G., & Glaser, E. (1964) *Critical thinking appraisal manual*. New York, NY: Harcourt Brace & World.

Wheatley, M. J. (1999). *Leadership and the new science* (2nd ed.). San Francisco, CA: Berrett-Koehler.

Yang, Y. T., & Meiners, M. R. (2014). Care coordination and the expansion of nursing scopes of practice. *Journal of Law, Medicine & Ethics, 42*(1), 93–103.

Zimmerman, B. (1998). Developing self-fulfilling cycles of academic regulation: An analysis of exemplary instructional models. In D. H. Schunk & B. J. Zimmerman (Eds.), *Self-regulated learning: From teaching to self-reflective practice* (pp. 1–19). New York, NY: Guilford Press.

Zimmerman, B. (2000). Attaining self-regulation: A social cognitive perspective. In M. Boekaerts, P. R. Pintrich, & M. Zeidner (Eds.), *Handbook of self-regulation* (pp. 13–39). San Diego, CA: Academic Press.

Zimmerman, B., & Schunk, D. S. (2001). *Self-regulated learning and academic thought.* Mahwah, NJ: Lawrence Erlbaum.

PART II

CARE COORDINATION CLINICAL REASONING CASE STUDIES

CHAPTER 6

CARE COORDINATION FOR A PATIENT IN PRIMARY COMMUNITY HEALTH

In this chapter, we use the Care Coordination Clinical Reasoning (CCCR) systems model, as described in Part I, and explain how the model can be used to reason about a case given the context of primary community health care. The case presented in this chapter illustrates how an advanced practice nurse works with a family who is in need of health and wellness services to promote quality-of-life outcomes. The provider/clinic is the point of access for patients/families. The advanced practice nurse provides care coordination through the application and use of critical-, creative-, systems-, and complexity-thinking processes to manage patient problems with an interprofessional team, which will design appropriate interventions and establish patient-centered outcomes. Depending on the nature of need involved in the case, referrals to other specialty or primary care providers, community services, and living environments are determined and considered in managing care coordination and transitions (Haas, Swan, & Haynes, 2014).

The CCCR systems model framework begins with the patient story, which is derived from gathering data and evidence from an interview, history, physical examination, and the health record. The advanced practice nurse then develops a patient-centered plan of care using the Outcome-Present State-Test (OPT) model worksheets. In order to do this, patient-centered systems-thinking skills are activated for complex patient stories and key questions are consistently used to reflect on the specific sections of the model (Pesut, 2008), as well as the dimensions and elements of care coordination.

LEARNING OUTCOMES

After completing this chapter, the reader should be able to:

1. Explain the components of a care coordination framework that are needed to manage the problems, interventions, and outcomes of people in the primary community health context

2. Describe the different thinking processes that support clinical reasoning skills and strategies for determining priorities in primary community health care coordination

3. Define the cognitive and metacognitive self-regulatory processes that support individual provider critical reflection related to levels and perspectives associated with clinical reasoning for primary community health care coordination

4. Describe how the communication and knowledge management between interprofessional health care team members are essential for care coordination to address patient and family needs in primary community health

5. Describe the critical meta-reflective processes that support team reflection, communication, and value-added impact related to levels and perspectives associated with the care coordination challenges and clinical reasoning required to navigate patient care plans in primary health contexts

THE PATIENT STORY

We begin with the history and story of a 60-year-old African American female, Dorothy Smith, recently admitted into the Program of All-Inclusive Care for the Elderly (PACE). She lives with her brother and sister-in-law, who are her primary care providers. Ms. Smith recently moved from another state in a different region of the United Sates where she lived with another brother who recently passed away. She never married and has no children. She came to PACE (a primary community health clinic) with complaints of physical and verbal abuse from both her brother and sister-in-law. She was evaluated in the emergency department of the local hospital 2 days after she was injured as a result of a fall caused by her care providers. From the accident, she had a laceration that resulted in cellulitis of the lower right leg. The provider in the emergency department prescribed an antibiotic ointment for the laceration and discharged her to home. This leg is now painful to touch, erythematous, and swollen around the laceration.

The patient also reports financial exploitation from her caregivers as evidenced by their absconding with her food stamps and disability checks without sharing any of the resources with her. She states that her brother is trying to have her declared incompetent and he became "very angry" when he found out that she decided on a "do not resuscitate" (DNR) status on her medical record. This patient reports increased anxiety, difficulty sleeping at night, and a decreased appetite. She was placed in a skilled nursing facility (SNF) after she reported the abuse. Her brother was notified of the allegations and that adult protective services (APS) was contacted.

The physical examination and functional assessment reveal that she is wheelchair bound, but independent in mobilizing herself in the home. She is able to feed herself after meals are prepared and set up. She requires assistance with toileting, bathing, and dressing. This patient smokes cigarettes and has a 45-pack-year history (1 pack per day for 45 years). She scores 18 out of 21 on the Mini-Mental State Exam (MMSE) with an orientation of eight out of 10, and a recall of two out of three. Clock draw was normal.

The patient's past medical history includes left hemiparesis after a cerebral vascular accident, which resulted in wheelchair dependency. She also has a history of hypertension, hyperlipidemia, gastroesophageal reflux disease (GERD), vitamin D deficiency, recurrent urinary tract infections, morbid obesity, eczema, bilateral cataracts, mild cognitive impairment, and depression. Current medications include Plavix, Flexiril, Benadryl, hydrochlorothiazide, lisinopril, ranitidine, Tylenol, vitamin D_3, naproxen, and Keflex.

PATIENT-CENTERED PLAN OF CARE USING OPT WORKSHEETS

Once the patient story is obtained from all possible sources, care planning and clinical reasoning follow using the OPT clinical reasoning web worksheet (Figure 6.1) to help determine relationships among issues and to highlight potential keystone issues. The OPT clinical reasoning web is a graphic representation of the functional relationships between and among diagnostic hypotheses derived from the analysis and synthesis regarding how each element and issue of the story relates to another. This activates critical and creative thinking. The visual diagram that results illustrates dynamics among issues, and a convergence helps to point out central issues that require nursing care. As one thinks about this case and begins to spin and weave a clinical reasoning web, relationships are identified among nursing diagnoses as they are jointly considered with medical conditions. The chronic medical condition in this case is a history of cerebrovascular accident (CVA) with comorbidities. Once the advanced practice nurse considers these medical diagnoses, the nursing care domains associated with them are identified. The complementary nursing domains and diagnoses most appropriate in this case are risk for injury, falls, and other directed violence.

To spin and weave the web, provider uses thinking processes to analyze and synthesize relationships among diagnostic hypotheses associated with a patient's health status. The visual representation and mapping of these relationships support the development of patient-centered systems thinking and connections between and among the medical and nursing diagnoses under consideration, given the patient story.

The steps to the creation of the OPT clinical reasoning web using the worksheet are as follows:

1. Place a general description of the patient in the respective middle circle—60-year-old African American female.
2. Place the major medical diagnoses in the respective middle circle—history of CVA with comorbidities.
3. Place the major nursing diagnoses in the respective middle circle—risk for injury, falls, and other directed violence.
4. Choose the nursing domains for which each medical and nursing diagnosis is appropriate—safety and protection, nutrition, coping and stress tolerance, health promotion, activity and rest, perception, and cognition.
5. Generate all the International Classification of Diseases (ICD)-10 codes that are appropriate for the particular patient and family story that coincide with the nursing domains—physical abuse (T76.11), cellulitis (L03.115), obesity (E66.9), vitamin D deficiency (E55.9), hyperlipidemia (E78.5), depression (F33.0), nicotine dependence (F17.203), GERD (K21.9), hypertension (I10), hemiplegia (I69.35), and mild cognitive impairment (G31.84).

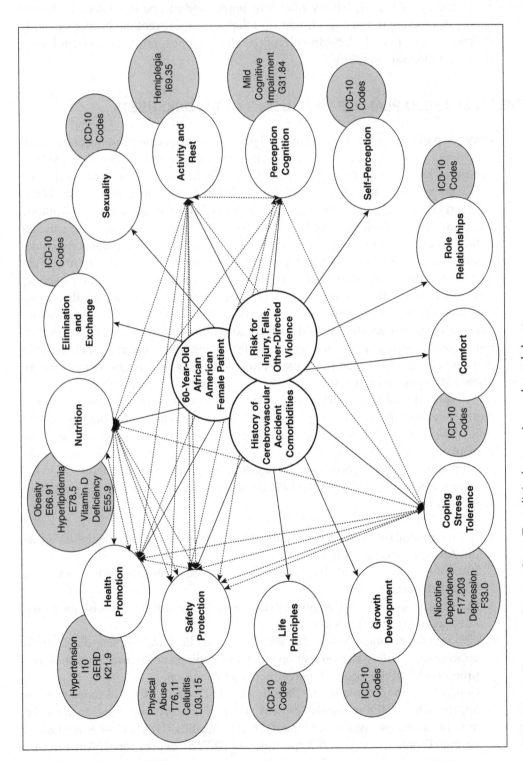

FIGURE 6.1 Outcome-Present State-Test clinical reasoning web worksheet.

GERD, gastroesophageal reflux disease; ICD-10, International Classification of Diseases, 10th edition.

6. Once the nursing domains, diagnoses, and ICD-10 codes are identified, reflect on the total web worksheet and concurrently consider and explain how each of the issues is or is not related to the other issues. Draw lines of relationship to spin and weave the web connections or associations among the ICD-10 codes/diagnoses. As you draw the lines, think out loud, justify the reasons for the connections, and explain specifically how the diagnoses may or may not be connected or related.

7. After you have spent some time connecting the relationships, determine which domain (domains) has the highest priority for care coordination and most efficiently and effectively represents the keystone nursing care needs of the patient by counting the arrows that connect the medical problems (ICD-10 codes). In this case, counting 14 lines pointing to or from the nursing domain of safety and protection represents the priority present state keystone issues.

8. Look once again at the sets of relationships and determine the theme or keystone that summarizes the patient-in-context or the patient story—the consequences of physical abuse and the promoters of infection/cellulitis are the keystone issues for this case.

The OPT clinical reasoning web worksheet in Figure 6.1 shows a template with the patient health care situation, medical diagnoses, and nursing diagnoses at the center. Around the outer edges of the web are nursing domains with ICD-10 codes derived from history and physical assessment associated with the patient story. The directional arrows that create the web effect represent connections, explanations, and functional relationships between and among the diagnostic possibilities. As one can see, the domains and ICD-10 codes with more connections converging on one of the circles display the priority problem or keystone, in this case safety and protection. A keystone issue is one or more central supporting element of the patient's story that help focus and determine a root cause or center of gravity of the system dynamics and help guide reasoning and care coordination based on an analysis (breaking things down into discrete parts) and synthesis (putting the parts together in a greater whole) of diagnostic possibilities as represented in the web. Some key questions to ask here are: How the clinical reasoning web reveals relationships between and among the identified diagnoses? To what degree do these relationships make practical clinical sense according to the evidence and patient story? Table 6.1 offers a summary of the connections highlighting the priority with the most connections.

After considering the full picture using the clinical reasoning web worksheet, the next step is to use an OPT clinical reasoning model worksheet to facilitate and structure the patient-centered systems thinking about the care coordination of the identified problems highlighted in Table 6.1. As the advanced practice nurse thinks about the patient, she or he will concurrently consider the frame, outcome state, and present state. Each aspect of the OPT clinical reasoning model contributes to the other. The OPT clinical reasoning model worksheet is a map of the structure designed to provide an illustrative representation and to guide thinking processes about relationships between and among competing issues and problems. Some questions that guide the use of the OPT clinical reasoning model are shown in Table 6.2 (Pesut, 2008).

TABLE 6.1 Relationships Among Nursing Domains, Medical Diagnoses, and Web Connections

NURSING DOMAINS	MEDICAL DIAGNOSES (ICD-10 CODES)	WEB CONNECTIONS
Safety/protection	Physical abuse T76.11 Cellulitis L03.115	14
Nutrition	Morbid obesity E66.9 Vitamin D deficiency E55.9 Hyperlipidemia E78.5	13
Coping/stress tolerance	Depression F33.0 Nicotine dependence F17.203	12
Perception/cognition	Mild cognitive impairment G31.84	12
Health promotion	GERD K21.9 Hypertension I10	11
Activity/rest	Hemiplegia I69.35	10

GERD, gastroesophageal reflux disease.

Source: World Health Organization (2015).

EXHIBIT 6.1 PATIENT-IN-CONTEXT STORY

Dorothy Smith is a 60-year-old African American female who presents with the complaint of ongoing abuse at home by family care providers.

Insomnia, anxiety, fearfulness, does not receive disability checks or food stamps from family, single, never married, no children

Cellulitis in right lower leg after tripping

Wheelchair bound for immobility and spasticity after CVA

Daily tobacco use

Ht: 5′ 6″, Wt: 244.8 lb., BMI: 39.5, BP: 132/84 mmHg, HR: 84 bpm, RR: 20, O_2 sat: 94% at rest

Elevated cholesterol and HbA1C

Decreased vitamin D

Abnormal urinalysis

BP, blood pressure; BMI, body mass index; HbA1c, glycosylated hemoglobin; HR, heart rate; Ht, height; O_2 sat, oxygen saturation; RR, respiratory rate; Wt, weight.

TABLE 6.2 Questions That Guide the Use of the OPT Model

Patient-in-context	What is the patient story?
Diagnostic cue/web logic	What diagnoses have you generated? What outcomes do you have in mind given the diagnoses? What evidence supports those diagnoses? How does a reasoning web reveal relationships among the identified problems (diagnoses)? What keystone issue(s) emerge?
Framing	How are you framing the situation?
Present state	How is the present state defined?
Outcome state	What are the desired outcomes? What are the gaps or complementary pairs (~) of outcomes and present states?
Test	What are the clinical indicators of the desired outcomes? On what scales will the desired outcomes be rated? How will you know when the desired outcomes are achieved? How are you defining your testing in this particular case?
Decision making (interventions)	What clinical decisions or interventions help to achieve the outcomes? What specific intervention activities will you implement? Why are you considering these activities?
Judgment	Given your testing, what is your clinical judgment? Based on your judgment, have you achieved the outcome or do you need to reframe the situation? How, specifically, will you take this experience and learning with you into the future as you reason about similar cases?

OPT, Outcome-Present State-test.
Adapted from Pesut (2008).

By writing each element on the worksheet, all the parts of the model become related to each other. As the health care provider moves from right to left, the model structures the plan of care. Critical thinking skills are used to consider the patient story and creative thinking is used to identify and reason about the keystone issues/themes/cues to determine the most significant evidence in the present state. Complexity thinking helps the provider to consider the outcomes desired and the gaps between the present and outcome states. Once interventions and tests are decided, the plan of care transitions to a care coordination model and team-centered systems thinking that consider patient and family preferences within the frame of the situation.

The patient-in-context story (Exhibit 6.1) is depicted on the far right-hand side in Figure 6.2. The advanced practice nurse notes relevant facts of the story, which in this case include the following: the patient demographics and characteristics; history of abuse by family care providers; psychosocial issues of insomnia, anxiety, and fearfulness; physical disabilities of immobility, injury, and cellulitis; and the fact that the patient is wheelchair bound because of immobility from a CVA. Assessment

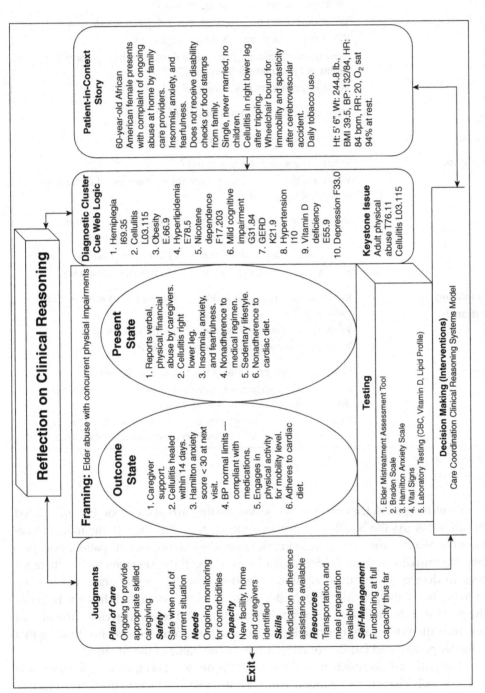

FIGURE 6.2 Outcome–Present State–Test clinical reasoning model for care coordination worksheet.

BMI, body mass index; BP, blood pressure; CBC, complete blood count; GERD, gastroesophageal reflux disease; Ht, height; HR, heart rate; O₂ sat, oxygen saturation; RR, respiratory rate; Wt, weight.

reveals obesity with normal vital signs and slightly decreased oxygen saturation at rest. Pertinent laboratory data include a complete metabolic panel and complete blood count (CBC) all within normal limits. Dorothy had an elevated cholesterol level of 181 mg/dL; elevated hemoglobin, A1C 5.9; decreased vitamin D, 11.1 ng/m and some white blood cells; 3+ occult blood; and protein in the urine. A key step at this juncture is to review and reflect on the patient story for accuracy and thoroughness to proceed with care planning for care coordination.

Moving to the left of the model worksheet, there is a place to list the diagnostic cluster cues on the web of medical diagnoses and ICD-10 codes (Exhibit 6.2). At the bottom of this box are placed the designated keystone issues or themes that fall under the most significant nursing domain—adult physical abuse (T76.11) and cellulitis (L03.115). Remember diagnostic cluster cue web logic is the use of inductive and deductive thinking skills. Some key questions to ask here are: What diagnoses were generated, is there evidence to support those diagnoses? Is the keystone issue appropriate given this patient story?

At the center and background of the worksheet are places to indicate the frame or theme that best represents the background issues regarding thinking about the patient story (Exhibit 6.3). The frame in this case is elder abuse with concurrent physical impairments. This frame helps organize the present state and the outcome state, illustrates the gaps, and provides insights about what tests need to be considered to fill the gap. Decision making and reflection surround the framing as the advanced practice nurse thinks of many things simultaneously. Reflective thinking is used to monitor thinking and behavior. Some key questions to ask here are: How

EXHIBIT 6.2 DIAGNOSTIC CLUSTER CUE WEB LOGIC

1. Hemiplegia I69.35
2. Cellulitis L03.115
3. Obesity E66.9
4. Hyperlipidemia E78.5
5. Nicotine dependence F17.203
6. Mild cognitive impairment G31.84
7. GERD K21.9
8. Hypertension I10
9. Vitamin D deficiency E55.9
10. Depression F33.0

KEYSTONE ISSUE/THEME

1. Adult physical abuse T76.11
2. Cellulitis L03.115

EXHIBIT 6.3 FRAMING

Elder abuse with concurrent physical impairments

EXHIBIT 6.4 PRESENT STATE

1. Verbal, physical, and financial abuse by caregivers
2. Cellulitis in right lower leg
3. Insomnia, anxiety, and fearfulness
4. Nonadherence to medical regimen
5. Sedentary lifestyle
6. Nonadherence to cardiac diet

EXHIBIT 6.5 OUTCOME STATE

1. Supportive safe care environment
2. Cellulitis healed within 14 days
3. Hamilton Anxiety Rating score less than 30 at next visit
4. BP normal limits—compliant with medications
5. Engages in physical activity for mobility level
6. Adheres to cardiac diet

am I framing the situation and does it agree with the patient's view of the situation? Given my disciplinary perspectives, what are the results I want to create for this person?

At the center of the sheet are spaces to place the present state (Exhibit 6.4) and outcome state (Exhibit 6.5) side by side. The present state in this case shows six primary health care problems related to the keystone issue: verbal, physical, and financial abuse by care givers; cellulitis in right lower leg; insomnia, anxiety, and fearfulness; nonadherence to medical regimen; sedentary lifestyle; and nonadherence to cardiac diet. The outcome state shows six matching goals to be achieved through care coordination: supportive safe care environment free from abuse; cellulitis healed within 14 days; Hamilton Anxiety Scale score less than 30 at next visit; BP normal limits—compliant with medications; engages in physical activity for mobility level; and adheres to cardiac diet. Putting the two states together creates a gap analysis that naturally shows where the patient is and what the goals are in terms of the patient's care. Some key questions to ask here are whether the outcomes are appropriate given the diagnoses, whether there are gaps between the outcomes and present state, and whether there are clinical indicators of the desired outcome state?

The gap between where the patient is and where the advanced practice nurse wants the patient to be is one way to create a test (Exhibit 6.6). Clinical decisions are choices made about interventions that will help the patient transition from the present state to a desired outcome state. As interventions are tested, the advanced practice nurse evaluates the degree to which outcomes are or are not being achieved. The tests chosen in this case include Elder Mistreatment Assessment Tool, Braden Scale, Hamilton Anxiety Rating Scale, vital signs, and laboratory testing (CBC, vitamin D, and lipid profile).

EXHIBIT 6.6 TESTING

1. Elder Mistreatment Assessment Tool
2. Braden Scale
3. Hamilton Anxiety Rating Scale
4. Vital signs
5. Laboratory testing (CBC, vitamin D, and lipid profile)

EXHIBIT 6.7 REFLECTION ON CLINICAL REASONING

What clinical decisions or interventions help to achieve the outcomes?

What specific intervention activities will you implement?

Why are you considering these activities?

Testing is concurrent and iterative as one gets closer and closer in successive increments toward goal achievement.

Some key questions to ask here are how the advanced practice nurse is defining *testing*? On what scales will the desired outcome be rated? How will the advanced practice nurse know when the desired targeted outcomes are achieved?

The reflection box at the top of Figure 6.2 (Exhibit 6.7) reminds the advanced practice nurse of the thinking strategies used for the patient situation. These strategies also help make explicit many of the relationships among ideas and issues associated with the patient problems. Examples of clinical reasoning reflection questions that could be used during patient-centered systems thinking are listed in Table 6.3.

Finally, the judgment space on the far left-hand side of the model (Exhibit 6.8) is the place to write in the results of the conclusions drawn from the CCCR model. The degree of gap or comparison of where the patient is, and where the health care team wants the patient to be, determines whether there is a gap in the evidence. Once there is evidence that fills that gap, the nurse has to attribute meaning to the data. Making judgments about clinical issues is about the meaning the advanced practice nurse attributes to the evidence derived from the test or gap analysis of present to desired state. Complexity thinking, team-centered systems thinking, and organization-centered systems-thinking skills are used by the care coordination team at this point to evaluate and judge the successes or deficits from the plan of care. Interprofessional team activity requires negotiation and communication regarding competing values of collaboration—creating, competing, and controlling—and involves managing shared knowledge; acknowledgment of values impacted; and the brokering, directing, coordinating, and monitoring of practice issues, interventions, and outcomes. The judgments are made by the team after the care coordination essential need outcomes are evaluated. Each of the items in the judgment column corresponds to an essential need addressed in the CCCR systems model

TABLE 6.3 Patient-Centered Systems-Thinking Reflection Questions

SELF-REGULATION ACTIVITIES	REFLECTION QUESTIONS
Monitoring thinking	I. **Reflect on the thinking processes you used with the care coordination of this case.** 1. The baseline needs I identify in this case are.... I think I can identify future adjustments in the plan of care by.... If I have difficulty I... 2. When I think about my feelings during the care coordination of this case, I describe them as...and I handle them by... 3. When I try to remember or understand important facts to develop the plan of care, coach, and educate the patient/family I... 4. As I look back on meaningful activities, the resources I could have spent: 　a. More time on... 　b. Less time on...
Monitoring the environment	II. **Reflect on the environmental circumstances you encountered in the care coordination of this case.** 5. When I prepare to carry out coaching and education activities for care coordination, I... 6. When I think about particular distractions to facilitating medical care services and supports for care coordination, I... 7. When I work and communicate with interprofessional partners for care coordination of this case, I... 8. If I had the chance to redo the care coordination activities, I would do...instead of...Because...
Monitoring behavior	III. **Reflect on your behaviors and reactions to the care coordination of this case.** 9. My impression of my performance in evaluating capacity, energy, support, readiness, and skills to organize and manage the plan of care, is.... 10. I make sure I will update the needs assessment and individualized plan of care by...and if I need to make changes, I... 11. I make sure I empower the patient/family for self-management of health care needs by...and if I need to make changes, I... 12. Reaction to care coordination of this case... 　a. My reaction to what I like about the care coordination of this case... 　b. My reaction to what I do not like about the care coordination of this case... Optional prompt: Other comments I have about the care coordination of this case...

Adapted from Kuiper, Pesut, and Kautz (2009).

(Figure 6.3). Some key questions to ask are: Given the testing, what are the clinical judgments? Have the outcomes been achieved? Does the situation need to be reframed?

Once the advanced practice nurse has experience coordinating care for primary community health patients, the cases become part of a clinical reasoning learning

EXHIBIT 6.8 JUDGMENTS RELATED TO CARE COORDINATION VARIABLES

PLAN OF CARE

Ongoing, to provide appropriate skilled caregiving

SAFETY

Safe when out of current situation

NEEDS

Ongoing monitoring for comorbidities

CAPACITY

New facility, home, and caregivers identified

SKILLS

Medication adherence assistance available

RESOURCES

Transportation and meal preparation available

SELF-MANAGEMENT

Functioning at full capacity thus far

history, which become prototypes or schemas for other similar cases. These schemas and experience build on each other over time and result in the development of pattern recognition for future clinical reasoning applications. If the scenario results in negative judgments, or progress is not being made to transition patients from present to desired states, the advanced practice nurse may have to reframe the situation, reconsider the keystone priority, and reconsider the care coordination activities for the problem to be solved and the outcome to be achieved. The key question to ask here is: How will this clinical learning experience impact future clinical reasoning about similar cases?

CARE COORDINATION USING CCCR MODEL WORKSHEETS

The next step in the nursing diagnostic reasoning process is to augment the plan of care to include activities related to interprofessional care planning using the CCCR systems model framework (Exhibit 6.9), which builds on the OPT model of clinical reasoning. The systems' dynamics and interactions between and among the patient issues determine the care needed and the services provided. The complexities in

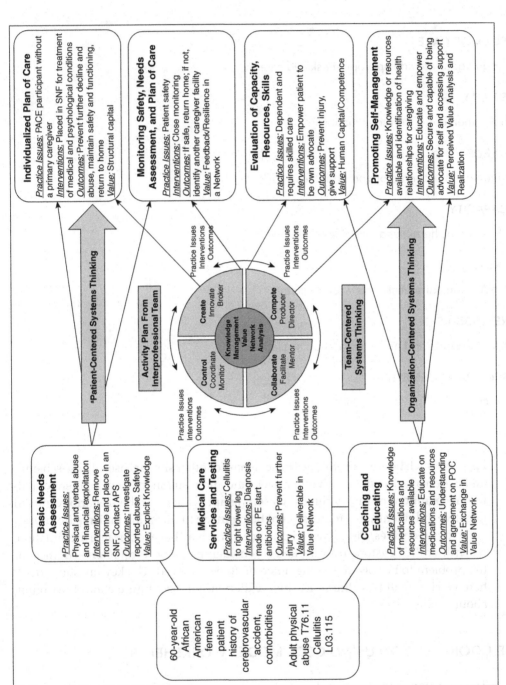

FIGURE 6.3 Care Coordination Clinical Reasoning systems model worksheet.

[a] Practice issues can be from any discipline: nursing, medicine, pharmacy, social work, and so on.

APS, adult protective services; PACE, Program of All-Inclusive Care for the Elderly; PE, physical examination; POC, plan of care; SNF, skilled nursing facility.

EXHIBIT 6.9 CARE COORDINATION CLINICAL REASONING DEFINITION

The authors define *care coordination clinical reasoning* as the application of critical, creative, systems, and complexity thinking to determine the practice issues, interdependencies, and interconnections of role relationships for collaborative work in service of caring for people to address problems, interventions, and outcomes through time and across health care contexts and services.

this case are the overlapping issues related to the physical abuse this patient is experiencing and the physical comorbidities in her health status. The CCCR systems model web (Figure 6.4) visually represents the complexities in this case along with the essential care coordination practice issues that need attention so as to organize thinking that focuses on the patient's and/or family's priority needs.

The CCCR systems model web (Exhibit 6.10) provides a blueprint for consideration of the care coordination practice issues so that clinicians can determine interventions, outcomes, and the value exchange that supports safe, high-quality care. This process involves patient-centered systems thinking, team-centered systems thinking, and organization-centered systems thinking to thoroughly and efficiently manage all aspects of patient and family cases. The steps to create the web for this case start at the center with the patient description and medical diagnoses (Dorothy Smith, a 60-year-old African American patient with a history of CVA and comorbidities), priority nursing domain (safety and protection), and ICD-10 codes (physical abuse T76.11, cellulitis L03.115), which show the overlap of patient issues that must be addressed by the advanced practice nurse and the care coordination interprofessional team.

Next, each large circle in this web represents the essential care coordination practice issues with evidence and defining characteristics for this patient story: needs assessment (physical and verbal abuse, including financial exploitation); individualized plan of care (PACE participant without a primary caregiver); medical care services and testing (needed for physical comorbidities and cellulitis); evaluation of capacity, resources, and skills (dependency requires a skilled level of care for some activities of daily living); monitoring and safety (safety concerns because of comorbidities that require monitoring); team collaboration (collaboration and communication among providers regarding reported abuse); coaching and educating (education regarding medications and available resources); and self-management (knowledge of available resources and identification of healthy relationship with the primary caregiver).

The provider then reflects on the total picture on the worksheet and begins to draw lines of relationship, connection, or association among the essential needs. As directional lines are drawn to create the web, functional relationships between and among the needs are recognized. Clinical reasoning and thinking processes are used to explain and justify the reasons for connecting these care coordination needs as central supporting elements in the patient's story based on an analysis and synthesis of possible priorities as represented in the web. The priority care coordination needs that would most efficiently and effectively represent the key issues of the patient that align with the patient story are addressed. A key question to ask here is

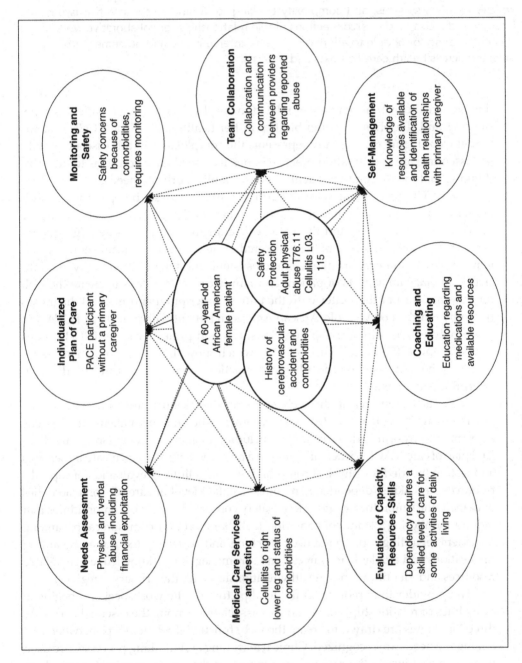

FIGURE 6.4 Care Coordination Clinical Reasoning systems model web.

PACE, Program of All-Inclusive Care for the Elderly.

EXHIBIT 6.10 CCCR SYSTEMS MODEL WEB DEFINITION

The Care Coordination Clinical Reasoning systems model web enables one to visually represent the complexities and essential care coordination practice issues that need attention so as to organize thinking that focuses on the patient's and/or family's priority needs within the context of services provided within and between health care delivery systems.

whether the CCCR systems model web provides a comprehensive consideration of the most pertinent evidence for care coordination practice issues.

The CCCR systems model worksheet (see Figure 6.3) is the next worksheet in the framework and it is designed to provide a graphic representation or visual map of the structure of the CCCR systems model and to help guide team-centered and organization-centered systems thinking. Some key questions to ask here are: What clinical decisions and interventions will help to achieve the outcomes identified on the OPT model of clinical reasoning (see Figure 6.2)? What specific interventions will the advanced practice nurse and/or the team implement? Why are providers considering these activities?

Writing each element on the worksheet shows how parts of the model relate to each other. In Figure 6.3, on the far left-hand side, there is space to write the description of the patient's health care situation, which was at the center of the CCCR systems model web. Three essential needs are placed in the first boxes to the right of the description and include basic needs assessment, medical care services and testing, and coaching and education. Each of the care coordination needs identified in this model includes practice issues, interventions, outcomes, and value specification.

From patient-centered systems-thinking processes used to create the OPT clinical reasoning model worksheets for this patient story, the identified basic needs practice issues include physical and verbal abuse and financial exploitation. Targeted interventions for the team would be to remove the patient from the home and place in an SNF. The documented desired outcomes would be safety and a thorough investigation of the reported abuse. A key question to ask is: Have the basic needs been identified given the frame of the situation? Consider the value impact analysis in this case using the questions from Table 6.4.

KNOWLEDGE MANAGEMENT AND VALUE ANALYSIS

The explicit value for role clarity, collaboration, and interaction of the team placed on the needs assessment is explicit knowledge. From Table 6.4, the value networking reflection question for basic needs is: What knowledge is codified and conveyed to others through dialogue, demonstration, or media? Name three knowledge classification systems that could be used to represent the patient characteristics in this case:

1.
2.
3.

TABLE 6.4 Value Definitions and Reflection Questions

Deliverable	The specific values or objects that are conveyed from one role or participant to another role or participant. What are the deliverables that you offer and expect of others?
Exchange	Two or more transactions between two or more roles or participants that evoke reciprocity. A process in which one role as agent receives resources from another role or agent and provides resources in return. What are the resource exchanges between roles or participants on your interprofessional health care team?
Explicit knowledge	The knowledge that is codified and conveyed to others through dialogue, demonstration, or media. What is the explicit knowledge shared among members of the team?
Feedback	The return of information about the impact of an activity. It can also mean the return of a portion of the output of a process as new input. What feedback is returned on activities or outputs in your care coordination activities? How does feedback influence team dynamics and goal attainment?
Human capital/ competence	The knowledge, skills, and competencies that reside in individuals who work in an organization or that are embedded in the organization's internal and external social networks. What human capital resources are needed in order for care coordination in your context to be successful?
Impact analysis	An assessment of how an input for a role is handled. What are the tangible/intangible costs, gains, or values from the input that generate a response or activity, or increase/decrease tangible assets?
Knowledge management	The degree to which the team facilitates and supports processes for creating, sustaining, sharing, and renewing organizational knowledge in order to generate social or economic gain or improve performance. Who is responsible and how is knowledge managed in the care coordination process?
Perceived value	The degree of value participants feel they receive from individual deliverables, which can come from roles, participants, or the network. What are the value-added dimensions of individual, collective, team, and organizational networks?
Resilience	The degree to which the network is able to reconfigure to respond to changing conditions and then return to the original form. What is the resilience capacity of the team and organization in which you work?
Structural capital	The infrastructure, routines, concepts, models, information systems, work systems, and business processes that support productivity and sustainability. To what degree do the structural capital and infrastructure support interprofessional teamwork and care coordination processes?
Systems thinking	An analysis and synthesis of the forces and interrelationships that shape the behavior of systems. To what degree do members of the team think about the system dynamics at the patient, group, team, or organizational levels?
Value realization	The degree to which tangible or intangible values turn the input into gains, benefits, capabilities, or assets that contribute to the success of an individual, group, organization, or network (Allee, 2008). To what degree do members of the team intentionally negotiate and manage competing values related to collaborating, creating, competing, and or controlling?

Adapted from Allee, Schwabe, and Babb (2015).

From team-centered systems-thinking processes used for the basic needs assessment, the identified medical care services and testing practice issues include cellulitis in the right lower leg. Targeted interventions for the team are making the correct diagnosis and starting antibiotics. The documented desired outcomes are to prevent further injury. A key question to ask is: Do the testing and interventions sufficiently manage the primary care needs? The explicit value for role clarity, collaboration, and interaction of the team placed on the medical care services and testing is to deliver evidence-based interventions based on the health care provider role. From Table 6.4, the value-networking reflection question for medical care services and testing of basic needs is: What is the specific value or object that is conveyed from one role or participant to another role or participant? Name three deliverables that are essential for the care coordination success of this case:

1.
2.
3.

Organization-centered systems thinking is used by the team to enhance coaching and to educate the patient and family. The identified coaching and educating practice issues include knowledge of medications and available resources. Targeted interventions for the team are delivering the education regarding medications and resources. The documented desired outcomes are to improve medication understanding and agreement on the plan of care. A key question to ask is: Do the content and methods for coaching and teaching match the patient's and family's cognitive abilities and understanding? From Table 6.4, the value-networking reflection question for educating and coaching involves evaluating the transactions between two or more roles or participants whereby one role as an agent receives resources from another role or agent and provides resources in return. The question would be: What is the exchange of resources and information between the providers and the patient and family regarding medication and available resources? Name three resources that could be exchanged between the providers and the patient in this case:

1.
2.
3.

The diagram at the center of the worksheet is the activity plan from the inter-professional team (Exhibit 6.11). The team engages in collaborating, creating, competing, and controlling dynamics through communication (Quinn, Bright, Faerman, Thompson, & McGrath, 2014; Quinn, Heynoski, Thomas, & Spreitzer, 2014; Quinn & Quinn, 2015; Quinn & Rohrbough, 1983) to manage essential areas of organizational culture to realize the intangible value exchanges used to develop and manage an activity plan that considers interventions from the individualized plan of care, monitoring processes, evaluation of patient and family capacity with regard to resources and skills, and promotion of self-management. For example, in terms of

EXHIBIT 6.11

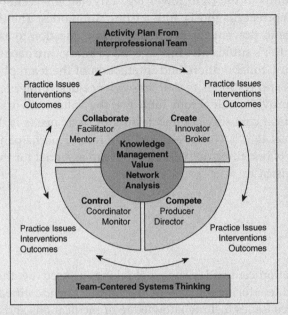

Key questions to consider for the four dimensions of the competing-values framework in the CCCR model are as follows:

- What are the desired outcomes in this case?
- What are the values I expect of myself and others?
- How are the feelings of the patient, family, and team considered in this case?
- What strategies could the team use to coordinate care?

collaboration, people must understand themselves and communicate honestly and effectively. Individuals mentor and develop others collaboratively and know how to participate and lead teams. Often this knowledge requires encouraging and managing constructive conflict. Competition enhances productivity and profitability. In this domain, vision and goal setting are the path to motivating self and others so that systems can be developed and organized to get results. Creating and promoting the adoption of new ideas or clinical innovations require attention to judicious use of power and ethics as well as championing new ideas and innovations through negotiating commitments and agreements for implementing and sustaining change. Control contributes to the development of stability and continuity as people work and manage across functions, organize information exchange, measure and monitor performance and quality, and enable compliance.

Key ingredients to team-centered systems thinking are that the members must be purpose centered, internally directed, other focused, and externally open to negotiation and communication surrounding competing values (Quinn, 2015; Quinn & Quinn, 2015). The activity plan from the interprofessional team in the CCCR model is guided by these principles and will promote the development of positive organizations and relationships. Each team member should be externally open to challenges, responsive to feedback, strive for higher performance, and cultivate the development of communities of practice. When this outcome is challenged and false fixed, some team members are valued more than others in the context of competitive versus collaborative goals. Being other influenced cultivates empathy, rapport, energy, and calmness. Together, the team members feel safe and secure enough to take risks and act with trust, integrity, and resilience. Creating such a culture supports a spirit of inquiry, learning, and experimentation, which results in higher performance. Such behavior requires the activation of a reflective self in contrast to automatic self-justification and reactive modes of being and communicating. In order to be a positive influence and bring a state of leadership to the team, each member of the team needs to be vigilant about being purpose centered, choosing goals that create focus, energy, and meaning for the team. A focused purpose-centered team is likely to attract and create resources related to the reasoning required to communicate across settings to achieve CCCR goals.

The activity plan from the interprofessional team iteratively visits the practice issues, which include communication among providers specific to this case and targeted interventions that are updated at team meetings across the contexts in which the providers are interacting, and documents the desired outcomes to maintain team support and to keep the team equally informed about patient status. A key question to ask is: Are the communication processes in place and do they promote information exchange between and among the interprofessional health team members? The explicit value for role clarity, collaboration, and interaction of the team placed on the activity plan from the interprofessional team is determined by knowledge management and value impact analysis. From Table 6.4, the value-networking reflection questions for the activity plan from the interprofessional team are: What are the tangible/intangible costs, gains, or values from the input that generate a response or activity, or that increase/decrease tangible assets? How does the team facilitate and support processes for collaborating, controlling, creating, and competing to sustain, share, and renew organizational knowledge in order to generate social or economic gain or improve performance? Name a cost, a gain, and a value that would be generated from the activity plan of the team for this case:

1.
2.
3.

To the far right of the CCCR system model worksheet are four essential care coordination needs that evolve from the activity plan from the interprofessional team stemming from patient-centered systems thinking, team-centered systems thinking, and organization-centered systems thinking. These needs include the individualized plan of care; monitoring safety, needs assessment, and plan of care; evaluation of capacity, resources, and skills; and promoting self-management. Each of these care coordination essentials is also defined by practice issues, interventions, outcomes, and values.

The patient-centered systems-thinking and team-centered systems-thinking activities are used for the individualized plan of care. The identified practice issues revolve around a PACE participant without a primary caregiver. Targeted interventions for the provider and the team are placing the patient in an SNF for treatment of medical and psychological conditions. The documented desired outcomes are to prevent further decline and abuse while maintaining safety and functioning. The ultimate goal is to return home. Key questions to ask are: Does the individualized plan of care include team collaboration? Is there any input that was not yet considered? Are there providers who were overlooked? The explicit value for role clarity, collaboration, and interaction of the provider and team placed on the individualized plan of care is on structural capital. From Table 6.4, the value-networking reflection question for the individualized plan of care is: What are the infrastructure, routines, concepts, models, information systems, work systems, and business processes that support productivity and have sustainability? Name three routines, systems, or processes that support and sustain the productivity of the care coordination in this case:

1.
2.
3.

From the patient-centered systems-thinking and team-centered systems-thinking processes used for monitoring safety, needs assessment, and plan of care, identified practice issues include patient safety. Targeted interventions for the team are close monitoring. The documented desired outcomes are to return to a safe environment whether it is home or a caregiver facility. A key question to ask is: Does the plan of care promote safety and meet the patient and family needs? The explicit value for role clarity, collaboration, and interaction of the team placed on monitoring safety, needs assessment, and plan of care is to obtain feedback and assess resilience in the network. From Table 6.4, the value-networking reflection questions for medical care services and testing basic needs are: What feedback is returned about activities or outputs? Was the network able to reconfigure to respond to changing conditions and then return to its original form? Name three areas of need and/or safety that were reassessed to determine whether the plan of care needed to be adjusted:

1.
2.
3.

Organization-centered systems-thinking processes, such as coaching and education, are used by the team to evaluate capacity, resources, and skills. The identified practice issues include the identification of patient dependency that requires skilled care. Targeted interventions for the team are to empower the patient to be his or her own advocate and to maintain as much independence as possible. The documented desired outcomes are to prevent injury and give support. A key question to ask is: Do the interventions in the plan of care require skilled help and/or can the patient and family manage care needs independently? The explicit value for role clarity, collaboration, and interaction of the team placed on evaluating capacity, resources, and skills is identifying human capital and competence. From Table 6.4, the value-networking reflection question for educating and coaching involves evaluating the transactions between two or more roles or participants in which one role as an agent receives resources from another role or agent and provides resources in return. The question would be: What is the exchange of resources and information between the providers and the patient and family regarding medication and available resources? Name three exchanges of resources, skills, or information with the patient that are essential to the care coordination success of this case:

1.
2.
3.

Organization-centered systems-thinking processes are used by the team to promote self-management. The identified practice issues include knowledge or resources available and identification of health relationships of caregiving. Targeted interventions for the team are to educate and empower the patient and family. The documented desired outcomes are to have the patient feel secure and capable of being an advocate for self and to access support. A key question to ask is: Are the patient and family able to identify the resources they need and self-manage to navigate the health care system? The explicit value for role clarity, collaboration, and interaction of the team placed on promoting self-management is perceived value realization. From Table 6.4, the value-networking reflection question for promoting self-management is: What is the level of value that roles or participants feel they receive from individual deliverables that can come from roles, participants, or the network? Name three examples of learned self-management that resulted from the care coordination of this case:

1.
2.
3.

With the use of the CCCR systems model, the advanced practice nurse and other providers address practice issues by using and developing evidence-based interventions, implementing measures of adherence, and evaluating processes and outcomes. This requires clinical reasoning at different levels of perspective—the individual patient needs, interprofessional team contributions, and attention to the systems in which people work and provide care. These practice issues, interventions, and outcomes for patient and family care coordination stem from the National Quality Forum (NQF, 2010a, 2010b) and the Agency for Healthcare Research and Quality (AHRQ, 2014).

As the center of attention for health care needs is managed by webs of relationships between and among providers, each interaction supports a specific value exchange as participants partner for successful outcomes (Allee, 2003). The dynamic relationships that occurred for this PACE patient among the advanced practice nurse, nursing staff, physician, pharmacist, and social worker were collaborative, trusting, dynamic, and interdependent. Application of the competing value competencies will relate to collaboration, creating, competing, and controlling, and help make explicit knowledge shared and managed to support innovation, coordination, and directing. Through the use of the electronic health record, connectivity impacted the value networking with greater access to knowledge and information. This process provided quick and effective feedback between team members for the complex needs this patient had related to physical abuse and multiple health problems.

CLINICAL JUDGMENTS AND CCCR

The final phase of the clinical reasoning process is to determine whether outcomes were met and whether care coordination activities were successful. The CCCR model of clinical reasoning is revisited for the final phase of care coordination, where judgments are made about achieving outcomes from the interprofessional team's activity plan (see Exhibit 6.8). The worksheet (see Figure 6.2) is revisited to make judgments about the care coordination essentials (needs; individualized plan of care; safety; capacity, resources, and skills; and self-management). Shifting to the next level of perspective, using team-centered and organization-centered systems-thinking activities, collaboration, and coordination of the plan of care, reveals ongoing planning and evaluation to provide skilled care for this patient. The patient is deemed safe when removed from the current home environment and comorbidities continue to be monitored. The new SNF provides safety and greater medication and dietary adherence. Transportation and meal preparation are available as well. These resources lead to the best possible functioning and independence for the patient until a new homecare provider can be arranged.

Some remaining questions may arise as the evaluation of outcomes occurs: Can the organizations provide continuing resources and reach care coordination outcomes for this patient? Were communication and the feedback loop effective between the health care providers, and patient and family? Did the complexity of the system hinder or enhance the achievement of outcomes? How do the competencies of the competing-values framework support interprofessional dialogue and reasoning about the care coordination of this particular case? The advanced practice nurse as the care coordinator views all the systems and is the key informant to communicate with the team regarding the efficiency and effectiveness of the processes for care outcomes. Judgments are made about whether the outcomes from case management have been achieved, and the information is recycled back to revise or enhance the plan of care.

The thinking processes used by the advanced practice nurse and other health care providers while implementing the CCCR systems model are promoted through monitoring of thinking, the environment, and behaviors for goal attainment (Zimmerman & Schunk, 2001). The courses of action chosen to manage issues and ensure that this patient remained safe revolve around behaviors and actions taken, thinking processes used, and environmental structuring. Critical reflective questions that can be used to prompt clinical reasoning to make judgments about the achievement of patient and family outcomes are shown in Table 6.5. Critical-, creative-, and systems-thinking processes are used for total care coordination, flow from

TABLE 6.5 Team-Centered and Organization-Centered Systems-Thinking Reflection Questions

SELF-REGULATION ACTIVITIES	REFLECTION QUESTIONS
Monitoring thinking	**I. Reflect on the thinking processes the team used to navigate organizational systems for care coordination of this case.** 1. The baseline needs identified by the team in this case are.... Adjustments in the plan of care for future successes include.... Difficulties were resolved by... 2. Team reactions during the care coordination of this case in regard to organizational systems could be described as...and they were handled by... 3. When the team was dealing with important facts to develop the plan of care, coach, and educate the patient/family about organizational systems they... 4. Looking back on meaningful activities, the resources the team could have spent: a. More time on... b. Less time on...
Monitoring the environment	**II. Reflect on the environmental circumstances you encountered in the care coordination of this case.** 5. When the team prepares to carry out coaching and education activities for care coordination, it... 6. When the team considers particular distractions in the organizations that impede medical care services and supports for care coordination, it... 7. When the team works and communicates with organizational partners for care coordination of this case, it... 8. If the team had the chance to redo the care coordination activities, it would do...instead of...because...
Monitoring behavior	**III. Reflect on your behaviors and reactions to the care coordination of this case.** 9. Impressions of the team performance in evaluating capacity, energy, support, readiness, and skills to organize and manage the plan of care within organizational systems are... 10. The team assures that it will update the needs assessment and individualized plan of care by...and if it needs to make changes, it... 11. The team makes sure that it empowers the patient/family to navigate through organizational systems for management of health care needs by...and if it needs to make changes, it... 12. The team reaction to care coordination of this case... a. Reaction to what it likes about the navigation of organizational systems to facilitate the care coordination of this case... b. Reaction to what it did not like about the navigation of organizational systems to facilitate the care coordination of this case... Optional prompt: Other comments about the care coordination of this case...

Adapted from Kuiper, Pesut, and Kautz (2009).

patient-centered systems (Table 6.3), team-centered systems thinking (Table 6.5), and organization-centered systems thinking (Table 6.5) for case management.

SUMMARY

The clinical reasoning challenge for primary community health begins with a description and understanding of the patient's story. The thinking strategies used in this case provided a safe and health-promoting environment for a patient who was being abused. As the providers practice self-monitoring, self-evaluation, and self-correction, successful strategies are employed, and flaws in thinking are corrected as they collaborate and align interventions for patient and family success. The OPT clinical reasoning model provides the foundation and structure for clinical reasoning and systems thinking within an individual patient and family situation. The OPT structure and process can be used at several levels for care planning by the provider, by the team, and by the organization to discern alignment and coordination of care activities. The CCCR systems model provides the structure for clinical reasoning for the care coordination essential needs and their related practice issues, interventions, outcomes, and values.

KEY CONCEPTS

1. Clinical reasoning for care coordination in primary community health can be promoted with a framework that includes structure, content, and process.
2. A supporting framework for CCCR extends case management using provider systems thinking and the OPT clinical reasoning model across levels of perspective that also include team-centered systems thinking and organization-centered systems thinking to align care coordination activities.
3. The process of CCCR involves critical reflection for the individual provider and the team.
4. Value-network analysis helps to define and describe the unique contributions that individual providers make to CCCR efforts supported through knowledge management and value-impact analysis.
5. A supporting framework for CCCR is completed by attending to the organization-centered systems thinking to make judgments about care coordination essentials.

STUDY QUESTIONS AND ACTIVITIES

1. Describe in your own words the benefits and processes of using the CCCR systems model in primary community health situations.
2. Using the CCCR systems model, identify the care coordination essential needs of cases in primary community health.
3. To what degree can you explicitly identify and describe the value exchanges associated with care coordination in primary community health situations?
4. How can an interprofessional team use the competencies of the competing values of collaboration, creating, competing, and controlling to ensure efficiency

and effectiveness of care coordination? How does your team negotiate roles of mentor, broker, director, and coordinator?

5. Identify all the possible standardized health care languages and communication strategies that could be considered in a primary community health case. Does language impact on communication and the patient outcomes? How does a discipline-specific framework influence the feedback, decisions, and outcomes in primary community health?

6. Identify the relationship between critical reflection and thinking strategies as they are applied to the three levels of system-thinking perspectives that are required—patient, team, and organization. What unique reflections are required to focus on team and organizational function in primary community health?

REFERENCES

Agency for Healthcare Research and Quality (AHRQ). (2014). *What is care coordination? Care coordination measures atlas update.* Rockville, MD: Author. Retrieved from http://www.ahrq.gov/professionals/prevention-chronic-care/improve/coordination/index.html

Allee, V. (2003). *The future of knowledge: Increasing prosperity through value networks.* Burlington, MA: Butterworth-Heinemann.

Allee, V. (2008). Value network analysis and value conversion of tangible and intangible assets. *Journal of Intellectual Capital, 9*(1), 5–24.

Allee, V., Schwabe, O., & Babb, M. K. (Eds.). (2015). *Value networks and the true nature of collaboration.* Tampa, FL: Megher–Kifer Press ValueNet Works and Verna Allee Associates.

Haas, S. A., Swan, B. A., & Haynes, T. S. (2014). *Care coordination and transition management core curriculum.* Pitman, NJ: American Academy of Ambulatory Care Nursing.

Kuiper, R., Pesut, D., & Kautz, D. (2009). Promoting the self-regulation of clinical reasoning skills in nursing students. *Open Nursing Journal, 3,* 76–85. Retrieved from http://www.ncbi.nlm.nih.gov/pmc/articles/PMC2771264

National Quality Forum (NQF). (2010a). *Preferred practices and performance measures for measuring and reporting care coordination: A consensus report.* Washington, DC: Author.

National Quality Forum (NQF). (2010b). *Quality connections: Care coordination.* Washington, DC: Author.

Pesut, D. J. (2008). Thoughts on thinking with complexity in mind. In C. Lindberg, S. Nash, & C. Lindberg (Eds.), *On the edge: Nursing in the age of complexity* (pp. 211–238). Bordentown, NJ: Plexus Press.

Quinn, R. (2015). *The positive organization: Breaking free from conventional cultures, constraints, and beliefs.* Oakland, CA: Berrett-Koehler.

Quinn, R., & Quinn, R. E. (2015). *Lift: Becoming a positive force in any situation.* San Francisco, CA: Berrett-Koehler.

Quinn, R. E., Bright, D., Faerman, S. R., Thompson, M. P., & McGrath, M. R. (2014). *Becoming a master manager: A competing values approach.* Hoboken, NJ: John Wiley & Sons.

Quinn, R. E., Heynoski, K., Thomas, M., & Spreitzer, G. M. (2014). *The best teacher in you: How to accelerate learning and change lives.* San Francisco, CA: Berrett-Koehler.

Quinn, R. E., & Rohrbough, J. (1983). A spatial model of effectiveness criteria: Towards a competing values approach to organizational analysis. *Management Science, 29,* 363–377.

World Health Organization (WHO). (2015). *Manual of the International Classification of Diseases and related health problems* (10th rev. ed.). Geneva, Switzerland: Author. Retrieved from http://www.icd10data.com

Zimmerman, B., & Schunk, D. S. (2001). *Self-regulated learning and academic thought*. Mahwah, NJ: Lawrence Erlbaum.

CHAPTER 7

CARE COORDINATION FOR A PSYCHOLOGICAL/MENTAL HEALTH PATIENT

In this chapter, we use the Care Coordination Clinical Reasoning (CCCR) systems model as described in Part I and explain how the model can be used to reason about a case given the context of psychological/mental health. The case presented in this chapter illustrates how the advanced practice nurse works with a family that is in need of mental health and wellness services to promote quality-of-life outcomes. The provider/clinic is the point of access for patients/families. The advanced practice nurse provides care coordination through the application and use of critical-, creative-, systems-, and complexity-thinking processes to manage patient problems with an interprofessional team to design appropriate interventions and establish patient-centered outcomes. Depending on the nature of need involved in the case, referrals to other specialty or primary care providers or community services and living environments are determined and considered in managing care coordination and transitions (Haas, Swan, & Haynes, 2014).

The CCCR systems model framework begins with the patient story, which is derived from gathering data and evidence from an interview, history, physical examination, and the health record. The advanced practice nurse then develops a patient-centered plan of care using the Outcome-Present State-Test (OPT) model worksheets. In order to do this, one activates patient-centered systems-thinking skills for complex patient stories and habitually uses key questions to reflect on the specific sections of the model (Pesut, 2008), as well as the dimensions and elements of care coordination.

LEARNING OUTCOMES

After completing this chapter, the reader should be able to:

1. Explain the components of a care coordination framework that are needed to manage the problems, interventions, and outcomes of people with psychological/mental health issues

2. Describe the different thinking processes that support clinical reasoning skills and strategies for determining priorities in psychological/mental health care coordination

3. Define the cognitive and metacognitive self-regulatory processes that support individual provider critical reflection related to levels and perspectives associated with clinical reasoning for psychological/mental health care coordination

4. Describe how the communication and knowledge management between interprofessional health care team members are essential for care coordination to address patient and family needs with psychological/mental health issues

5. Describe the critical meta-reflective processes that support team reflection related to levels and perspectives associated with the care coordination challenges and clinical reasoning required to navigate patient-care plans with psychological/mental health issues

THE PATIENT STORY

We begin with the history and story of a 14-year-old White male, David Simms, who has a history of attention deficit hyperactivity disorder (ADHD) and bipolar disorder. David lives with his parents, who are his primary care providers, and one brother. His parents have concerns about his escalating mood swings, impulsivity, and aggression toward them, his stepparents, his brother, and select peers at school. His parents divorced when he was 8 years old and his mother has primary custody of him and his 11-year-old brother. He and his brother spend almost every weekend with their father and stepmother. He is able to identify one close friend at school.

David's behavior problems started 1 year ago after he was hit by a car while riding his bicycle. He was thrown from the bicycle and hit the pavement head first. He was wearing a helmet at the time and it cracked on impact. His mother relates that "he does not listen to me and sometimes when I tell him to do things or try talking to him; he just stares off into space." About 3 months ago, his mother found marijuana and drug paraphernalia in his bedroom. When confronted about the drug behavior, he firmly denied that he was using the marijuana and indicated that he "was holding it for a friend." His parents describe that he had "normal" developmental maturation and had been an average student in school. During the past 2 years, he has barely been passing his classes.

During the interview, David had an angry affect and showed poor eye contact. He cooperated with the nurse practitioner, but adamantly stated, "I don't want to be here." His daily oral medications include Depakote 500 mg twice a day, Zyprexa 5 mg at bedtime, and Adderall XR 40 mg every morning.

PATIENT-CENTERED PLAN OF CARE USING OPT WORKSHEETS

Once the story is obtained from all possible sources, care planning and reasoning proceeds using the OPT clinical reasoning web worksheet (Figure 7.1), which helps determine relationships among issues and highlights potential keystone issues. The OPT clinical reasoning web is a graphic representation of the functional relationships between and among diagnostic hypotheses derived from the analysis and

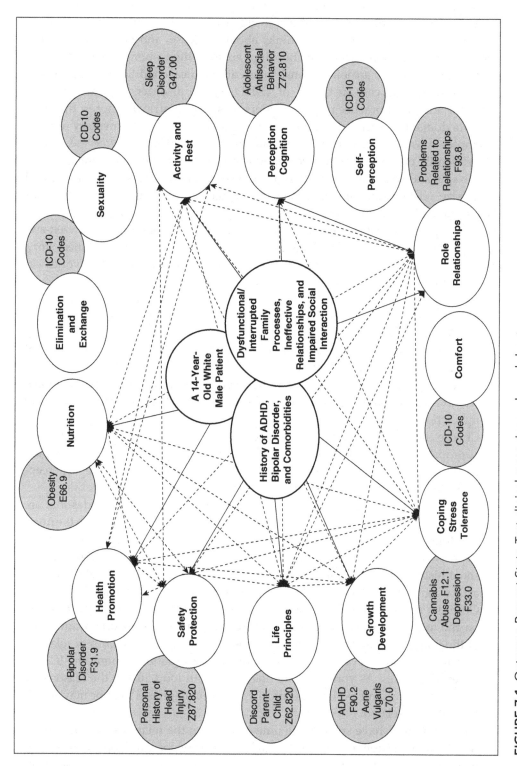

FIGURE 7.1 Outcome-Present State-Test clinical reasoning web worksheet.

ADHD, attention deficit hyperactivity disorder; ICD-10, International Classification of Diseases, 10th edition.

synthesis regarding how each element of the story and issues relate to one another. This activates critical and creative thinking. The visual diagram that results illustrates dynamics among issues and a convergence helps to point out central issues that require nursing care. As one thinks about this case, and begins to spin and weave a clinical reasoning web, relationships are identified among nursing domains and diagnoses as they are jointly considered with medical conditions. The psychiatric conditions in this case are history of ADHD, bipolar disorder, and comorbidities. Once the advanced practice nurse considers these psychiatric diagnoses, the nursing care domains associated with them are identified. The complementary nursing diagnoses most impacted in this case are dysfunctional family processes, interrupted family processes, ineffective relationships, and impaired social interaction.

To spin and weave the web, the provider uses thinking processes to analyze and synthesize relationships among diagnostic hypotheses associated with a patient's health status. The visual representation and mapping of these relationships supports the development of patient-centered systems thinking and connections between and among the medical and nursing diagnoses under consideration given the patient story.

The steps to the creation of the OPT clinical reasoning web using the worksheet are as follows:

1. Place a general description of the patient in the respective middle circle—14-year-old White adolescent male.
2. Place the major medical diagnoses in the respective middle circle—history of ADHD and bipolar disorder with comorbidities.
3. Place the major nursing diagnoses in the respective middle circle—dysfunctional and interrupted family processes, ineffective relationships, and impaired social interaction.
4. Choose the nursing domains for which each medical and nursing diagnosis is appropriate—nutrition, health promotion, safety and protection, life principles, growth and development, coping and stress tolerance, role relationships, perception and cognition, activity and rest.
5. Generate all the International Classification of Diseases (ICD)-10 codes that are appropriate for the particular patient and family story that coincide with the nursing domains—problems related to relationships (F93.8), cannabis abuse (F12.1), depression (F33.0), discord parent–child (Z62.820), sleep disorder (G47.00), personal history of head injury (Z87.820), bipolar disorder (F31.9), ADHD (F90.2), acne vulgaris (L70.0), obesity (E66.9), adolescent antisocial behavior (Z72.810).
6. Once the nursing domains, diagnoses, and ICD-10 codes are identified, reflect on the total web worksheet and concurrently consider and explain how each of the issues is related or not related to the other issues. Draw lines of relationship to spin and weave the web connections or associations among the ICD-10 codes/diagnoses. As you draw the lines, think out loud, justify the reasons for the connections, and explain specifically how the diagnoses may or may not be connected or related.
7. After you nurse have spent some time connecting the relationships, determine which domain/domains have the highest priority for care coordination and most efficiently and effectively represent the keystone nursing care needs of the patient by counting the arrows that connect the medical problems (ICD-10

TABLE 7.1 Relationships Among Nursing Domains, Medical Diagnoses, and Web Connections

NURSING DOMAINS	MEDICAL DIAGNOSES (ICD-10 CODES)	WEB CONNECTIONS
Role relationships	Problems related to relationships F93.8	11
Activity/rest	Sleep disorder G47.00	10
Coping/stress tolerance	Cannabis abuse F12.1 Depression F33.0	9
Life principles	Discord parent–child Z62.820	9
Safety protection	Personal history of head injury Z87.820	9
Health promotion	Bipolar disorder F31.9	9
Nutrition	Obesity E66.9	9
Growth development	ADHD F90.2 Acne vulgaris L70.0	7
Perception cognition	Adolescent antisocial behavior Z72.810	4

ADHD, attention deficit hyperactivity disorder.

Source: World Health Organization (2015).

codes). In this case, counting 11 lines (Table 7.1) pointing to or from the nursing domain of role relationships represents the priority present state keystone issues.

8. Look once again at the sets of relationships and determine the theme or keystone that summarizes the patient-in-context or the patient story—the problems related to relationships is the keystone issue for this case.

The OPT clinical reasoning web worksheet in Figure 7.1 shows a template with the patient health care situation, medical diagnoses, and nursing diagnoses at the center. Around the outer edges of the web are nursing domains with ICD-10 codes derived from history and physical assessment associated with the patient story. The directional arrows that create the web effect represent connections, explanations, and functional relationships between and among the diagnostic possibilities. As one can see, the domains and ICD-10 codes with more connections converging on one of the circles display the priority problem or keystone, in this case, problems related to relationships. A keystone issue is one or more central supporting element of the patient's story that helps focus and determine a root cause or center of gravity of the system dynamics and helps guide reasoning and care coordination based on an analysis (breaking things down into discrete parts) and synthesis (putting the parts together in a greater whole) of diagnostic possibilities as represented in the web. Some key questions to ask here are: How does the clinical reasoning web reveal relationships between and among the identified diagnoses? To what degree do these relationships make practical clinical sense according to the evidence and

TABLE 7.2 Questions That Guide the Use of the OPT Model

Patient-in-context	What is the patient story?
Diagnostic cue/web logic	What diagnoses have you generated?
	What outcomes do you have in mind given the diagnoses?
	What evidence supports those diagnoses?
	How does a reasoning web reveal relationships among the identified problems (diagnoses)?
	What keystone issue(s) emerge?
Framing	How are you framing the situation?
Present state	How is the present state defined?
Outcome state	What are the desired outcomes?
	What are the gaps or complementary pairs (~) of outcomes and present states?
Test	What are the clinical indicators of the desired outcomes?
	On what scales will the desired outcomes be rated?
	How will you know when the desired outcomes are achieved?
	How are you defining your testing in this particular case?
Decision making (interventions)	What clinical decisions or interventions help to achieve the outcomes?
	What specific intervention activities will you implement?
	Why are you considering these activities?
Judgment	Given your testing, what is your clinical judgment?
	Based on your judgment, have you achieved the outcome or do you need to reframe the situation?
	How, specifically, will you take this experience and learning with you into the future as you reason about similar cases?

OPT, Outcome-Present State-Test.

Adapted from Pesut (2008).

patient story? Table 7.1 shows a summary of the connections highlighting the priority with the most connections.

After considering the full picture using the clinical reasoning web worksheet, the next step is to use an OPT clinical reasoning model worksheet to facilitate and structure the patient-centered systems thinking about the care coordination of the identified problems highlighted in Table 7.1. As the advanced practice nurse thinks about the patient, she or he will concurrently consider the frame, outcome state, and present state. Each aspect of the OPT clinical reasoning model contributes to the other. The OPT clinical reasoning model worksheet is a map of the structure designed to provide an illustrative representation and guide thinking processes about relationships between and among competing issues and problems. Some questions that guide the use of the OPT clinical reasoning model are shown in Table 7.2 (Pesut, 2008).

By writing each element on the worksheet, all the parts of the model become related to each other. As the health care provider moves from right to left, the model structures the plan of care. Critical thinking skills are used to consider the patient story and

EXHIBIT 7.1 PATIENT-IN-CONTEXT STORY

David Simms is a 14-year-old White male who presents with parents reporting escalating mood swings, impulsivity, and aggression.

He was hit by a car while riding his bike 1 year ago. Helmet was worn but cracked after impact.

Diagnosis of ADHD and recently diagnosed with bipolar disorder. Marijuana and paraphernalia found in his bedroom 3 months ago. He denies use, reporting he was "holding it for a friend."

Ht: 5′ 6″, Wt: 188 lb., BMI: 30.34

BP: 120/74 mmHg, HR: 88 bpm, RR: 20

BMI, body mass index; BP, blood pressure; HR, heart rate; Ht, height; RR, respiration rate; Wt, weight.

creative thinking is used to identify and reason about the keystone issues/themes/cues to determine the most significant evidence in the present state. Complexity thinking helps the provider to consider the outcomes desired and the gaps between the present and outcome state. Once interventions and tests are decided, the plan of care transitions over to a care coordination model and team-centered systems thinking, which considers patient and family preferences within the frame of the situation.

The patient-in-context story (Exhibit 7.1) is depicted on the far right-hand side of Figure 7.2. The advanced practice nurse notes relevant facts of the story, which in this case include the patient demographics and characteristics; history of escalating mood swings, impulsivity, and aggression. He had an auto accident that resulted in a head injury and he has a diagnosis of ADHD and bipolar disorder. He also has a history of marijuana use. Assessment reveals an overweight 14-year-old with normal vital signs. Pertinent laboratory values show therapeutic levels of Valproic (108 mcg/mL), positive urine drug screen for amphetamines and tetrahydrocannabinol, and a normal lipid panel while taking Zyprexa.

A key step at this juncture is to review and reflect on the patient story for accuracy and thoroughness before proceeding with care planning for care coordination.

Moving to the left, there is a place to list the diagnostic cluster cues on the web of medical diagnoses and ICD-10 codes (Exhibit 7.2). At the bottom of this box is placed the designated keystone issue or themes that fall under the most significant nursing domain—problems related to relationships F93.8. Remember diagnostic cluster cue web logic is the use of inductive and deductive thinking skills. Some key questions to ask here are: What diagnoses were generated? Is there evidence to support those diagnoses? Is the keystone issue appropriate given this patient story?

In the center and background of the worksheet are places to indicate the frame or theme that best represents the background issues regarding thinking about the patient story (Exhibit 7.3). The frame of this case is a White adolescent male with an angry affect, poor eye contact, stating, "I don't want to be here." This frame (White adolescent male with psychological/mental health issues) helps to organize the present state and outcome state, illustrates the gaps, and provides insights about

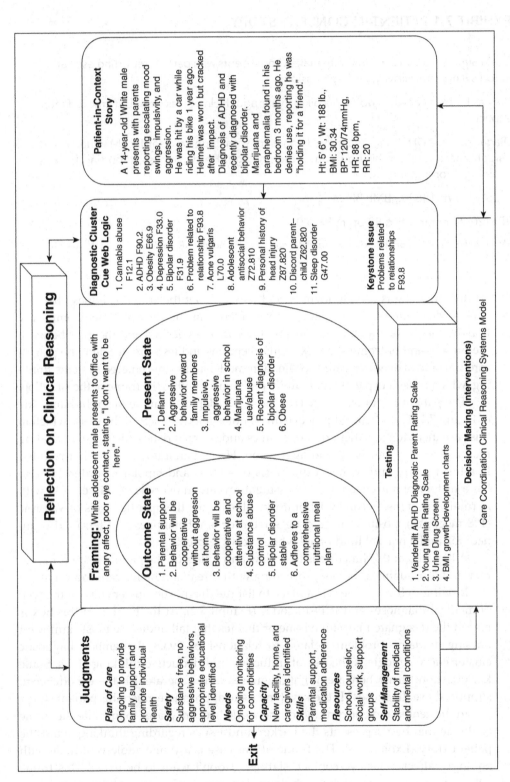

FIGURE 7.2 Outcome-Present State-Test clinical reasoning model for care coordination worksheet.

ADHD, attention deficit hyperactivity disorder; BMI, body mass index; BP, blood pressure; HR, heart rate; Ht, height; RR, respiration rate; Wt, weight.

EXHIBIT 7.2 DIAGNOSTIC CLUSTER CUE WEB LOGIC

1. Cannabis abuse F12.1
2. ADHD cellulitis L90.2
3. Obesity E66.9
4. Depression E33.0
5. Bipolar disorder F31.9
6. Problem related to relationship F93.8
7. Acne vulgaris L70.0
8. Adolescent antisocial behavior Z72.810
9. Personal history of head injury Z87.820
10. Discord parent–child Z62.820
11. Sleep disorder G47.00

KEYSTONE ISSUE/THEME

1. Problems related to relationship F93.8

EXHIBIT 7.3 FRAMING

A White adolescent male presents to office with angry affect, poor eye contact, stating, "I don't want to be here."

EXHIBIT 7.4 PRESENT STATE

1. Defiant
2. Aggressive behavior toward family members
3. Impulsive, aggressive behavior in school
4. Marijuana use/abuse
5. Recent diagnosis of bipolar disorder
6. Obese

what tests need to be considered to fill the gap. Decision making and reflection surround the framing as the advanced practice nurse thinks of many things simultaneously. Reflective thinking is used to monitor thinking and behavior. Some key questions to ask here are: How am I framing the situation? Does the frame agree with the patient's view of the situation? Given my disciplinary perspectives, what are the results I want to create for this person?

At the center of the sheet are spaces to place the present state (Exhibit 7.4) and outcome state (Exhibit 7.5) side by side. The present state in this case shows six primary health care problems related to the keystone issue: defiant attitude, aggressive behavior toward family members, impulsive and aggressive behavior in school, marijuana use/abuse, recent diagnosis of bipolar disorder, and obesity. The outcome state shows six matching goals to be achieved through care coordination: parental support, behavior will be cooperative without aggression at home, behavior will be cooperative and attentive at school, no drug use, bipolar disorder is stable, and adheres to comprehensive nutritional meal plan. Putting the two states together creates a gap analysis that naturally shows where the patient is and what the goals are in terms of the patient's care. A key question to ask here is: If the outcomes are appropriate given the diagnoses, are there gaps between the outcomes and present state and are there clinical indicators of the desired outcome state?

The gap between where the patient is and where the advanced practice nurse wants the patient to be is one way to create a test (Exhibit 7.6). Clinical decisions are choices made about interventions that will help the patient transition from present state to a desired outcome state. As interventions are tested, the advanced practice nurse evaluates the degree to which outcomes are or are not being achieved. The tests chosen in this case include: Vanderbilt ADHD Diagnostic Parent Rating Scale, Young Mania Rating Scale, urine drug screen, and body mass index (BMI) and growth-development charts.

Testing is concurrent and iterative as one gets closer and closer successive increments toward goal achievement. Some key questions to ask here are: How is the advanced practice nurse defining *testing*? On what scales will the desired outcome be rated? How will the advanced practice nurse know when the desired targeted outcomes are achieved?

EXHIBIT 7.5 OUTCOME STATE

1. Parental support
2. Behavior will be cooperative without aggression at home
3. Behavior will be cooperative and attentive at school
4. Control of substance use
5. Bipolar disorder stable
6. Adheres to comprehensive nutritional meal plan

EXHIBIT 7.6 TESTING

1. Vanderbilt ADHD Diagnostic Parent Rating Scale
2. Young Mania Rating Scale
3. Urine drug screen
4. Body mass index (BMI) and growth-development charts

The reflection box at the top of Figure 7.3 (Exhibit 7.7) reminds the advanced practice nurse of the thinking strategies used for the patient situation. These strategies also help make explicit many of the relationships among ideas and issues associated with the patient problems. Examples of clinical reasoning reflection questions that could be used during patient-centered systems thinking are listed in Table 7.3.

Finally, the judgment space on the far left-hand side of the model (Exhibit 7.8) is the place to write in the results of the conclusions drawn from the CCCR model. The degree of gap or comparison of where the health care team wants the patient to be determines whether there is a gap in the evidence. Once there is evidence that fills that gap, the nurse has to attribute meaning to the data. Making judgments about clinical issues is about the meaning the advanced practice nurse attributes to the evidence derived from the test or gap analysis of present to desired state. Complexity thinking, team-centered systems thinking, and organization-centered systems thinking skills are used by the care coordination team at this point to evaluate and judge the successes or deficits from the plan of care. Interprofessional team activity requires negotiation and communication about competing values of collaboration—creating, competing, and controlling—and involves managing shared knowledge; acknowledgment of values impacted; and brokering, directing, coordinating, and monitoring of practice issues, interventions, and outcomes. The judgments made in this case are made by the team after the care coordination essential needs outcomes are evaluated. Each of the items in the judgment column corresponds to an essential need addressed in the CCCR systems model (Figure 7.4). Some key questions to ask, given the testing, are: What are the clinical judgments? Have the outcomes been achieved? Does the situation need to be reframed?

Once the advanced practice nurse has experience coordinating care for patients with psychiatric mental health issues, the cases become part of a clinical reasoning learning history that become prototypes or schemas for other similar cases. These schemas and experience build on each other over time and result in the development of pattern recognition for future clinical reasoning applications. If the scenario results in a negative judgment or progress is not being made to transition patients from present to desired states, the advanced practice nurse may have to reframe the situation, reconsider the keystone priority, and reconsider the care coordination activities for the problem to be solved and the outcome to be achieved. The key question to ask here is: How will this clinical learning experience impact future reasoning about similar cases?

CARE COORDINATION USING CCCR MODEL WORKSHEETS

The next step in the nursing diagnostic reasoning process is to augment the plan of care to include activities related to interprofessional care planning using the CCCR systems model framework (Exhibit 7.9), which builds on the OPT model of clinical reasoning. The systems dynamics and interactions between and among the patient issues determine the care needed and the services provided. The complexities in this case are the overlapping issues related to the emotional problems he is experiencing and the psychological comorbidities interfering with patient and family

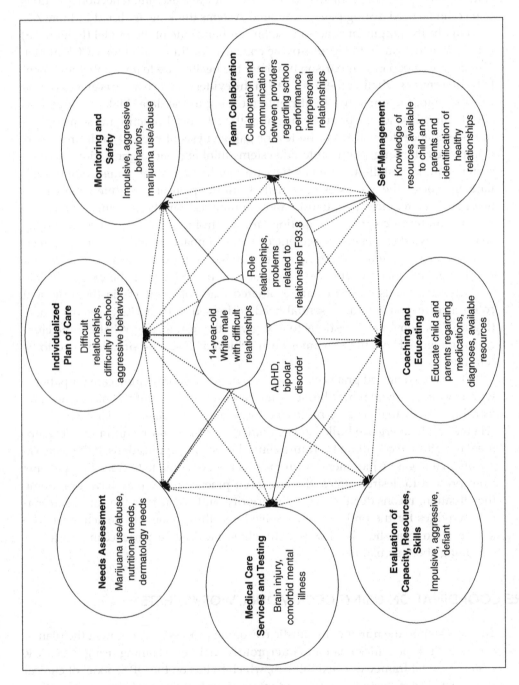

FIGURE 7.3 Care Coordination Clinical Reasoning systems model web.

ADHD, attention deficit hyperactivity disorder.

EXHIBIT 7.7 REFLECTION ON CLINICAL REASONING

What clinical decisions or interventions help to achieve the outcomes?

What specific intervention activities will you implement?

Why are you considering these activities?

TABLE 7.3 Patient-Centered Systems-Thinking Reflection Questions

SELF-REGULATION ACTIVITIES	REFLECTION QUESTIONS
Monitoring thinking	I. **Reflect on the thinking processes you used with the care coordination of this case.** 1. The baseline needs I identify in this case are.... I think I can identify future adjustments in the plan of care by.... If I have difficulty, I... 2. When I think about my feelings during the care coordination of this case, I describe them as...and I handle them by... 3. When I try to remember or understand important facts to develop the plan of care, coach, and educate the patient/family, I... 4. As I look back on meaningful activities, the resources I could have spent: 　a. More time on... 　b. Less time on...
Monitoring the environment	II. **Reflect on the environmental circumstances you encountered in the care coordination of this case.** 5. When I prepare to carry out coaching and education activities for care coordination, I... 6. When I think about particular distractions to facilitating medical care services and supports for care coordination, I... 7. When I work and communicate with interprofessional partners for care coordination of this case, I... 8. If I had the chance to redo the care coordination activities, I would do...instead of...because...
Monitoring behavior	III. **Reflect on your behaviors and reactions to the care coordination of this case.** 9. My impression of my performance in evaluating capacity, energy, support, readiness, and skills to organize and manage the plan of care, is... 10. I make sure I will update the needs assessment and individualized plan of care by...and if I need to make changes, I... 11. I make sure I empower the patient/family for self-management of health care needs by...and if I need to make changes, I... 12. Reaction to care coordination of this case... 　a. My reaction to what I like about the care coordination of this case... 　b. My reaction to what I do not like about the care coordination of this case... Optional prompt: Other comments I have about the care coordination of this case...

Adapted from Kuiper, Pesut, and Kautz (2009).

EXHIBIT 7.8 JUDGMENTS RELATED TO CARE COORDINATION VARIABLES

PLAN OF CARE

Ongoing, to provide family support and promote individual health

SAFETY

Drug free, no aggressive behaviors, appropriate educational level identified

NEEDS

Ongoing monitoring for comorbidities

CAPACITY

Home and caregivers identified

SKILLS

Parental support, medication adherence

RESOURCES

School counselor, social work, support groups

SELF-MANAGEMENT

Stability of medical and mental conditions

processes. The CCCR systems model web (Figure 7.3) visually represents the complexities in this case along with the essential care coordination practice issues that need attention so as to organize thinking that focuses on the patient's and/or family's priority needs.

The CCCR systems model web (Exhibit 7.10) provides a blueprint for consideration of the care coordination practice issues so clinicians can determine interventions, outcomes, and the value exchange that supports safe, high-quality care. This process involves patient-centered systems thinking, team-centered systems thinking, and organization-centered systems thinking to thoroughly and efficiently manage all aspects of the case. The steps to create the web for this case start in the center with the patient description and medical diagnoses (David Simms, a 14-year-old White male with ADHD and bipolar disorder), priority nursing domain (role relationships), and ICD-10 codes (problems related to relationships F93.8), which shows the overlap of patient issues that must be addressed by the advanced practice nurse and the care coordination interprofessional team.

Next, each large circle in this web represents the essential care coordination practice issues with evidence and defining characteristics for this patient story: needs assessment (marijuana use/abuse, nutritional needs, dermatology needs); individualized plan of care (difficult relationships, difficulty in school, aggressive behaviors);

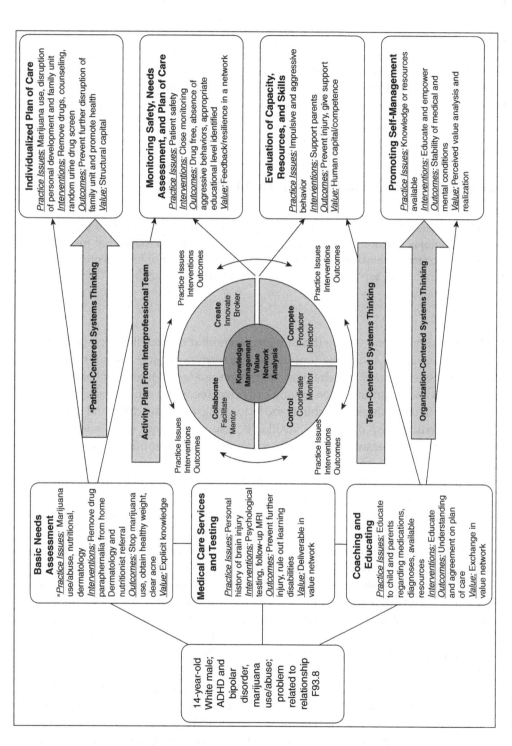

FIGURE 7.4 Care Coordination Clinical Reasoning systems model worksheet.

[a] Practice issues can be from any discipline: nursing, medicine, pharmacy, social work, and so on.

ADHD, attention deficit hyperactivity disorder.

EXHIBIT 7.9 CARE COORDINATION CLINICAL REASONING DEFINITION

The authors define *care coordination cinical reasoning* as the application of critical, creative, systems, and complexity thinking to determine the practice issues, interdependencies, and interconnections of role relationships for collaborative work in service of caring for people to address problems, interventions, and outcomes through time and across health care contexts and services.

EXHIBIT 7.10 CCCR SYSTEMS MODEL WEB DEFINITION

The Care Coordination Clinical Reasoning systems model web enables one to visually represent the complexities and essential care coordination practice issues that need attention so as to organize thinking that focuses on the patient's and/or family's priority needs within the context of services provided within and between health care delivery systems.

medical care services and testing (brain injury, comorbid mental illness); evaluation of capacity, resources, and skills (impulsive, aggressive, defiant); monitoring and safety (impulsive, aggressive behaviors, marijuana use/abuse); team collaboration (collaboration and communication among providers regarding school performance, interpersonal relationships); coaching and educating (educate child and parents regarding medications, diagnoses, available resources); and self-management (knowledge of resources available to child and parents and identification of healthy relationships).

The provider then reflects on the total picture on the worksheet and begins to draw lines of relationship, connection, or association among the essential needs. As directional lines are drawn to create the web, functional relationships between and among the needs are recognized. Clinical reasoning and thinking processes are used to explain and justify the reasons for connecting these care coordination needs as central supporting elements in the patient's story, based on an analysis and synthesis of possible priorities as represented in the web. The priority care coordination needs that would most efficiently and effectively represent the key issues of the patient that align with the patient story are addressed. A key question to ask here is: Does the CCCR systems model web provide a comprehensive consideration of the most pertinent evidence for care coordination practice issues?

The CCCR systems model worksheet (see Figure 7.4) is the next worksheet in the framework and is designed to provide a graphic representation or visual map of the structure of the CCCR systems model and to help guide team-centered systems and organization-centered systems thinking. Some key questions to ask here are: What clinical decisions and interventions will help to achieve the outcomes identified in the OPT model of clinical reasoning (see Figure 7.2)? What specific interventions will the advanced practice nurse and/or the team implement? Why are providers considering these activities?

Writing each element on the worksheet shows how parts of the model relate to each other. In Figure 7.4, on the far left-hand side, there is space to write the description of the patient's health care situation found at the center of the CCCR systems model web. Three essential needs are placed in the first boxes to the right of the description and include basic needs assessment, medical care services and testing, and coaching and education. Each of the care coordination needs identified in this model include practice issues, interventions, outcomes, and value specification.

From the patient-centered systems-thinking processes used to create the OPT clinical reasoning model worksheets for this patient story the identified basic needs practice issues include marijuana use/abuse, nutritional needs, and dermatology issues. Targeted interventions for the team would be to remove the drug paraphernalia from the home and obtain referrals for dermatology and nutrition. The documented desired outcomes would be to stop marijuana use, obtain a healthy weight, and clear acne. A key question to ask here is: Have the basic needs been identified given the frame of the situation? Consider the value-impact analysis in this case using the questions from Table 7.4.

KNOWLEDGE MANAGEMENT AND VALUE ANALYSIS

The explicit value for role clarity, collaboration, and interaction of the team placed on the needs assessment is explicit knowledge. From Table 7.4, the value-networking reflection question for basic needs is: What knowledge is codified and conveyed to others through dialogue, demonstration, or media? Name three knowledge classification systems that could be used to represent the patient characteristics in this case:

1.
2.
3.

From team-centered systems-thinking processes used for the basic needs assessment, the identified medical care services and testing practice issues include personal history of brain injury. Targeted interventions for the team are psychological testing and a follow-up MRI. The documented desired outcomes are to prevent further injury and rule out learning disabilities. A key question to ask is: Do the testing and interventions sufficiently manage the primary care needs? The explicit value for role clarity, collaboration, and interaction of the team placed on the medical care services and testing is to deliver evidence-based interventions based on the health care provider role. From Table 7.4, the value-networking reflection question for medical care services and testing basic needs is: What is the specific value or object that is conveyed from one role or participant to another role or participant? Name three deliverables that are essential for the care coordination success of this case:

1.
2.
3.

TABLE 7.4 Value Definitions and Reflection Questions

Deliverable	The specific values or objects that are conveyed from one role or participant to another role or participant. What are the deliverables that you offer and expect of others?
Exchange	Two or more transactions between two or more roles or participants that evoke reciprocity. A process in which one role as agent receives resources from another role or agent and provides resources in return. What are the resource exchanges between roles or participants on your interprofessional health care team?
Explicit knowledge	The knowledge that is codified and conveyed to others through dialogue, demonstration, or media. What is the explicit knowledge shared among members of the team?
Feedback	The return of information about the impact of an activity. It can also mean the return of a portion of the output of a process as new input. What feedback is returned about activities or outputs in your care coordination activities? How does feedback influence team dynamics and goal attainment?
Human capital/ competence	The knowledge, skills, and competencies that reside in individuals who work in an organization or that are embedded in the organization's internal and external social networks. What human capital resources are needed in order for care coordination in your context to be successful?
Impact analysis	An assessment of how an input for a role is handled. What are the tangible/intangible costs, gains, or values from the input that generate a response or activity, or increase/decrease tangible assets?
Knowledge management	The degree to which the team facilitates and supports processes for creating, sustaining, sharing, and renewing organizational knowledge in order to generate social or economic gain or improve performance. Who is responsible and how is knowledge managed in the care coordination process?
Perceived value	The degree of value participants feel they receive from individual deliverables that can come from roles, participants, or the network. What are the value-added dimensions of individual, collective, team, and organizational networks?
Resilience	The degree to which the network is able to reconfigure itself to respond to changing conditions and then return to its original form. What is the resilience capacity of the team and organization in which you work?
Structural capital	The infrastructure, routines, concepts, models, information systems, work systems, and business processes that support productivity and sustainability. To what degree do the structural capital and infrastructure support interprofessional teamwork and care coordination processes?
Systems thinking	An analysis and synthesis of the forces and interrelationships that shape the behavior of systems. To what degree do the members of the team think about the system dynamics at the patient, group, team, or organizational levels?
Value realization	The degree to which tangible or intangible values turn the input into gains, benefits, capabilities, or assets that contribute to the success of an individual, a group, an organization, or a network (Allee, 2008). To what degree do the members of the team intentionally negotiate and manage competing values related to collaborating, creating, competing, and/or controlling?

Adapted from Allee, Schwabe, and Babb (2015).

Organization-centered systems thinking is used by the team to enhance coaching and educating the patient and family. The identified coaching and educating practice issues include education of the child and parents regarding medications, diagnoses, and available resources. Targeted interventions for the team are to educate patient and family. The documented desired outcomes are to improve understanding and agreement on the plan of care. A key question to ask is: Do the content and methods for coaching and teaching match the patient and family cognitive abilities and understanding? From Table 7.4, the value-networking reflection question for educating and coaching involves evaluating the transactions between/among two or more roles or participants in which one role as an agent receives resources from another role or agent and provides resources in return. The question would be: What is the exchange of resources and information between the providers and the patient and family regarding medication and available resources? Name three resources that could be exchanged between the providers and patient in this case:

1.
2.
3.

The diagram in the center of the worksheet is the activity plan from the interprofessional team (Exhibit 7.11). The team engages in collaborating, creating, competing, and controlling dynamics through communication (Quinn, Bright, Faerman, Thompson, & McGranth, 2014; Quinn, Heynoski, Thomas, & Spreitzer, 2014; Quinn & Rohrbough, 1983; Quinn & Quinn, 2015) to manage essential areas of organizational culture to realize the intangible value exchanges used to develop and manage an activity plan, which considers interventions from the individualized plan of care, monitoring processes, evaluation of patient and family capacity with regard to resources and skills, and promotion of self-management. For example, in terms of collaboration, people must understand themselves and communicate honestly and effectively. Individuals mentor and develop others collaboratively, and know how to participate and lead teams. Often this knowledge requires encouraging and managing constructive conflict. Competition enhances productivity and profitability. In this domain vision and goal setting is a path to motivating self and others so that systems can be developed and organized to get results. Creating and promoting the adoption of new ideas or clinical innovations requires attention to judicious use of power and ethics as well as championing new ideas and innovations through negotiating commitments and agreements for implementing and sustaining change. Control contributes to the development of stability and continuity as people work and manages across functions, organize information exchange, measure and monitor performance and quality, and enable compliance.

To foster team-centered systems thinking members must be purpose centered, internally directed, other focused, and externally open to negotiation and communication surrounding competing values (Quinn, 2015; Quinn & Quinn,

EXHIBIT 7.11

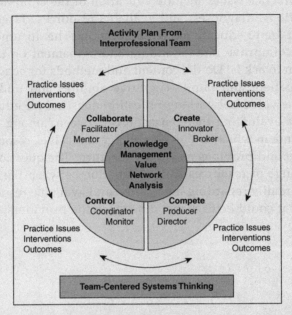

Key questions to consider for the four dimensions of the competing-values framework in the CCCR model are:

- What are the desired outcomes in this case?
- What are the values I expect of myself and others?
- How are the feelings of the patient, family, and team considered in this case?
- What strategies could the team use to coordinate care?

2015). The activity plan from the interprofessional team in the CCCR model is guided by these principles and will promote the development of positive organizations and relationships. Each team member should be externally open to challenges, responsive to feedback, strive for higher performance, and cultivate the development of communities of practice. When this outcome is challenged and false fixed, some team members are valued more than others in the context of competitive versus collaborative goals. Being other influenced cultivates empathy, rapport, energy, and calmness. Together, the team members feel safe and secure enough to take risks and act with trust, integrity, and resilience. Creating such a culture supports a spirit of inquiry, learning, and experimentation, which results in higher performance. Such behavior requires the activation of a reflective self in contrast to automatic self-justification and reactive modes of being and communicating. In order to be a positive influence and bring a state of leadership to the team, each member of the team needs to be vigilant about being purpose centered, choosing goals that create focus, energy, and meaning for the team. A focused, purpose-centered team is likely to attract and create resources related to the reasoning required to communicate across settings to achieve CCCR goals.

The activity plan from the interprofessional team iteratively visits the practice issues that include communication among providers specific to this case, targeted interventions that are updated at team meetings across the contexts in which the providers are interacting, and documents the desired outcomes to maintain team support and to keep the team equally informed about patient status. A key question to ask is: Are the communication processes in place and do they promote information exchange between and among the interprofessional health team members? The explicit value for role clarity, collaboration, and interaction of the team placed on the activity plan from the interprofessional team is determined by knowledge management and value impact analysis. From Table 7.4, the value-networking reflection questions for the activity plan from the interprofessional team are: What are the tangible/intangible costs, gains, or values from the input that generate a response or activity, or increase/decrease tangible assets? How does the team facilitate and support processes for collaborating, controlling, creating, and competing to sustain, share, and renew organizational knowledge in order to generate social or economic gain or improve performance? Name a cost, gain, and value that would be generated from the activity plan of the team for this case:

1.
2.
3.

To the far right of the CCCR system model worksheet are four essential care coordination needs that evolve from the activity plan from the interprofessional team stemming from patient-centered systems thinking, team-centered systems thinking, and organization-centered systems thinking. These needs include the individualized plan of care; monitoring safety, needs assessment, and plan of care; evaluation of capacity, resources, and skills; and promoting self-management. Each of these care coordination essentials are defined as well by practice issues, interventions, outcomes, and values.

The patient-centered systems-thinking and team-centered systems-thinking activities are used for the individualized plan of care. The identified practice issues revolve around a young man with marijuana use with disruption of personal development and the family unit. Targeted interventions for the provider and team are to remove drugs from the home, counsel the patient, and do random drug screens. The documented desired outcomes are to prevent further disruption of the family unit and promote psychological and physical health in the patient. Some key questions to ask are: Does the individualized plan of care include team collaboration? Is there any input that was not yet considered, or are there providers who were overlooked? The explicit value for role clarity, collaboration, and interaction of the provider and team placed on the individualized plan of care is on structural capital. From Table 7.4, the value-networking reflection question for the individualized plan of care is: What are the infrastructure, routines, concepts, models, information systems, work systems, and business processes that support productivity and have sustainability? Name three routines, systems, or processes that support and sustain the productivity of the care coordination in this case:

1.
2.
3.

From the patient-centered systems-thinking and team-centered systems-thinking processes used for monitoring safety, needs assessment, and plan of care, identified practice issues include patient safety. Close monitoring is a targeted intervention for the team. The documented desired outcomes are to return to a drug-free safe environment in the home, the absence of aggressive behaviors, and identification of an appropriate educational level. A key question to ask is: Does the plan of care promote safety and meet the patient and family needs? The explicit value for role clarity, collaboration, and interaction of the team placed on monitoring safety, needs assessment, and plan of care is to obtain feedback and assess resilience in the network. From Table 7.4, the value-networking reflection questions for medical care services and testing of basic needs are: What feedback is returned about activities or outputs? Was the network able to reconfigure to respond to changing conditions and then return to original form? Name three areas of need and/or safety that were reassessed to determine whether the plan of care needed to be adjusted:

1.
2.
3.

Organization-centered systems-thinking processes such as coaching and education, are used by the team to evaluate capacity, resources, and skills. The identified practice issues include the identification of impulsive and aggressive behavior. Targeted interventions for the team are to support the patient and parents. The documented desired outcomes are to prevent injury and give support. A key question to ask is: Do the interventions in the plan of care require skilled help and/or can the patient and family manage care needs independently? The explicit value for role clarity, collaboration, and interaction of the team placed on evaluating capacity, resources, and skills is identifying human capital and competence. From Table 7.4, the value-networking reflection question for educating and coaching involves evaluating the transactions between two or more roles or participants in which one role as an agent receives resources from another role or agent and provides resources in return. The question would be: What is the exchange of resources and information between the providers and the patient and family regarding medication and available resources? Name three exchanges of resources, skills, or information with the patient that are essential to the care coordination success of this case:

1.
2.
3.

Organization-centered systems-thinking processes, such as coaching and education, are used by the team from to promote self-management. The identified practice issues include knowledge or available resources. Targeted interventions for the team are to educate and empower the patient and family. The documented desired outcomes are to stabilize both the medical and mental conditions. A key question to ask is: Are the patient and family able to identify the resources they need and to navigate the health care system? The explicit value for role clarity, collaboration, and interaction of the team placed on promoting self-management is perceived-value realization. From Table 7.4, the value-networking reflection question for promoting self-management is: What is the level of value that roles or participants feel they receive from individual deliverables, which can come from roles, participants, or the network? Name three examples of learned self-management that resulted from the care coordination of this case:

1.
2.
3.

With the use of the CCCR systems model, the advanced practice nurse and other providers address practice issues by using and developing evidence-based interventions, implementing measures of adherence, and evaluating processes and outcomes. This requires clinical reasoning at different levels of perspective—the individual patient needs, interprofessional team contributions, and attention to the systems in which people work and provide care. These practice issues, interventions, and outcomes for patient and family care coordination stem from the National Quality Forum (NQF, 2010a, 2010b) and Agency for Healthcare Research and Quality (AHRQ, 2014).

As the center of attention for health care needs is managed by webs of relationships between and among providers, each interaction supports a specific value exchange as participant's partner for successful outcomes (Allee, 2003). The dynamic relationships that occurred for this patient among the advanced practice nurse, nursing staff, physician, pharmacist, and social worker were collaborative, trusting, dynamic, and interdependent. Application of the competing-value competencies will relate to collaboration, creating, competing, and controlling, and help make explicit knowledge shared and managed to support innovation, coordination, and directing. Through the use of the electronic health record, connectivity impacted the value networking with greater access to knowledge and information. This process provided quick and effective feedback among team members for the complex needs this patient had related to psychological comorbidities problems.

CLINICAL JUDGMENTS AND CCCR

The final phase of the clinical reasoning process is to determine whether outcomes were met and whether care coordination activities were successful. The OPT model of clinical reasoning is revisited for the final phase of care coordination, where judgments are made about achieving outcomes from the interprofessional team activity plan (see Exhibit 7.8). The worksheet (see Figure 7.2) is revisited to make judgments about the care coordination essentials (needs, individualized plan of care; safety; capacity, resources, and skills; and self-management). Shifting to the next level of perspective, using team-centered systems and organization-centered systems-thinking activities, collaboration and coordination of the plan of care reveal ongoing planning and evaluation to provide appropriate family support and physical and mental health support for individual health. The goal is to provide a safe home environment, which is drug free, with no aggressive behaviors, and an appropriate educational level for the patient. The appropriate home and caregivers should be identified. Parental support is needed to educate about skills to handle the behaviors of the child and maintain medication adherence. Resources identified for this case would be the school counselor, social worker, and support groups. These resources lead to the best possible functioning and independence for the patient in self-management of medical and mental conditions.

Some remaining questions may arise as the evaluation of outcomes occurs, such as: Can the organizations provide continuing resources and reach care coordination outcomes for this patient? Were communication and the feedback loop effective between the health care providers and patient and family? Did the complexity of the system hinder or enhance the achievement of outcomes? How do the competencies of the competing-values framework support the interprofessional dialogue and reasoning about the care coordination of this particular case? The advanced practice nurse as care coordinator views all the systems and is the key informant to communicate with the team regarding the efficiency and effectiveness of the processes for care outcomes. Judgments are made about whether the outcomes from case management have been achieved, and the information is recycled back to revise or enhance the plan of care.

The thinking processes used by the advanced practice nurse and other health care providers while implementing the CCCR systems model are promoted through monitoring of thinking, the environment, and behaviors for goal attainment (Zimmerman & Schunk, 2001). The courses of action chosen to manage issues and ensure that this patient remained safe revolve around behaviors and actions taken, thinking processes used, and environmental structuring. Critical reflective questions that can be used to prompt clinical reasoning to make judgments about the achievement of patient and family outcomes are shown in Table 7.5. Critical-, creative-, and systems-thinking processes are used for total care coordination, flow from patient-centered systems thinking (Table 7.3), team-centered systems thinking (Table 7.5), and organization-centered systems thinking (Table 7.5) for case management.

TABLE 7.5 Team-Centered and Organization-Centered Systems-Thinking Reflection Questions

SELF-REGULATION ACTIVITIES	REFLECTION QUESTIONS

Monitoring thinking	I. **Reflect on the thinking processes the team used to navigate organizational systems for care coordination of this case.**
	1. The baseline needs identified by the team in this case are.... Adjustments in the plan of care for future successes include.... Difficulties were resolved by...
	2. Team reactions during the care coordination of this case in regard to organizational systems could be described as... and they were handled by...
	3. When the team was dealing with important facts to develop the plan of care, coach, and educate the patient/family about organizational systems, it ...
	4. Looking back on meaningful activities, the resources the team could have spent:
	   a. More time on...
	   b. Less time on...

Monitoring the environment	II. **Reflect on the environmental circumstances you encountered in the care coordination of this case.** 5. When the team prepares to carry out coaching and education activities for care coordination, it... 6. When the team considers particular distractions in the organizations that impede medical care services and supports for care coordination, it... 7. When the team works and communicates with organizational partners for care coordination of this case, it... 8. If the team had the chance to redo the care coordination activities, it would do... instead of... because...

Monitoring behavior	III. **Reflect on your behaviors and reactions to the care coordination of this case.**
	9. Impressions of the team performance in evaluating capacity, energy, support, readiness, and skills to organize and manage the plan of care within organizational systems are...
	10. The team assures that it will update the needs assessment and individualized plan of care by... and if it needs to make changes, it...
	11. The team makes sure it empowers the patient/family to navigate through organizational systems for management of health care needs by... and if it needs to make changes, it...
	12. The team reaction to care coordination of this case...
	   a. Reaction to what it likes about the navigation of organizational systems to facilitate the care coordination of this case...
	   b. Reaction to what it did not like about the navigation of organizational systems to facilitate the care coordination of this case...
	Optional prompt: Other comments about the care coordination of this case...

Adapted from Kuiper, Pesut, and Kautz (2009).

SUMMARY

The clinical reasoning challenge for psychological/mental health begins with a description and understanding of the patient's story. The thinking strategies used in this case provided a safe and health-promoting environment for a patient who was being aggressive and disruptive to the family unit. As the providers practice self-monitoring, self-evaluation, and self-correction, successful strategies are employed, and flaws in thinking are corrected as they collaborate and align interventions for patient and family success. The OPT clinical reasoning model provides the foundation and structure for clinical reasoning and systems thinking within an individual patient and family situation. The OPT structure and process can be used at several levels for care planning by the provider, by the team, and by the organization to discern alignment and coordination of care activities. The CCCR systems model provides the structure for clinical reasoning for the care coordination of essential needs and their related practice issues, interventions, outcomes, and values.

KEY CONCEPTS

1. Clinical reasoning for care coordination with psychological/mental health can be promoted with a framework that includes structure, content, and process.
2. A supporting framework for CCCR extends case management using patient-centered systems thinking and the OPT clinical reasoning model across levels of perspective that also include team-centered systems thinking and organization-centered systems thinking to align care coordination activities.
3. The process of CCCR involves critical reflection for the individual provider and team.
4. Value-network analysis helps to define and describe the unique contributions that individual providers make to CCCR efforts supported through knowledge management and value-impact analysis.
5. A supporting framework for CCCR is completed by attending to the organization-centered systems thinking to make judgments about care coordination essentials.

STUDY QUESTIONS AND ACTIVITIES

1. Describe in your own words the benefits and processes of using the CCCR systems model with psychological/mental health cases.
2. Using the CCCR systems model, identify the care coordination of essential needs for cases involving psychological/mental health.
3. To what degree can you explicitly identify and describe the value exchanges associated with care coordination in psychological/mental health situations?
4. How can an interprofessional team use the competencies of the competing values of collaboration, creating, competing, and controlling to ensure efficiency

and effectiveness of care coordination? How does your team negotiate roles of mentor, broker, director, and coordinator?

5. Identify all the possible standardized health care languages and communication strategies that could be considered in a psychological/mental health case. Does language impact on communication and the patient outcomes? How does a discipline-specific framework influence the feedback, decisions, and outcomes with psychological/mental health?

6. Identify the relationship between critical reflection and thinking strategies as they are applied to the three levels of system-thinking perspectives that are required—patient, individual provider, team, and organization. What unique reflections are required to focus on team and organizational function with psychological/mental health?

REFERENCES

Agency for Healthcare Research and Quality (AHRQ). (2014). *What is care coordination? Care coordination measures atlas update.* Rockville, MD: Author. Retrieved from http://www.ahrq.gov/professionals/prevention-chronic-care/improve/coordination/index.html

Allee, V. (2003). *The future of knowledge: Increasing prosperity through value networks.* Burlington, MA: Butterworth-Heinemann.

Allee, V. (2008). Value network analysis and value conversion of tangible and intangible assets. *Journal of Intellectual Capital, 9*(1), 5–24.

Allee, V., Schwabe, O., & Babb, M. K. (Eds.). (2015). *Value networks and the true nature of collaboration.* Tampa, FL: Megher–Kifer Press Value Net Works and Verna Allee Associates.

Haas, S. A., Swan, B. A., & Haynes, T. S. (2014). *Care coordination and transition management core curriculum.* Pitman, NJ: American Academy of Ambulatory Care Nursing.

Kuiper, R., Pesut, D., & Kautz, D. (2009). Promoting the self-regulation of clinical reasoning skills in nursing students. *Open Nursing Journal, 3*, 76–85. Retrieved from http://www.ncbi.nlm.nih.gov/pmc/articles/PMC2771264

National Quality Forum (NQF). (2010a). *Preferred practices and performance measures for measuring and reporting care coordination: A consensus report.* Washington, DC: Author.

National Quality Forum (NQF). (2010b). *Quality connections: Care coordination.* Washington, DC: Author.

Pesut, D. J. (2008). Thoughts on thinking with complexity in mind. In C. Lindberg, S. Nash, & C. Lindberg (Eds.), *On the edge: Nursing in the age of complexity* (pp. 211–238). Bordentown, NJ: Plexus Press.

Quinn, R. (2015). *The positive organization: Breaking free from conventional cultures, constraints, and beliefs.* Oakland, CA: Berrett-Koehler.

Quinn, R., & Quinn, R. E. (2015). *Lift: Becoming a positive force in any situation.* San Francisco, CA: Berrett-Koehler.

Quinn, R. E., Bright, D., Faerman, S. R., Thompson, M. P., & McGrath, M. R. (2014). *Becoming a master manager: A competing values approach.* Hoboken, NJ: John Wiley & Sons.

Quinn, R. E., Heynoski, K., Thomas, M., & Spreitzer, G. M. (2014). *The best teacher in you: How to accelerate learning and change lives.* San Francisco, CA: Berrett-Koehler.

Quinn, R. E., & Rohrbough, J. (1983). A spatial model of effectiveness criteria: Towards a competing values approach to organizational analysis. *Management Science, 29*, 363–377.

World Health Organization (WHO). (2015). *Manual of the International Classification of Diseases and related health problems* (10th rev. ed.). Geneva, Switzerland: Author. Retrieved from http://www.icd10data.com

Zimmerman, B., & Schunk, D. S. (2001). *Self-regulated learning and academic thought*. Mahwah, NJ: Lawrence Erlbaum.

CHAPTER 8

CARE COORDINATION FOR A PATIENT IN ACUTE CARE

In this chapter, we use the Care Coordination Clinical Reasoning (CCCR) systems model as described in Part I and explain how the model can be used to reason about an acute care case. The case presented in this chapter illustrates how an advanced practice nurse works with a patient who requires admission to an acute care unit after being seen in the emergency department because of new-onset confusion. The emergency department is the first point of access for the patient. The advanced practice nurse provides care coordination through the application and use of critical-, creative-, systems-, and complexity-thinking processes to manage patient problems with an interprofessional team to design appropriate interventions and establish patient-centered outcomes. Depending on the nature of need involved in the case, referrals to other specialty or primary care providers are determined (Haas, Swan, & Haynes, 2014).

The CCCR systems model framework begins with the patient story, which is derived from gathering data and evidence from an interview, history, physical examination, and the health record. The advanced practice nurse then develops a patient-centered plan of care using the Outcome-Present State-Test (OPT) model worksheets. In order to do this, one activates patient-centered systems-thinking skills for complex patient stories and consistently uses key questions to reflect on the specific sections of the model (Pesut, 2008), as well as the dimensions and elements of care coordination.

LEARNING OUTCOMES

After completing this chapter, the reader should be able to:

1. Explain the components of a care coordination framework that are needed to manage the problems, interventions, and outcomes of acute care patients managing health care issues
2. Describe the different thinking processes that support clinical reasoning skills and strategies for determining priorities and desired outcomes for the acute care patient
3. Define the cognitive and metacognitive self-regulatory processes that support individual provider critical reflection related to levels and perspectives associated with clinical reasoning for the acute care patient and care coordination

4. Describe how the communication and knowledge management between inter-professional health care team members are essential for care coordination to address acute care patient needs
5. Describe the critical meta-reflective processes that support team reflection and value-added impact related to levels and perspectives associated with the care coordination challenges and clinical reasoning required to navigate acute care patient care plans

THE PATIENT STORY

We begin with the history and story of an 87-year-old male, Tony Brown, who presents with new-onset confusion, right-side weakness, slurred speech, and altered mental status. All the symptoms resolved during transport to the emergency department prior to any interventions. Mr. Brown's friend called 911 because he was confused and had difficulty using his right side. These symptoms lasted 45 minutes. On arrival to the emergency department, Mr. Brown had a CT scan of the head and was medicated with 325 mg of aspirin.

Mr. Brown reports a similar episode occurred in 2007, with a negative workup. In 2011, warfarin was changed to a novel anticoagulation agent because there was difficulty in managing the international normalized ratio (INR). The patient denied excessive alcohol intake on admission and had a negative CAGE questionnaire assessment (an acronym formed from the first letters of the most significant words used in the four questions in the questionnaire [Cut/Annoyed/Guilty/Eye-opener]). During his hospital stay he developed delirium tremens. It is noted that Mr. Brown has a poor support system and as no familial relationships. Mr. Brown also admits to poor medication compliance and often misses several doses of the anticoagulant per week.

His past medical history includes the comorbidities of transient ischemic attack, chronic atrial fibrillation, nonischemic cardiomyopathy, and hyperlipidemia. He drinks alcohol and is nonadherent with his medication regimen. Current medications include colchicine, dabigatran, hydrochlorothiazide, and pravastatin.

The physical examination reveals a height of 5' 11", weight of 95.39 kg, body mass index (BMI) of 29.4, blood pressure of 148/66 mmHg, heart rate of 87 beats per minute, temperature of 96.3°F, and a respiratory rate of 16 breaths per minute. His oxygen saturation was 100% on room air. Other laboratory values are as follows: EKG shows atrial fibrillation with left axis deviation and no ST- or T-wave elevations or depressions; CT scan of the head shows appropriate age-related atrophy without hemorrhage, mass effect, or edema.

PATIENT-CENTERED PLAN OF CARE USING OPT WORKSHEETS

Once the story is obtained from all possible sources, care planning and reasoning proceeds using the OPT clinical reasoning web worksheet (Figure 8.1), which helps

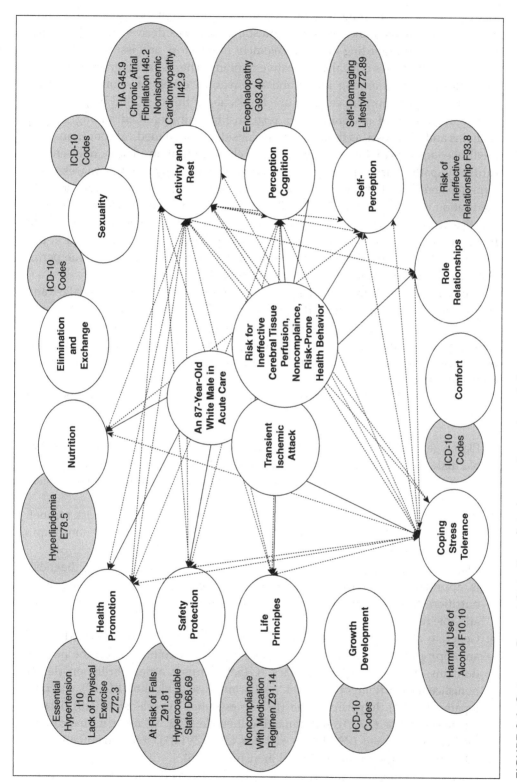

FIGURE 8.1 Outcome-Present State-Test clinical reasoning web worksheet.

ICD-10, International Classifications of Diseases, 10th edition; TIA, transient ischemic attack.

determine relationships among issues and highlights potential keystone issues. The OPT clinical reasoning web offers a graphic representation of the functional relationships between and among diagnostic hypotheses derived from the analysis and synthesis regarding how each element of the story and issues relate to one another. This activates critical and creative thinking. The visual diagram that results illustrates dynamics among issues and a convergence helps to point out central issues that require nursing care. As one thinks about this case, and begins to spin and weave a clinical reasoning web, relationships are identified among nursing domains and diagnoses as they are jointly considered with medical conditions. The medical conditions in this case are history of chronic atrial fibrillation, nonischemic cardiomyopathy, harmful use of alcohol, encephalopathy, hyperlipidemia, essential hypertension, lack of physical exercise, self-damaging lifestyle, noncompliance with medication regimen, risk for falls, and a hypercoagulable state. Once the advanced practice nurse considers these diagnoses, the nursing care domains associated with them are identified. The complementary nursing diagnoses most impacted in this case are risk for ineffective relationships, risk for ineffective cerebral tissue perfusion, noncompliance, and risk-prone health behavior.

To spin and weave the web, the provider uses thinking processes to analyze and synthesize relationships among diagnostic hypotheses associated with a patient's health status. The visual representation and mapping of these relationships supports the development of patient-centered systems thinking and connections between and among the medical and nursing diagnoses under consideration, given the patient story.

The steps to the creation of the OPT clinical reasoning web using the worksheet are as follows:

1. Place a general description of the patient in the respective middle circle—87-year-old male presents to the emergency department with new-onset confusion.
2. Place the major medical diagnoses in the respective middle circle—transient ischemic attack.
3. Place the major nursing diagnoses in the respective middle circle—risk for ineffective relationships, risk for ineffective cerebral tissue perfusion, noncompliance, and risk-prone health behavior.
4. Choose the nursing domains for which each medical and nursing diagnosis is appropriate—activity/rest, coping/stress tolerance, perception/cognition, nutrition, health promotion, self-perception, life principles, safety protection, and role relationships.
5. Generate all the International Classification of Diseases (ICD)-10 codes that are appropriate for the particular patient story that coincide with the nursing domains—transient ischemic attack (G45.9), chronic atrial fibrillation (I48.2), nonishcemic cardiomyopathy (I142.9), harmful use of alcohol (F10.10), encephalopathy (G93.4), hyperlipidemia (E78.5), essential hypertension (I10), lack of physical exercise (Z72.3), self-damaging lifestyle (Z72.89), noncompliance with medication regimen (Z91.14), at risk for falls (Z91.81), hypercoagulable state (D68.69), and risk for ineffective relationship (F93.8).
6. Once the nursing domains, diagnoses, and ICD-10 codes are identified, reflect on the total web worksheet and concurrently consider and explain how each of

the issues is or is not related to the other issues. Draw lines of relationship to spin and weave the web connections or associations among the ICD-10 codes/diagnoses. As you draw the lines, think out loud, justify the reasons for the connections, and explain specifically how the diagnoses may or may not be connected or related.

7. After you have spent some time connecting the relationships, determine which domain/domains have the highest priority for care coordination and most efficiently and effectively represent the keystone nursing care needs of the patient by counting the arrows that connect the medical problems (ICD-10 codes). In this case, counting 15 lines (Table 8.2) that point to or from the nursing domain of activity/rest represents the priority, present-state keystone issues.

8. Look once again at the sets of relationships and determine the theme or key-stone that summarizes the patient-in-context or the patient story—the problems related to transient ischemic attack from chronic atrial fibrillation and noncompliance with anticoagulation medications are the keystone issues for this case.

The OPT clinical reasoning web worksheet in Figure 8.1 shows a template with the patient health care situation, medical diagnoses, and nursing diagnoses at the center. Around the outer edges of the web are nursing domains with ICD-10 codes derived from history and physical assessment associated with the patient story. The directional arrows create the web effect and represent connections, explanations, and functional relationships between and among the diagnostic possibilities. As one can see, the domains and ICD-10 codes with more connections converging on one of the circles display the priority problem or keystones, in this case activity/rest. A keystone issue is one or more central supporting elements of the patient's story that help focus and determine a root cause or center of gravity of the system dynamics and help guide reasoning and care coordination based on an analysis (breaking things down into discrete parts) and synthesis (putting the parts together in a greater whole) of diagnostic possibilities as represented in the web. A key question to ask here is: How does the clinical reasoning web reveal relationships between and among the identified diagnoses and to what degree do these relationships make practical clinical sense according to the evidence and patient story? Table 8.1 shows a summary of the connections highlighting the priority with the most connections.

After considering the full picture using the clinical reasoning web worksheet, the next step is to use an OPT clinical reasoning model worksheet to facilitate and structure the patient-centered systems thinking about the care coordination of the identified problems highlighted in Table 8.1. As the advanced practice nurse thinks about the patient, she or he will concurrently consider the frame, outcome state, and present state. Each aspect of the OPT clinical reasoning model contributes to the other. The OPT clinical reasoning model worksheet is a map of the structure designed to provide a representation and guide thinking processes about relationships between and among competing issues and problems. Some questions that guide the use of the OPT clinical reasoning model are shown in Table 8.2 (Pesut, 2008).

TABLE 8.1 Relationships Among Nursing Domains, Medical Diagnoses, and Web Connections

NURSING DOMAINS	MEDICAL DIAGNOSES (ICD-10 CODES)	WEB CONNECTIONS
Activity/rest	Transient ischemic attack G45.9 Chronic atrial fibrillation I48.2 Nonischemic cardiomyopathy II42.9	15
Coping/stress tolerance	Harmful use of alcohol F10.10	13
Perception/cognition	Encephalopathy G93.4	6
Health promotion	Essential hypertension I10 Lack of physical exercise Z72.3	6
Self-perception	Self-damaging lifestyle Z72.89	6
Life principles	Noncompliance with medication regimen Z91.14	5
Safety/protection	At risk for falls Z91.81 Hypercoagulable state D68.69	5
Nutrition	Hyperlipidemia E78.5	4
Role relationships	Risk for ineffective relationship (nursing diagnosis)	3

Source: World Health Organization (2015).

By writing each element on the worksheet, all the parts of the model become related to each other. As the health care provider moves from right to left, the model structures the plan of care. Critical thinking skills are used to consider the patient story and creative thinking is used to identify and reason about the keystone issues/themes/cues to determine the most significant evidence in the present state. Complexity thinking helps the provider to consider the outcomes desired and the gaps between the present and outcomes states. Once interventions and tests are decided, the plan of care transitions over to a care coordination model and team-centered systems thinking which considers patient preferences within the frame of the situation.

The patient-in-context story (Exhibit 8.1) is depicted on the far right-hand side of Figure 8.2. The advanced practice nurse notes relevant facts of the story, which in this case include the patient demographics and characteristics: 87-year-old male who lives alone without social support. He has diagnoses of chronic atrial fibrillation, nonischemic cardiomyopathy, harmful use of alcohol, encephalopathy, hyperlipidemia, essential hypertension, lack of physical exercise, self-damaging lifestyle, noncompliance with medication regimen, risk for falls, and hypercoagulable state. He currently has had a transient ischemic attack complicated by delirium tremens while in the hospital. His initial treatment was with an aspirin and his symptoms subsided during transport to the emergency department. He

TABLE 8.2 Questions That Guide the Use of the OPT Model

Patient-in-context	What is the patient story?
Diagnostic cue/web logic	What diagnoses have you generated?
	What outcomes do you have in mind given the diagnoses?
	What evidence supports those diagnoses?
	How does a reasoning web reveal relationships among the identified problems (diagnoses)?
	What keystone issue(s) emerge?
Framing	How are you framing the situation?
Present state	How is the present state defined?
Outcome state	What are the desired outcomes?
	What are the gaps or complementary pairs (~) of outcomes and present states?
Test	What are the clinical indicators of the desired outcomes?
	On what scales will the desired outcomes be rated?
	How will you know when the desired outcomes are achieved?
	How are you defining your testing in this particular case?
Decision making (interventions)	What clinical decisions or interventions help to achieve the outcomes?
	What specific intervention activities will you implement?
	Why are you considering these activities?
Judgment	Given your testing, what is your clinical judgment?
	Based on your judgment, have you achieved the outcome or do you need to reframe the situation?
	How, specifically, will you take this experience and learning with you into the future as you reason about similar cases?

OPT, Outcome-Present State-Test.
Adapted from Pesut (2008).

EXHIBIT 8.1 PATIENT-IN-CONTEXT STORY

Tony Brown is an 87-year-old male with new-onset confusion from a transient ischemic attack. Symptoms of confusion and right-sided weakness subsided during transport to the hospital. He developed delirium tremens while in the acute care unit. He admits to harmful alcohol intake and noncompliance with his medication regimen. He lives alone and has no support system.

Prescribed medications include dabigatran, hydrochlorothiazide, and pravastatin.

BP: 148/66 mmHg, O_2 sat: 100%, temperature: 96.38°F, pulse: 87, respiration: 16, BMI: 29.4, CT of the head is negative, and EKG shows no significant changes

BMI, body mass index; BP, blood pressure, O_2 sat: Oxygen saturation.

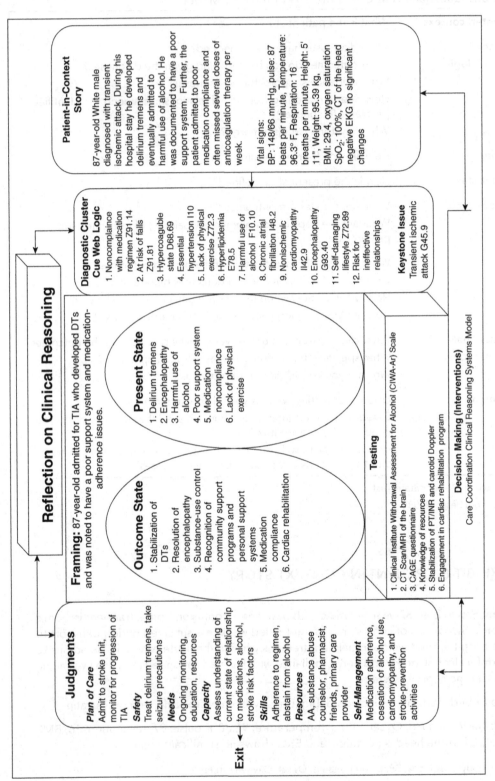

FIGURE 8.2 Outcome–Present State–Test clinical reasoning model for care coordination worksheet.

AA, Alcoholics Anonymous; BMI, body mass index; DTs, delirium tremens; INR, international normalized ratio; PT, prothrombin time; TIA, transient ischemic attack.

has essential hypertension, nonischemic cardiomyopathy, harmful consumption of alcohol, and noncompliance with his medication regimen. Because of the lack of social support, he has no resources to rely on for day-to-day care activities and medical-needs management. The acute care nurse practitioner will pull the acute care team together to promote his health and manage his chronic comorbidities while in the hospital. Significant laboratory data show no acute changes on the CT scan of the head or the EKG. A key point at this juncture is to review and reflect on the patient story for accuracy and thoroughness to proceed with care planning for care coordination.

Moving to the left of the figure, there is a place to list the diagnostic cluster cues on the web of medical diagnoses and ICD-10 codes (Exhibit 8.2). At the bottom of this box is placed the designated keystone issues or themes that fall under the most significant nursing domain—transient ischemic attack G45.9. Remember diagnostic cluster cue web logic is the use of inductive and deductive thinking skills. Some key questions to ask here are: What diagnoses were generated? Is there evidence to support those diagnoses? Is the keystone issue appropriate, given this patient story?

In the center and background of the worksheet are places to indicate the frame or theme that best represents the background issues regarding thinking about the patient story (Exhibit 8.3). The frame of this case is an 87-year-old male who presents

EXHIBIT 8.2 DIAGNOSTIC CLUSTER CUE WEB LOGIC

1. Noncompliance with medication regimen Z91.14
2. At risk for falls Z91.81
3. Hypercoagulable state D68.69
4. Essential hypertension I10
5. Lack of physical exercise Z72.3
6. Hyperlipidemia E78.5
7. Harmful use of alcohol F10.10
8. Chronic atrial fibrillation I48.2
9. Nonischemic cardiomyopathy I142.9
10. Encephalopathy G93.40
11. Self-damaging lifestyle Z72.89
12. Risk for ineffective relationships

KEYSTONE ISSUE/THEME

Transient ischemic attach G45.9

EXHIBIT 8.3 FRAMING

An 87-year-old male presents to the emergency department with new-onset confusion, right-sided weakness, and delirium tremens; no support system; medication-adherence issues.

EXHIBIT 8.4 PRESENT STATE

1. Delirium tremens
2. Encephalopathy
3. Harmful use of alcohol
4. Poor support system
5. Medication-compliance issues
6. Lack of physical exercise

EXHIBIT 8.5 OUTCOME STATE

1. Stabilization of delirium tremens
2. Resolution of encephalopathy
3. Alcohol-use cessation
4. Community support programs and personal support system
5. Medication compliance
6. Cardiac rehabilitation

to the emergency department with new-onset confusion, right-sided weakness, delirium tremens, medication adherence issues, and lack of a support system. This frame helps to organize the present state, outcome state, illustrates the gaps, and provides insights about what tests need to be considered to fill the gap. Decision making and reflection surround the framing as the advanced practice nurse thinks of many things simultaneously. Reflective thinking is used to monitor thinking and behavior. Key questions to ask here are: How am I framing the situation and does it agree with the patient's view of the situation? Given my disciplinary perspectives, what are the results I want to create for this person?

At the center of the sheet are spaces to place the present state (Exhibit 8.4) and outcome state (Exhibit 8.5) side by side. The present state in this case shows six primary health care problems related to the keystone issue: delirium tremens, encephalopathy, harmful use of alcohol, poor support system, medication-compliance issues, and lack of physical exercise.

The outcome state shows six matching goals to be achieved through care coordination: stabilization of delirium tremens, resolution of encephalopathy, permanent cessation of alcohol, recognition of community and personal support programs, medication compliance, and cardiac rehabilitation. Putting the two states together creates a gap analysis that naturally shows where the patient is and what the goals are in terms of the patient's care. Some key questions to ask here: Are the outcomes appropriate given the diagnoses? Are there gaps between the outcomes and present state? Are there clinical indicators of the desired outcome state?

EXHIBIT 8.6 TESTING

1. CIWA-Ar scale
2. CT scan/MRI of the head
3. CAGE questionnaire
4. Knowledge of resources
5. Doppler studies
6. Stabilization of PT/INR
7. Engagement in cardiac rehabilitation

EXHIBIT 8.7 REFLECTION ON CLINICAL REASONING

What clinical decisions or interventions help to achieve the outcomes?
What specific intervention activities will you implement?
Why are you considering these activities?

The gap between where the patient is and where the advanced practice nurse wants the patient to be is one way to create a test (Exhibit 8.6). Clinical decisions are choices made about interventions that will help the patient's transition from present state to a desired outcome state. As interventions are tested, the advanced practice nurse evaluates the degree to which outcomes are or are not being achieved. The tests chosen in this case include: Clinical Institute Withdrawal Assessment for Alcohol (CIWA) scale, CT and MRI of the head, CAGE questionnaire, knowledge of resources, Doppler studies, stabilization of PT/INR, and engagement in cardiac rehabilitation. Testing is concurrent and iterative as one gets closer and closer to goal achievement. Some key questions to ask here are: How is the advanced practice nurse defining *testing*? On what scales will the desired outcome be rated? How will the advanced practice nurse know when the desired targeted outcomes are achieved?

The reflection box at the top of Figure 8.2 (Exhibit 8.7) reminds the advanced practice nurse of the thinking strategies used for the patient situation. These strategies also help make explicit many of the relationships among ideas and issues associated with the patient's problems. Examples of reflection questions that support and engage patient-centered systems thinking are listed in Table 8.3.

Finally, the judgment space on the far left-hand side of the model (Exhibit 8.8) is the place to write in the results of the conclusions drawn from the CCCR model. The degree of gap or comparison of where the patient is, and where the health care team wants the patient to be, will determine whether there is a gap in the evidence. Once there is evidence that fills that gap, the nurse has to attribute meaning to the data. Making judgments about clinical issues is about the meaning the advanced

TABLE 8.3 Patient-Centered Systems-Thinking Reflection Questions

SELF-REGULATION ACTIVITIES	REFLECTION QUESTIONS

Monitoring thinking	I. **Reflect on the thinking processes you used with the care coordination of this case.**
	1. The baseline needs I identify in this case are.... I think I can identify future adjustments in the plan of care by.... If I have difficulty I...
	2. When I think about my feelings during the care coordination of this case, I describe them as...and I handle them by...
	3. When I try to remember or understand important facts to develop the plan of care, coach, and educate the patient/family, I...
	4. As I look back on meaningful activities, the resources I could have spent:
	   a. More time on...
	   b. Less time on...

Monitoring the environment	II. **Reflect on the environmental circumstances you encountered in the care coordination of this case.** 5. When I prepare to carry out coaching and education activities for care coordination, I... 6. When I think about particular distractions to facilitating medical care services and supports for care coordination, I... 7. When I work and communicate with interprofessional partners for care coordination of this case, I... 8. If I had the chance to redo the care coordination activities, I would do...instead of...because...

Monitoring behavior	III. **Reflect on your behaviors and reactions to the care coordination of this case.**
	9. My impression of my performance in evaluating capacity, energy, support, readiness, and skills to organize and manage the plan of care, is...
	10. I make sure I will update the needs assessment and individualized plan of care by...and if I need to make changes, I...
	11. I make sure I empower the patient/family for self-management of health care needs by...and if I need to make changes, I...
	12. Reaction to care coordination of this case...
	   a. My reaction to what I like about the care coordination of this case...
	   b. My reaction to what I do not like about the care coordination of this case...
	Optional prompt: Other comments I have about the care coordination of this case...

Adapted from Kuiper, Pesut, and Kautz (2009).

EXHIBIT 8.8 JUDGMENTS RELATED TO CARE COORDINATION VARIABLES

PLAN OF CARE

Admit to the stroke unit, monitor for progression of TIA

SAFETY

Treat delirium tremens, seizure precautions

NEEDS

Ongoing monitoring, education, resources

CAPACITY

Assess understanding of current state relationship to medications, alcohol, stroke risk factors

SKILLS

Adhere to regimen, abstain from alcohol

RESOURCES

Alcoholics Anonymous, substance abuse counselor, pharmacist, friends, primary care provider

SELF-MANAGEMENT

Medication adherence, cessation of alcohol, and cardiomyopathy and stroke prevention activities

practice nurse attributes to the evidence derived from the test or gap analysis of the present to the desired state. Complexity thinking, team-centered systems thinking, and organization-centered systems-thinking skills are used by the care coordination team at this point to evaluate and judge the successes or deficits from the plan of care. Interprofessional team activity requires negotiation of the competing values of collaboration—creating, competing, and controlling—and involves managing shared knowledge; acknowledging values impacted; and the brokering, directing, coordinating, and monitoring of practice issues, interventions, and outcomes. The judgments made in this case are made by the team after the care coordination essential needs outcomes are evaluated. Each of the items in the judgment column corresponds to an essential need addressed in the CCCR systems model (Figure 8.3). Some key questions to ask given the testing are: What are the clinical judgments? Have the outcomes been achieved, or does the situation need to be reframed?

Once the advanced practice nurse has experience coordinating care for acute care patients, the cases become part of a clinical reasoning learning history that

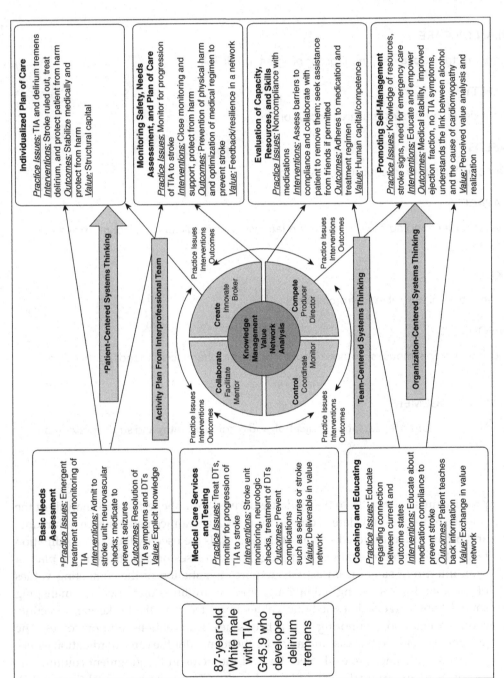

FIGURE 8.3 Care Coordination Clinical Reasoning systems model worksheet.

[a] Practice issues can be from any discipline: nursing, medicine, pharmacy, social work, and so on.

DTs, delirium tremens; TIA, transient ischemic attack.

become prototypes or schemas for other similar cases. These schemas and experience build on each other over time and result in the development of pattern recognition for future clinical reasoning applications. If the scenario results in a negative judgment, or progress is not being made to transition patients from present to desired states, the advanced practice nurse may have to reframe the situation, reconsider the keystone priority, reconsider the care coordination activities, and/or consult with members of the interprofessional team for the problem to be solved, and the outcome to be achieved. The key question to ask here is: How will this clinical learning experience impact future reasoning about similar cases?

CARE COORDINATION USING CCCR MODEL WORKSHEETS

The next step in the nursing diagnostic reasoning process is to augment the plan of care to include activities related to interprofessional care planning using the CCCR systems model framework (Exhibit 8.9) that builds on the OPT model of clinical reasoning. The systems dynamics and interactions between and among the patient issues determine the care needed and the services provided. The complexities in this case are the issues related to Mr. Brown's lack of social support, substance abuse, noncompliance with medications, and comorbidities in his health status. The CCCR systems model web (Figure 8.4) visually represents the complexities in this case along with the essential care coordination practice issues that need attention to organize thinking that focuses on the patient's priority needs.

The CCCR systems model web (Exhibit 8.10) provides a blueprint for consideration of the care coordination practice issues so clinicians can determine interventions, outcomes, and the value exchange that supports safe, high-quality care. This process involves patient-centered systems thinking, team-centered systems thinking, and organization-centered systems thinking to thoroughly and efficiently manage all aspects of patient cases. The steps to create the web for this case start in the center with the patient description and medical diagnoses (Tony Brown, an 87-year-old male with transient ischemic attack and delirium tremens), priority nursing domain (activity/rest), and ICD-10 code (transient ischemic attack G45.9), which show the overlap of patient issues that must be addressed by the advanced practice nurse and the care coordination interprofessional team.

Next, each large circle in this web represents the essential care coordination practice issues, with evidence and defining characteristics for this patient story:

EXHIBIT 8.9 CARE COORDINATION CLINICAL REASONING DEFINITION

The authors define *care coordination clinical reasoning* as the application of critical, creative, systems, and complexity thinking to determine the practice issues, interdependencies, and interconnections of role relationships for collaborative work in service of caring for people to address problems, interventions, and outcomes through time and across health care contexts and services.

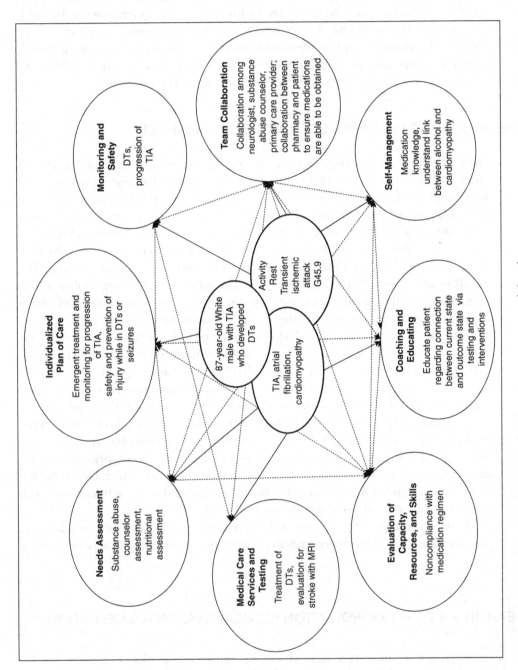

FIGURE 8.4 Care Coordination Clinical Reasoning systems model web.

DTs, delirium tremens; TIA, transient ischemic attack.

EXHIBIT 8.10 CCCR SYSTEMS MODEL WEB DEFINITION

The Care Coordination Clinical Reasoning systems model web enables one to visually represent the complexities and essential care coordination practice issues that need attention so as to organize thinking that focuses on the patient's and/or family's priority needs within the context of services provided within and between health care delivery systems.

needs assessment (substance abuse, counselor assessment, nutritional assessment); individualized plan of care (emergent treatment and monitoring for progression of transient ischemic attack, safety, and prevention of injury while in delirium tremens and/or seizures); medical care services and testing (treatment of delirium tremens, evaluation for stroke with MRI); evaluation of capacity, resources, and skills (noncompliance with medication regimen); monitoring and safety (delirium tremens, progression of transient ischemic attack); team collaboration (collaboration among neurologist, substance abuse counselor, primary care provider, pharmacist, and the patient); coaching and educating (educate of patient regarding connection between current state and outcome state via testing and interventions); and self-management (medication knowledge, understand link between alcohol and cardiomyopathy).

The provider then reflects on the total picture on the worksheet and begins to draw lines of relationship, connection, or association among the essential needs. As directional lines are drawn to create the web, functional relationships between and among the needs are recognized. Clinical reasoning and thinking processes are used to explain and justify the reasons for connecting these care coordination needs as central supporting elements in the patient's story, based on an analysis and synthesis of possible priorities as represented in the web. The priority care coordination needs that would most efficiently and effectively represent the key issues of the patient are addressed that align with the patient story. A key question to ask is: Does the CCCR systems model web provide a comprehensive consideration of the most pertinent evidence for care coordination practice issues?

The CCCR systems model worksheet (see Figure 8.3) is the next worksheet in the framework designed to provide a graphic representation or visual map of the structure of the CCCR systems model to help guide team-centered systems and organization-centered systems thinking. Some key questions to ask are: What clinical decisions and interventions will help to achieve the outcomes identified on the OPT model of clinical reasoning (see Figure 8.2)? What specific interventions will the clinicians and members of the team implement? Why are providers considering these activities?

Writing each element on the worksheet shows how parts of the model relate to each other. In Figure 8.3, on the far left-hand side, there is space to write the description of the patient's health care situation, which was at the center of the CCCR systems model web. Three essential needs are placed in the first boxes to the right of the description and include basic needs assessment, medical care services and testing, and coaching and education. Each of the care coordination needs identified in this model include practice issues, interventions, outcomes, and value specification.

From patient-centered systems-thinking processes used to create the OPT clinical reasoning model worksheets for this patient story, the identified basic needs practice issues include emergent treatment and monitoring of transient ischemic attack. Targeted interventions for the team would be to admit to the stroke unit, perform neurovascular checks, and medicate to prevent seizures. The documented desired outcomes would be resolution of transient ischemic attack symptoms and delirium tremens. A key question to ask is: Have the basic needs been identified given the frame of the situation? Consider the value-impact analysis in this case using the questions from Table 8.4.

KNOWLEDGE MANAGEMENT AND VALUE ANALYSIS

The explicit value for role clarity, collaboration, and interaction of the team placed on the needs assessment is explicit knowledge. From Table 8.4, the value-networking reflection question for basic needs is: What knowledge is codified and conveyed to others through dialogue, demonstration, or media? Name three knowledge classification systems that could be used to represent the patient characteristics in this case:

1.
2.
3.

From team-centered systems-thinking processes used for the basic needs assessment, the identified medical care services and testing practice issues include treat delirium tremens, monitor for progression of transient ischemic attack to stroke. Targeted interventions for the team are stroke unit monitoring, neurologic checks, and treatment of delirium tremens. The documented desired outcomes are to prevent complications such as seizures or stroke. A key question to ask is: Do the testing and interventions sufficiently manage the primary care needs? The explicit value for role clarity, collaboration, and interaction of the team placed on the medical care services and testing is to deliver evidence-based interventions based on the health care provider role. From Table 8.4, the value-networking reflection question for medical care services and testing basic needs is: What is the specific value or object that is conveyed from one role or participant to another role or participant? Name three deliverables that are essential for the care coordination success of this case:

1.
2.
3.

Organization-centered systems thinking is used by the team to enhance coaching and educating the patient. The identified coaching and educating practice issues include educating the patient regarding the connection between current and outcome states. Targeted intervention for the team is to educate the patient about medication compliance to prevent stroke. The documented desired

TABLE 8.4 Value Definitions and Reflection Questions

Deliverable	The specific values or objects that are conveyed from one role or participant to another role or participant. What are the deliverables that you offer and expect of others?
Exchange	Two or more transactions between two or more roles or participants that evoke reciprocity. A process in which one role as agent receives resources from another role or agent and provides resources in return. What are the resource exchanges between roles or participants on your interprofessional health care team?
Explicit knowledge	The knowledge that is codified and conveyed to others through dialogue, demonstration, or media. What is the explicit knowledge shared among members of the team?
Feedback	The return of information about the impact of an activity. It can also mean the return of a portion of the output of a process as new input. What feedback is returned about activities or outputs in your care coordination activities? How does feedback influence team dynamics and goal attainment?
Human capital/ Competence	The knowledge, skills, and competencies that reside in individuals who work in an organization or that are embedded in the organization's internal and external social networks. What human capital resources are needed in order for care coordination in your context to be successful?
Impact analysis	An assessment of how an input for a role is handled. What are the tangible/intangible costs, gains, or values from the input that generate a response or activity, or increase/decrease tangible assets?
Knowledge management	The degree to which the team facilitates and supports processes for creating, sustaining, sharing, and renewing organizational knowledge in order to generate social or economic gain or improve performance. Who is responsible and how is knowledge managed in the care coordination process?
Perceived value	The degree of value participants feel they receive from individual deliverables, which can come from roles, participants, or the network. What are the value-added dimensions of individual, collective, team, and organizational networks?
Resilience	The degree to which the network is able to reconfigure itself to respond to changing conditions and then return to its original form. What is the resilience capacity of the team and organization in which you work?
Structural capital	The infrastructure, routines, concepts, models, information systems, work systems, and business processes that support productivity and sustainability. To what degree do the structural capital and infrastructure support interprofessional teamwork and care coordination processes?

(continued)

TABLE 8.4 Value Definitions and Reflection Questions *(continued)*

Systems thinking	An analysis and synthesis of the forces and interrelationships that shape the behavior of systems? To what degree do the members of the team think about the system dynamics at the patient, group, team, or organizational levels?
Value realization	The degree to which tangible or intangible values turn the input into gains, benefits, capabilities, or assets that contribute to the success of an individual, a group, an organization, or a network (Allee, 2008). To what degree do members of the team intentionally negotiate and manage competing values related to collaborating, creating, competing, and/or controlling?

Adapted from Allee, Schwabe, and Babb (2015).

outcomes are to have the patient teach back information. A key question to ask is: Do the content and methods for coaching and teaching match the patient's cognitive abilities and understanding? From Table 8.4, the value-networking reflection question for educating and coaching involves evaluating the transactions between two or more roles or participants, where one role as an agent receives resources from another role or agent and provides resources in return. The question would be: What is the exchange of resources and information between the providers and the patient regarding medication and available resources? Name three resources that could be exchanged between the providers and patient in this case:

1.

2.

3.

The diagram in the center of the worksheet is the activity plan from the interprofessional team (Exhibit 8.11). The team engages in collaborating, creating, competing, and controlling dynamics through communication (Quinn, Bright, Faerman, Thompson, & McGrath, 2014; Quinn, Heynoski, Thomas, & Spreitzer, 2014; Quinn & Quinn, 2015; Quinn & Rohrbough, 1983) to manage essential areas of organizational culture to realize the intangible value exchanges used to develop and manage an activity plan, which considers interventions from the individualized plan of care, monitoring processes, evaluation of patient and family capacity with regard to resources and skills, and promotion of self-management. For example, in terms of collaboration, people must understand themselves and communicate honestly and effectively. Individuals mentor and develop others collaboratively and know how to participate and lead teams. Often this knowledge requires encouraging and managing constructive conflict. Competition enhances productivity and profitability. In this domain, vision and goal setting are paths to motivating self and others so that systems can be developed and organized to get results. Creating and promoting the adoption of new ideas or clinical innovations requires attention to judicious use of power and ethics as well as championing new ideas and innovations through negotiating commitments and agreements

EXHIBIT 8.11

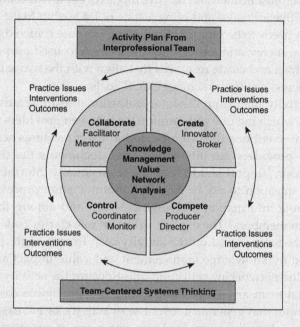

Key questions to consider for the four dimensions of the competing-values framework in the CCCR model are as follows:

- What are the desired outcomes in this case?
- What are the values I expect of myself and others?
- How are the feelings of the patient, family, and team considered in this case?
- What strategies could the team use to coordinate care?

for implementing and sustaining change. Control contributes to the development of stability and continuity as people work and manage across functions, organize information exchange, measure and monitor performance and quality, and enable compliance.

Key ingredients to team-centered systems thinking are that the members must be purpose centered, internally directed, other focused, and externally open to negotiation and communication surrounding competing values (Quinn, 2015; Quinn & Quinn, 2015). The activity plan from the interprofessional team in the CCCR model is guided by these principles and will promote the development of positive organizations and relationships. Each team member should be externally open to challenges, feedback and freedom from labels, higher performance, and the cultivation and development of communities of practice. When this outcome is challenged and false fixed, some team members are valued more than others in the context of competitive versus collaborative goals. Being other influenced cultivates empathy, rapport, energy, and calmness. Together, the team members feel safe and secure enough to take risks and act with trust, integrity, and resilience. Creating such a culture supports a spirit of inquiry, learning, and experimentation, which results in higher performance. Such behavior requires the activation of a reflective self in contrast to automatic self-justification and reactive modes of being and communicating. In order to be a positive influence and bring a state of leadership to the team, each member of the team needs to be vigilant about being purpose centered, choosing goals that create focus, energy, and meaning for the team. A focused purpose-centered team is likely to attract and create resources that align with the reasoning required to communicate across settings to achieve CCCR goals.

The activity plan from the interprofessional team iteratively visits the practice issues, which include communication between providers specific to this case, targeted interventions that are updated at team meetings across the contexts in which the providers are interacting, and documents the desired outcomes to maintain team support and to keep the team equally informed about patient status. A key question to ask is: Are the communication processes in place and do they promote information exchange between and among the interprofessional health team members? The explicit value for role clarity, collaboration, and interaction of the team placed on the activity plan from the interprofessional team is determined by knowledge management and value-impact analysis. From Table 8.4, the value-networking reflection questions for the activity plan from the interprofessional team are: What are the tangible/intangible costs, gains, or values from the input that generate a response or activity, or increase/decrease tangible assets? How does the team facilitate and support processes for collaborating, controlling, creating, and competing to sustain, share, and renew organizational knowledge in order to generate social or economic gain or improve performance? Name a cost, gain, and value that would be generated from the activity plan of the team for this case:

1.
2.
3.

To the far right of the CCCR system model worksheet are four essential care coordination needs that evolve from the activity plan from the interprofessional team stemming from patient-centered systems thinking, team-centered systems thinking, and organizational-centered systems thinking. These needs include the individualized plan of care; monitoring safety, needs assessment, and plan of care; evaluation of capacity, resources, and skills; and promoting self-management. Each of these care coordination essentials is also defined by practice issues, interventions, outcomes, and values.

The patient-centered systems-thinking and team-centered systems-thinking activities are used for the individualized plan of care. The identified practice issues revolve around the transient ischemic attack and delirium tremens. Targeted interventions for the provider and team are to rule out a stroke, treat the delirium tremens, and protect the patient from harm that would occur with seizures. The documented desired outcomes are to stabilize the patient medically and protect from harm. Some key questions to ask here are: Does the individualized plan of care include team collaboration? Is there any input that was not yet considered? Are there providers who were overlooked? The explicit value for role clarity, collaboration, and interaction of the provider and team placed on the individualized plan of care is on structural capital. From Table 8.4, the value-networking reflection question for the individualized plan of care is: What are the infrastructure, routines, concepts, models, information systems, work systems, and business processes that support productivity and have sustainability? Name three routines, systems, or processes that support and sustain the productivity of the care coordination in this case:

1.
2.
3.

From the patient-centered systems-thinking and team-centered systems-thinking processes used for monitoring safety, needs assessment, and plan of care, identified practice issues include monitoring for the progression of transient ischemic attack to stroke. Targeted interventions for the team are to closely monitor, support, and protect from harm. The documented desired outcomes are to prevent physical harm and optimize the medical regimen to prevent stroke. A key question to ask is: Does the plan of care promote safety and meet the patient needs? The explicit value for role clarity, collaboration, and interaction of the team placed on monitoring safety, needs assessment, and plan of care is to obtain feedback and assess resilience in the network. From Table 8.4, the value-networking reflection questions for medical care services and testing basic needs are: What feedback is returned about activities or outputs? Was the network able to reconfigure itself to respond to changing conditions and then return to its original form? Name three areas of need and/or safety that were reassessed to determine whether the plan of care needed to be adjusted:

1.
2.
3.

Organization-centered systems-thinking processes, such as coaching and education, are used by the team to evaluate capacity, resources, and skills. The identified practice issues include Mr. Brown's noncompliance with medications. Targeted interventions for the team are to assess barriers to compliance and collaborate with the patient to remove them, and also to seek assistance from friends, if they can be identified. The documented desired outcomes are to comply with medication and the treatment regimen. Some key questions to ask here are: Do the interventions in the plan of care require skilled help? Can the patient manage care needs independently? The explicit value for role clarity, collaboration, and interaction of the team placed on evaluating capacity, resources, and skills is identifying human capital and competence. From Table 8.4, the value-networking reflection question for educating and coaching involves evaluating the transactions between two or more roles or participants in which one role as an agent receives resources from another role or agent and provides resources in return. The key question would be: What is the exchange of resources and information between the providers and the patient regarding medication and available resources? Name three exchanges of resources, skills, or information with the patient that are essential to the care coordination success of this case:

1.
2.
3.

Organization-centered systems-thinking processes, such as coaching and education, are used by the team to promote self-management. The identified practice issues include knowledge of resources available to the patient, stroke signs, and when emergency care is needed. Targeted interventions for the team are to educate and to empower the patient. The documented desired outcomes are to stabilize of medical conditions, improve ejection fraction, eliminate any neurologic transient ischemic symptom, and to understand the link between alcohol and cause of cardiomyopathy. A key question to ask here is: Is the patient able to identify the resources he needs and to navigate the health care system? The explicit value for role clarity, collaboration, and interaction of the team placed on promoting self-management is perceived value realization. From Table 8.4, the value-networking reflection question for promoting self-management is: What is the level of value that roles or participants feel they receive from individual deliverables, which can come from roles, participants, or the network? Name three examples of learned self-management that resulted from the care coordination of this case:

1.
2.
3.

With the use of the CCCR systems model, the advanced practice nurse and other providers address practice issues by using and developing evidence-based interventions, implementing measures of adherence, and evaluating processes and outcomes. This requires clinical reasoning at different levels of perspective—the individual patient needs, interprofessional team contributions, and attention to the systems in which people work and provide care. These practice issues, interventions, and outcomes for patient care coordination stem from the National Quality Forum (NQF, 2010a, 2010b) and Agency for Healthcare Research and Quality (AHRQ, 2014).

As the center of attention for health care needs is managed by webs of relationships between and among providers, each interaction supports a specific value exchange as participant's partner for successful outcomes (Allee, 2003). For this acute care patient who will return home alone, the dynamic relationships that occurred among the advanced practice nurse, intensive care nursing staff, physician, substance abuse counselor, and pharmacist were collaborative, trusting, and interdependent. Application of the competing-value competencies will relate to collaboration, creating, competing, and controlling, and help make explicit knowledge shared and managed to support innovation, coordination, and directing. Through the use of the electronic health record, connectivity impacted the value networking with greater access to knowledge and information. This process provided quick and effective feedback among team members for the complex needs this patient had related to complications from chronic atrial fibrillation, transient ischemic attack, and alcoholism.

CLINICAL JUDGMENTS AND CCCR

The final phase of the clinical reasoning process is to determine whether outcomes were met and whether care coordination activities were successful. The CCCR model of clinical reasoning is revisited for the final phase of care coordination, where judgments are made about achieving outcomes from the interprofessional team activity plan (see Exhibit 8.8). The worksheet (see Figure 8.2), is revisited to make judgments about the care coordination essentials (needs, individualized plan of care; safety; capacity, resources, skills, self-management). Shifting to the next level of perspective, using team-centered systems and organization-centered systems-thinking activities, collaboration and coordination of the plan of care reveal ongoing planning and evaluation to provide appropriate patient support during this exacerbation of neurologic symptoms from a transient ischemic attack. The goal is to provide a supportive environment with the appropriate resources for this single 87-year-old male. His transient ischemic attack should be treated and discharge planning should include resource personnel to help him manage his chronic illnesses. The patient will need education about abstaining from alcohol, and about taking antistroke medications, cardiomyopathy medications, and the role of rehabilitation. These resources lead to the best possible management and safety for this patient with chronic atrial fibrillation and alcoholic cardiomyopathy.

Some remaining questions may arise as the evaluation of outcomes occurs, such as: Can the organization provide continuing resources and reach care coordination outcomes for this patient? Were communication and the feedback loop effective between the health care providers and the patient? Did the complexity of the system hinder or enhance the achievement of outcomes? How do the competencies of the competing-values framework support the interprofessional dialogue and reasoning about the care coordination of this particular case? How do members of the team share and manage knowledge in service of care coordination? The advanced practice nurse as care coordinator views all the systems and is the key informant to communicate with the team regarding the efficiency and effectiveness of the processes for care outcomes. Judgments are made about whether the outcomes from case management have been achieved, and the information is recycled back to revise or enhance the plan of care.

The thinking processes used by the advanced practice nurse and other health care providers while implementing the CCCR systems model are promoted through monitoring of thinking, the environment, and behaviors for goal attainment (Zimmerman & Schunk, 2001). The courses of action chosen to manage issues and ensure that this patient remained safe revolve around behaviors and actions taken, thinking processes used, and environmental structuring. Critical reflective questions that can be used to prompt clinical reasoning to make judgments about the achievement of patient outcomes are shown in Table 8.5. Critical-, creative-, and systems-thinking processes are used for total care coordination, flow from patient-centered systems (see Table 8.3), team-centered systems thinking (Table 8.5), and organization-centered systems thinking (Table 8.5) for case management.

TABLE 8.5 Team-Centered and Organization-Centered Systems-Thinking Reflection Questions

SELF-REGULATION ACTIVITIES	REFLECTION QUESTIONS

Monitoring thinking	I. **Reflect on the thinking processes the team used to navigate organizational systems for care coordination of this case.**
	 1. The baseline needs identified by the team in this case are.... Adjustments in the plan of care for future successes include.... Difficulties were resolved by...
	 2. Team reactions during the care coordination of this case in regard to organizational systems could be described as...and they were handled by...
	 3. When the team was dealing with important facts to develop the plan of care, coach, and educate the patient/family about organizational systems, it...
	 4. Looking back on meaningful activities, the resources the team could have spent:
	   a. More time on...
	   b. Less time on...

Monitoring the environment	II. **Reflect on the environmental circumstances you encountered in the care coordination of this case.** 5. When the team prepares to carry out coaching and education activities for care coordination, it... 6. When the team considers particular distractions in the organizations that impede medical care services and supports for care coordination, it... 7. When the team works and communicates with organizational partners for care coordination of this case, it... 8. If the team had the chance to redo the care coordination activities, it would do...instead of...because...

Monitoring Behavior	III. **Reflect on your behaviors and reactions to the care coordination of this case.**
	 9. Impressions of the team performance in evaluating capacity, energy, support, readiness, and skills to organize and manage the plan of care within organizational systems are...
	 10. The team assures that it will update the needs assessment and individualized plan of care by...and if it needs to make changes, it...
	 11. The team makes sure it empowers the patient/family to navigate through organizational systems for management of health care needs by...and if it needs to make changes, it...
	 12. The team reaction to care coordination of this case...
	   a. Reaction to what it likes about the navigation of organizational systems to facilitate the care coordination of this case...
	   b. Reaction to what it did not like about the navigation of organizational systems to facilitate the care coordination of this case...
	 Optional prompt: Other comments about the care coordination of this case...

Adapted from Kuiper, Pesut, and Kautz (2009).

SUMMARY

The clinical reasoning challenge for acute care begins with a description and under-standing of the patient's story. The thinking strategies used in this case provided a safe and health-promoting environment for an elderly male patient with declining neurologic and cardiac health. As the providers practice self-monitoring, self-eval-uation, and self-correction, successful strategies are employed, and flaws in think-ing are corrected as they collaborate and align interventions for patient success. The OPT clinical reasoning model provides the foundation and structure for clinical reasoning and systems thinking within an individual patient situation. The OPT structure and process can be used at several levels for care planning by the provider, by the team, and by the organization to discern alignment and coordination of care activities. The CCCR systems model provides the structure for clinical reasoning for the care coordination essential needs and their related practice issues, interventions, outcomes, and values.

KEY CONCEPTS

1. Clinical reasoning for care coordination with an acute care patient with chronic health problems can be promoted with a framework that includes structure, con-tent, and process.
2. A supporting framework for care coordination clinical reasoning extends case management using patient-centered systems thinking and the OPT clinical reasoning model across levels of perspective that also include team-centered systems thinking and organization-centered systems thinking to align care coor-dination activities.
3. The process of CCCR involves critical reflection for the individual provider and team.
4. Value-network analysis helps to define and describe the unique contributions that individual providers make to CCCR efforts enhanced through knowledge man-agement and value-impact analysis.
5. A supporting framework for CCCR is completed by attending to the organization-centered systems thinking to make judgments about care coordina-tion essentials.

STUDY QUESTIONS AND ACTIVITIES

1. Describe in your own words the benefits and processes of using the CCCR sys-tems model with acute care cases.
2. Using the CCCR systems model, identify the care coordination essential needs of cases in acute care.
3. To what degree can you explicitly identify and describe the value exchanges associated with care coordination in acute care situations?
4. How can an interprofessional team use the competencies of the competing val-ues of collaboration, creating, competing, and controlling to ensure efficiency

and effectiveness of care coordination? How does your team negotiate roles of mentor, broker, director, and coordinator?

5. Identify all the possible standardized health care languages and communication strategies that could be considered in an acute care case. Does language impact on communication and the patient outcomes? How does a discipline-specific framework influence the feedback, decisions, and outcomes with acute care?

6. Identify the relationship between critical reflection and thinking strategies as they are applied to the three levels of system-thinking perspectives that are required—patient, individual provider, team, and organization. What unique reflections are required to focus on team and organizational function with acute care?

REFERENCES

Agency for Healthcare Research and Quality (AHRQ). (2014). *What is care coordination? Care coordination measures atlas update*. Rockville, MD: Author. Retrieved from http://www .ahrq.gov/professionals/prevention-chronic-care/improve/coordination/index.html

Allee, V. (2003). *The future of knowledge: Increasing prosperity through value networks*. Burlington, MA: Butterworth-Heinemann.

Allee, V. (2008). Value network analysis and value conversion of tangible and intangible assets. *Journal of Intellectual Capital, 9*(1), 5–24.

Allee, V., Schwabe, O., & Babb, M. K (eds.). (2015). *Value networks and the true nature of collaboration*. Tampa, FL: Megher-Kifer Press Value Net Works and Verna Allee Associates.

Haas, S. A., Swan, B. A., & Haynes, T. S. (2014). *Care coordination and transition management core curriculum*. Pitman, NJ: American Academy of Ambulatory Care Nursing.

Kuiper, R., Pesut, D., & Kautz, D. (2009). Promoting the self-regulation of clinical reasoning skills in nursing students. *Open Nursing Journal, 3*, 76–85. Retrieved from http://www .ncbi.nlm.nih.gov/pmc/articles/PMC2771264

National Quality Forum (NQF). (2010a). *Preferred practices and performance measures for measuring and reporting care coordination: A consensus report*. Washington, DC: Author.

National Quality Forum (NQF). (2010b). *Quality connections: Care coordination*. Washington, DC: Author.

Pesut, D. J. (2008). Thoughts on thinking with complexity in mind. In C. Lindberg, S. Nash, and C. Lindberg (Eds.), *On the edge: Nursing in the age of complexity* (pp. 211–238). Bordentown, NJ: Plexus Press.

Quinn, R. (2015). *The positive organization: Breaking free from conventional cultures, constraints, and beliefs*. Oakland, CA: Berrett-Koehler.

Quinn, R., & Quinn, R. E. (2015). *Lift: Becoming a positive force in any situation*. San Francisco, CA: Berrett-Koehler.

Quinn, R. E., Bright, D., Faerman, S. R., Thompson, M. P., & McGrath, M. R. (2014). *Becoming a master manager: A competing values approach*. Hoboken, NJ: John Wiley & Sons.

Quinn, R. E., Heynoski, K., Thomas, M., & Spreitzer, G. M. (2014). *The best teacher in you: How to accelerate learning and change lives*. San Francisco, CA: Berrett-Koehler.

Quinn, R. E., & Rohrbough, J. (1983). A spatial model of effectiveness criteria: Towards a competing values approach to organizational analysis. *Management Science, 29*, 363–377.

World Health Organization (WHO). (2015). *Manual of the International Classification of Diseases and related health problems* (10th rev. ed.). Geneva, Switzerland: Author. Retrieved from http://www.icd10data.com

Zimmerman, B., & Schunk, D. S. (2001). *Self-regulated learning and academic thought.* Mahwah, NJ: Lawrence Erlbaum.

CHAPTER 9

CARE COORDINATION FOR A VETERAN/MILITARY PATIENT

In this chapter, we use the Care Coordination Clinical Reasoning (CCCR) systems model as described in Part I and explain how the model can be used to reason about a case given an acute care context with a military patient. The advanced practice nurse is working with a patient who is in need of support services to promote quality outcomes with chronic pulmonary disease and comorbidities. The provider/ clinic is the point of access for the patient. The advanced practice nurse provides care coordination through the application and use of critical-, creative-, systems-, and complexity-thinking processes to manage patient problems with an interprofessional team to design appropriate interventions and establish patient-centered outcomes. Depending on the nature of need involved in the case, referrals to other specialty or primary care providers, community services, and living environments are determined and considered in managing care coordination and transitions (Haas, Swan, & Haynes, 2014).

The CCCR systems model framework begins with the patient story, which is derived from gathering data and evidence from an interview, history, physical examination, and the health record. The advanced practice nurse then develops an individual plan of care using the Outcome-Present State-Test (OPT) model worksheets. In order to do this, one activates the patient-centered systems-thinking skills for complex patient stories and habitually uses key questions to reflect on the specific sections of the model (Pesut, 2008), as well as the dimensions and elements of care coordination.

LEARNING OUTCOMES

After completing this chapter, the reader should be able to:

1. Explain the components of a care coordination framework that are needed to manage the problems, interventions, and outcomes of a military patient navigating health issues
2. Describe the different thinking processes that support clinical reasoning skills and strategies for determining priorities and desired outcomes for the military patient

3. Define the cognitive and metacognitive self-regulatory processes that support individual provider critical reflection related to levels and perspectives associated with clinical reasoning for the military patient and care coordination

4. Describe how the communication and knowledge management among interprofessional health care team members are essential for care coordination to address patient needs as a veteran

5. Describe the critical meta-reflective processes that support team reflection related to levels and perspectives associated with the care coordination challenges and clinical reasoning required to navigate patient care plans with military patients

THE PATIENT STORY

We begin with the history and story of a 64-year-old Vietnam veteran, Ralph Wiseman, who presents with complaints of increasing shortness of breath over the past 2 days. He is being seen in the veteran's clinic by a family nurse practitioner to manage his chronic health problems. Mr. Wiseman was brought into an emergency department 11 days ago by the emergency medical system with similar symptoms. His oxygen saturations were in the 70% range, which was treated with an Albuteral nebulizer. He was discharged home on Zithromax. His symptoms abated until 2 days ago when the shortness of breath worsened and he developed "chest discomfort" that he describes as an "8" on a scale of 1 to 10. The pain is sharp and stabbing, which is different from the chest pain he experienced prior to having a coronary stent placement in the past.

At present, he has a one- to two-word dyspnea and has had minimal oral intake for the past 24 hours. He has a right lateral foot ulcer that "has been there for months." The ulcer does give him pain but it improves when he dangles his foot. He denies fever, chills, change in cough, increase in sputum production, or change in sputum consistency. He smokes one pack of cigarettes per day with a 49-pack-year history. He denies recreational drug use but drinks several cups of caffeinated coffee daily. He does not exercise and has a poor sleep pattern of 4 to 6 hours of interrupted sleep nightly. He is single with no family support. He has a technical degree and worked as a mechanic until he was disabled with lung disease. He was exposed to Agent Orange during the war.

His past medical history includes the comorbidities of chronic obstructive pulmonary disease, for which he has had several hospitalizations over the past 5 years for exacerbations of symptoms, coronary artery disease with stent placement, hypertension, hyperlipidemia, and depression. He has a history of alcohol abuse with delirium tremens but has not taken a drink in 20 years. The current peripheral vascular disease related to the foot ulcer is going to be treated with vascular surgery in 1 month.

Current medications include Albuteral nebulizer treatments, Symbicort, tiotropium, theophylline, and prednisone. He also takes one 81-mg aspirin per day. His influenza vaccination is up to date but he has never had the pneumococcal or herpes zoster vaccine.

The physical examination reveals a height of 5' 10", weight of 64.04 kg, body mass index (BMI) of 20.3, blood pressure of 89/47 mmHg, heart rate of 118 beats per minute, temperature of 99.8°F, and a respiratory rate of 24 breaths per minute. His oxygen saturation is 100% on 4 L BiPAP (bilevel positive airway pressure), and the arterial blood gases show a pH of 7.467, pO_2 of 124.8 mmHg, pCO_2 of 33.5 mmHg, base excess of 0.7 mEq/L, and HCO_3 of 24.2 mEq/L.

Other laboratory values are as follows—white blood count: $14.2/mm^3$, hemoglobin: 11.3 g/dL, hematocrit: 34.2%, mean corpuscular volume: 93.4 mcm^3, platelet count: $151/mm^3$, neutrophils: 82%, lymphocytes: 3%, monocytes: 13%, complete metabolic panel within normal limits, and cardiac enzymes negative. The electrocardiogram shows sinus tachycardia and the chest x-ray reveals hyperinflated lung fields with a possible right lower lobe infiltrate.

PATIENT-CENTERED PLAN OF CARE USING OPT WORKSHEETS

Once the story is obtained from all possible sources, care planning and reasoning proceed using the OPT clinical reasoning web worksheet (Figure 9.1), which helps determine relationships among issues and highlights potential keystone issues. The OPT clinical reasoning web is a graphic representation of the functional relationships between and among diagnostic hypotheses derived from the analysis and synthesis regarding how each element of the story and issues relate to one another. This activates critical and creative thinking. The visual diagram that results illustrates dynamics among issues and a convergence helps to point out central issues that require nursing care. As one thinks about this case, and begins to spin and weave a clinical reasoning web, relationships are identified among nursing domains and diagnoses as they are jointly considered with medical conditions. The medical conditions in this case are history of chronic obstructive pulmonary disease, coronary artery disease, hypertension, hyperlipidemia, history of alcohol abuse, depression, and peripheral vascular disease. Once the advanced practice nurse considers these diagnoses, the nursing care domains associated with them are identified. The complementary nursing diagnoses most impacted in this case are ineffective breathing pattern and impaired gas exchange.

To spin and weave the web, the provider uses thinking processes to analyze and synthesize relationships among diagnostic hypotheses associated with a patient's health status. The visual representation and mapping of these relationships support the development of systems thinking and making connections between and among the medical and nursing diagnoses under consideration given the patient story.

The steps to the creation of the OPT clinical reasoning web using the worksheet are as follows:

1. Place a general description of the patient in the respective middle circle—64-year-old Vietnam veteran exposed to Agent Orange in the war.
2. Place the major medical diagnoses in the respective middle circle—chronic obstructive pulmonary disease, respiratory alkalosis, coronary artery disease, and peripheral artery disease.
3. Place the major nursing diagnoses in the respective middle circle—ineffective breathing pattern and impaired gas exchange.
4. Choose the nursing domains for which each medical and nursing diagnosis is appropriate—health promotion, nutrition, elimination and exchange, activity/

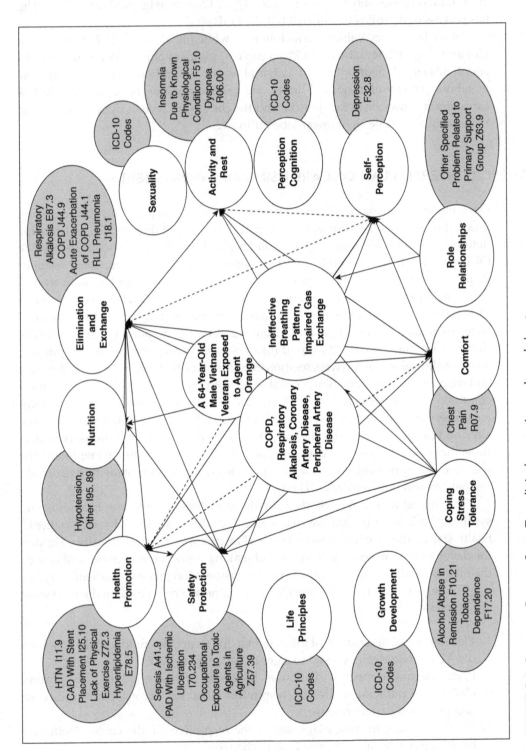

FIGURE 9.1 Outcome-Present State-Test clinical reasoning web worksheet.

CAD, coronary artery disease; COPD, chronic obstructive pulmonary disease; HTN, hypertension; ICD-10, International Classification of Diseases, 10th edition; PAD, peripheral artery disease; RLL, right lower lobe.

rest, self-promotion, role relationships, comfort, coping/stress tolerance, and safety/protection.

5. Generate all the International Classification of Diseases (ICD)-10 codes that are appropriate for the particular patient story that coincide with the nursing domains— respiratory alkalosis (E87.3), chronic obstructive pulmonary disease (J44.9), acute exacerbation of chronic obstructive pulmonary disease (J44.1), right lower lobe pneumonia (J18.1), sepsis (A41.9), peripheral artery disease with ischemic ulceration (I70.234), occupational exposure to toxic agents in agriculture (Z57.39), chest pain (R07.9), depression (F32.8), hypertension (I11.9), coronary artery disease with stent placement (I25.10), lack of exercise (Z72.3), hyperlipidemia (E78.5), alcohol abuse in remission (F10.21), tobacco dependence (F17.20), dyspnea (R06.00), insomnia caused by known psychological condition (F51.0), hypotension (I95.89), and other specified problem related to primary support group (Z63.9).

6. Once the nursing domains, diagnoses, and ICD-10 codes are identified, reflect on the total web worksheet and concurrently consider and explain how each of the issues is or is not related to the other issues. Draw lines of relationship to spin and weave the web connections or associations among the ICD-10 codes/diagnoses. As you draws the lines, think out loud, justify the reasons for the connections, and explain specifically how the diagnoses may or may not be connected or related.

7. After you have spent some time connecting the relationships, determine which domain/domains have the highest priority for care coordination and most efficiently and effectively represent the keystone nursing care needs of the patient by counting the arrows that connect the medical problems (ICD-10 codes). In this case, counting nine lines (Table 9.1) pointing to or from the nursing domain of elimination and exchange represents the priority present-state keystone issues.

8. Look once again at the sets of relationships and determine the theme or keystone that summarizes the patient-in-context or the patient story—the problems related to elimination and exchange from acute exacerbation of COPD and right lower lobe pneumonia are the keystone issues for this case.

The OPT clinical reasoning web worksheet in Figure 9.1 shows a template with the patient health care situation, medical diagnoses, and nursing diagnoses at the center. Around the outer edges of the web are nursing domains with ICD-10 codes derived from history and physical assessment associated with the patient story. The directional arrows create the web effect and represent connections, explanations, and functional relationships between and among the diagnostic possibilities. As one can see, the domains and ICD-10 codes with more connections converging on one of the circles display the priority problem or keystones, in this case elimination and exchange. A keystone issue is one or more central supporting elements of the patient's story that help focus and determine a root cause or center of gravity of the system dynamics and help guide reasoning and care coordination based on an analysis (breaking things down into discrete parts) and synthesis (putting the parts together in a greater whole) of diagnostic possibilities as represented in the web. A key question to ask here is: How does the clinical reasoning web reveal relationships between and among the identified diagnoses and to what degree do these relationships make practical clinical sense according to the evidence and patient story? Table 9.1 shows a summary of the connections highlighting the priority with the most connections.

TABLE 9.1 Relationships Among Nursing Domains, Medical Diagnoses, and Web Connections

NURSING DOMAINS	MEDICAL DIAGNOSES (ICD-10 CODES)	WEB CONNECTIONS
Elimination and exchange	Respiratory alkalosis E87.3 COPD J44.9 Acute exacerbation of COPD J44.1 Right lower lobe pneumonia J18.1	9
Safety and protection	Sepsis A41.9 Peripheral artery disease with ischemic ulceration I70.234 Occupational exposure to toxic agents in agriculture Z57.39	7
Comfort	Chest pain R07.9	7
Self-perception	Depression F32.8	7
Health promotion	Hypertension I11.9 Coronary artery disease with stent placement I25.10 Lack of physical exercise Z72.3 Hyperlipidemia E78.5	7
Coping/stress tolerance	Alcohol abuse in remission F10.21 Tobacco dependence F17.20	6
Activity/rest	Dyspnea R06.00 Insomnia due to known physiological condition F51.0	5
Nutrition	Hypotension I95.89	3
Role relationships	Other specified problems related to primary support Z63.9	2

COPD, chronic obstructive pulmonary disease.

Source: World Health Organization (2015).

After considering the full picture using the clinical reasoning web worksheet, the next step is to use the OPT clinical reasoning model worksheet to facilitate and structure the individual patient-centered systems thinking about the care coordination of the identified problems highlighted in Table 9.1. As the advanced practice nurse thinks about the patient, she or he will concurrently consider the frame, outcome state, and present state. Each aspect of the OPT clinical reasoning model contributes to the other. The OPT clinical reasoning model worksheet is a map of the structure designed to provide an illustrative representation and to guide thinking processes about relationships between and among competing issues and problems.

Some questions that guide the use of the OPT clinical reasoning model are shown in Table 9.2 (Pesut, 2008).

TABLE 9.2 Questions That Guide the Use of the OPT Model

Patient-in-context	What is the patient story?
Diagnostic cue/ web logic	What diagnoses have you generated?
	What outcomes do you have in mind given the diagnoses?
	What evidence supports those diagnoses?
	How does a reasoning web reveal relationships among the identified problems (diagnoses)?
	What keystone issue(s) emerge?
Framing	How are you framing the situation?
Present state	How is the present state defined?
Outcome state	What are the desired outcomes?
	What are the gaps or complementary pairs (~) of outcomes and present states?
Test	What are the clinical indicators of the desired outcomes?
	On what scales will the desired outcomes be rated?
	How will you know when the desired outcomes are achieved?
	How are you defining your testing in this particular case?
Decision making (interventions)	What clinical decisions or interventions help to achieve the outcomes?
	What specific intervention activities will you implement?
	Why are you considering these activities?
Judgment	Given your testing, what is your clinical judgment?
	Based on your judgment, have you achieved the outcome or do you need to reframe the situation?
	How, specifically, will you take this experience and learning with you into the future as you reason about similar cases?

OPT, Outcome-Present State-Test.
Adapted from Pesut (2008).

By writing each element on the worksheet, all the parts of the model become related to each other. As the health care provider moves from right to left, the model structures the plan of care. Critical thinking skills are used to consider the patient story, and creative thinking is used to identify and reason about the keystone issues/themes/cues to determine the most significant evidence in the present state. Complexity thinking helps the provider to consider the outcomes desired and the gaps between the present and outcomes states. Once interventions and tests are decided, the plan of care transitions over to a care coordination model and team-centered systems thinking that consider patient preferences within the frame of the situation.

The patient-in-context story (Exhibit 9.1) is on the far right-hand side, as depicted in Figure 9.2. The advanced practice nurse notes relevant facts of the story, which in this case include the patient demographics and characteristics: 64-year-old Vietnam veteran male who lives alone and without social support. He has diagnoses of chronic obstructive pulmonary disease, coronary artery disease, nicotine dependence, alcohol abuse in remission, peripheral artery disease, and exposure to Agent Orange in the war. He currently has right lower lobe pneumonia complicated by

EXHIBIT 9.1 PATIENT-IN-CONTEXT STORY

Ralph Wiseman is a 64-year-old male Vietnam veteran with increasing shortness of breath for 2 days. Recent emergency department visit via ambulance resulted in treatment with Zithromax and symptoms improved.

Starting 2 days ago, the dyspnea recurred and he currently has respiratory alkalosis requiring BiPAP. Other treatments include intravenous fluid bolus for hypotension and intravenous broad spectrum antibiotics. Oral steroids were added for acute exacerbation of chronic pulmonary disease and sepsis.

BP: 89/47 mmHg, O$_2$ sat: 100%, Temperature: 99.8°F, WBC: 14.2 mm^3, CXR: right lower lobe infiltrate

BiPAP, bilevel positive airway pressure; BP, blood pressure; CXR, chest x-ray; O$_2$ sat, oxygen saturation; WBC, white blood cell.

sepsis and respiratory alkalosis. His initial treatment with Zithromax was not long standing. Respiratory distress reoccurs as well as sepsis, which requires intravenous fluids and antibiotics. Oral steroids are used to treat airway inflammation from the infection and aggravation of the chronic obstructive pulmonary disease. The peripheral ulcer is also considered a source of the sepsis. His continued respiratory infection has placed him in the caseload of the veteran's clinic nurse practitioner, who is to assist him in adhering to the therapeutic regimen to promote pulmonary health. Significant laboratory data show hypotension and oxygen dependency caused by chronic obstructive pulmonary disease and respiratory infection in the right lower lobe. A key point at this juncture is to review and reflect on the patient story for accuracy and thoroughness to be able to proceed with care planning for care coordination.

Moving to the left of the worksheet, there is a place to list the diagnostic cluster cues on the web of medical diagnoses and ICD-10 codes (Exhibit 9.2). At the bottom of this box are placed the designated keystone issues or themes that fall under the most significant nursing domain—chronic obstructive pulmonary disease J44.9 and right lower lobe pneumonia J18.1. Remember diagnostic cluster cue web logic is the use of inductive and deductive thinking skills. Some key questions to ask here are: What diagnoses were generated? Is there evidence to support those diagnoses? Is the keystone issue appropriate given this patient story?

At the center and background of the worksheet are places to indicate the frame or theme that best represents the background issues regarding thinking about the patient story (Exhibit 9.3). The frame of this case is a 64-year-old Vietnam veteran who presents to the emergency department with dyspnea and shortness of breath. This frame helps one to organize the present state, outcome state, illustrates the gaps, and provides insights about what tests need to be considered to fill the gap. Decision making and reflection surround the framing as the advanced practice nurse thinks of many things simultaneously. Reflective thinking is used to monitor thinking and behavior. Key questions to ask here are How am I framing the situation and does it agree with the patient view of the situation? Given my disciplinary perspectives, what are the results I want to create for this person?

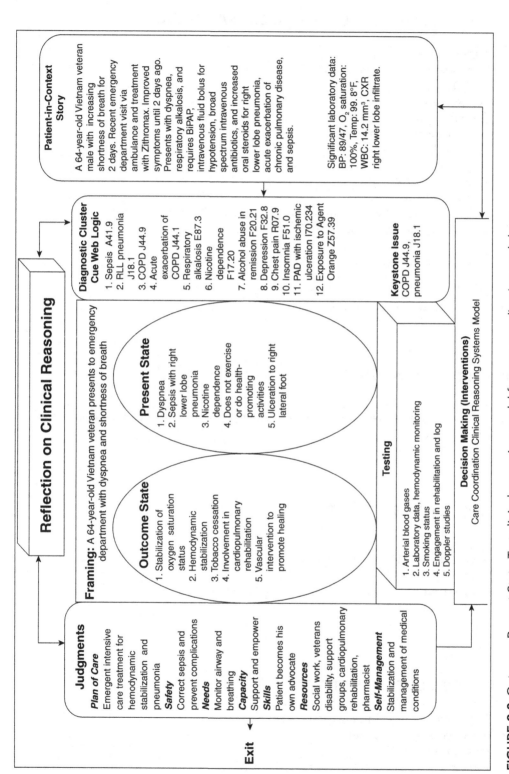

FIGURE 9.2 Outcome-Present State-Test clinical reasoning model for care coordination worksheet.

BiPAP, bilevel positive airway pressure; BP, blood pressure; COPD, chronic obstructive pulmonary disease; CXR, chest x-ray; O₂ sat, oxygen saturation; PAD, peripheral artery disease; RLL, right lower lobe; WBC, white blood cell.

EXHIBIT 9.2 DIAGNOSTIC CLUSTER CUE WEB LOGIC

1. Sepsis A41.9
2. Right lower lobe pneumonia J18.1
3. COPD J44.9
4. Acute exacerbation of COPD J44.1
5. Respiratory alkalosis E87.3
6. Nicotine dependence F17.20
7. Alcohol abuse in remission F20.21
8. Depression F32.8
9. Chest pain R07.9
10. Insomnia F51.0
11. Peripheral artery disease with ischemic ulceration I70.234
12. Exposure to Agent Orange Z57.39

KEYSTONE ISSUE/THEME

COPD J44.9 with pneumonia J18.1

COPD, chronic obstructive pulmonary disease.

EXHIBIT 9.3 FRAMING

A 64-year-old Vietnam veteran presents to emergency department with dyspnea and shortness of breath.

EXHIBIT 9.4 PRESENT STATE

1. Dyspnea
2. Sepsis with right lower lobe pneumonia
3. Nicotine dependence
4. Does not exercise or do health-promoting activities
5. Ulceration to right lateral foot

EXHIBIT 9.5 OUTCOME STATE

1. Stabilization of oxygen saturation status
2. Hemodynamic stabilization
3. Tobacco cessation
4. Involvement in cardiopulmonary rehabilitation
5. Vascular intervention to promote healing

EXHIBIT 9.6 TESTING

1. Arterial blood gases
2. Laboratory data, hemodynamic monitoring
3. Smoking status
4. Engagement in rehabilitation and log
5. Doppler studies

EXHIBIT 9.7 REFLECTION ON CLINICAL REASONING

What clinical decisions or interventions help to achieve the outcomes?

What specific intervention activities will you implement?

Why are you considering these activities?

At the center of the sheet are spaces to place the present state (Exhibit 9.4) and out-come state (Exhibit 9.5) side by side. The present state in this case shows five primary health care problems related to the keystone issue: dyspnea, sepsis with right lower lobe pneumonia, nicotine dependence, does not exercise or do health-promoting activities, and ulceration to right lateral foot. The outcome state shows five matching goals to be achieved through care coordination: stabilization of oxygen saturation status, hemody-namic stabilization, tobacco cessation, involvement in cardiopulmonary rehabilitation, and vascular intervention to promote health of the foot ulcer. Putting the two states together creates a gap analysis that naturally shows where the patient is and what the goals are in terms of the patient's care. Some key questions to ask here are: Are the out-comes appropriate given the diagnoses? Are there gaps between the outcomes and the present state? Are there clinical indicators of the desired outcome state?

The gap between where the patient is and where the advanced practice nurse wants the patient to be is one way to create a test (Exhibit 9.6). Clinical decisions are choices made about interventions that will help the patient transition from the pres-ent state to a desired outcome state. As interventions are tested, the advanced prac-tice nurse evaluates the degree to which outcomes are or are not being achieved. The tests chosen in this case include arterial blood gases, laboratory tests, hemody-namic monitoring, smoking status, rehabilitation log, and Doppler studies.

Testing is concurrent and iterative as one gets closer and closer in successive increments toward goal achievement. Some key questions to ask here are: How is the advanced practice nurse defining *testing*? On what scales will the desired out-come be rated? How will the advanced practice nurse know when the desired tar-geted outcomes are achieved?

The reflection box at the top of Figure 9.2 (Exhibit 9.7) reminds the advanced practice nurse of the thinking strategies used for the patient situation. These strate-gies also help make explicit many of the relationships among ideas and issues asso-ciated with the patient problems. Examples of reflection questions that support and engage patient-centered systems thinking are listed in Table 9.3.

TABLE 9.3 Patient-Centered Systems-Thinking Reflection Questions

SELF-REGULATION ACTIVITIES	REFLECTION QUESTIONS

Monitoring thinking	I. **Reflect on the thinking processes you used with the care coordination of this case.**
	
	1. The baseline needs I identify in this case are.... I think I can identify future adjustments in the plan of care by.... If I have difficulty, I...
	
	2. When I think about my feelings during the care coordination of this case, I describe them as...and I handle them by...
	
	3. When I try to remember or understand important facts to develop the plan of care, coach, and educate the patient/family, I...
	
	4. As I look back on meaningful activities, the resources I could have spent:
	   a. More time on...
	   b. Less time on...

Monitoring the environment	II. **Reflect on the environmental circumstances you encountered in the care coordination of this case.** 5. When I prepare to carry out coaching and education activities for care coordination, I... 6. When I think about particular distractions to facilitating medical care services and supports for care coordination, I... 7. When I work and communicate with interprofessional partners for care coordination of this case, I... 8. If I had the chance to redo the care coordination activities, I would do...instead of...because ...

Monitoring behavior	III. **Reflect on your behaviors and reactions to the care coordination of this case.**
	
	9. My impression of my performance in evaluating capacity, energy, support, readiness, and skills to organize and manage the plan of care, is...
	
	10. I make sure I will update the needs assessment and individualized plan of care by...and if I need to make changes, I...
	
	11. I make sure I empower the patient/family for self-management of health care needs by...and if I need to make changes, I...
	
	12. Reaction to care coordination of this case...
	   a. My reaction to what I like about the care coordination of this case...
	   b. My reaction to what I do not like about the care coordination of this case...
	
	Optional prompt: Other comments I have about the care coordination of this case...

Adapted from Kuiper, Pesut, and Kautz (2009).

Finally, the judgment space on the far left-hand side of the model (Exhibit 9.8) is the place to write in the results of the conclusions drawn from the CCCR model. Based on the degree of gap or comparison of where the patient is, and where the health care team wants the patient to be, there may or may not be an evidence gap. Once there is evidence that fills that gap, the nurse has to attribute meaning to the

EXHIBIT 9.8 JUDGMENTS RELATED TO CARE COORDINATION VARIABLES

PLAN OF CARE

Emergent intensive care treatment for hemodynamic stabilization

SAFETY

Resolve sepsis and prevent complications

NEEDS

Monitor airway

CAPACITY

Support patient and empower

SKILLS

Patient becomes his own advocate

RESOURCES

Social work, veteran's disability, support groups, cardiopulmonary rehabilitation, and pharmacist

SELF-MANAGEMENT

Stabilization and management of medical conditions

data. Making judgments about clinical issues is about the meaning the advanced practice nurse attributes to the evidence derived from the test or gap analysis of present to desired state. Complexity thinking, team-centered systems-thinking, and organization-centered systems-thinking skills are used by the care coordination team at this point to evaluate and judge the successes or deficits from the plan of care. Interprofessional team activity requires negotiation of the competing values of collaboration—creating, competing, and controlling—and involves managing shared knowledge; acknowledgment of values impacted; and the brokering, directing, coordinating, and monitoring of practice issues, interventions, and outcomes. The judgments made in this case are made by the team after the care coordination essential need outcomes are evaluated. Each of the items in the judgment column corresponds to an essential need addressed in the CCCR systems model (Figure 9.3). Some key questions to ask here are: Given the testing, what are the clinical judgments? Have the outcomes been achieved? Does the situation need to be reframed?

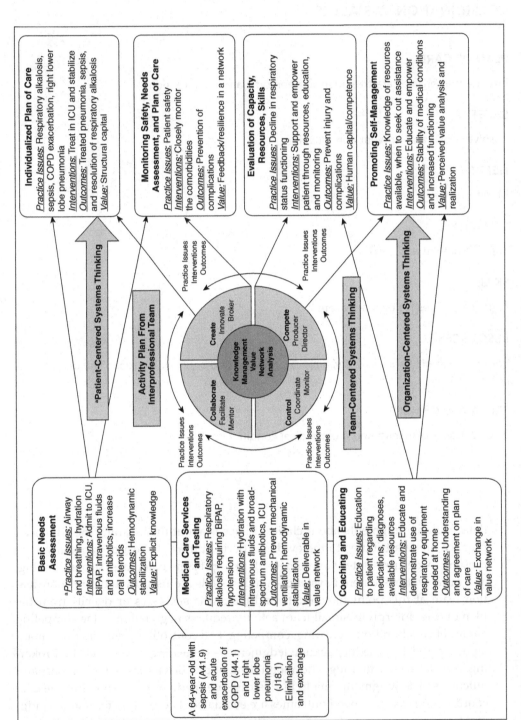

FIGURE 9.3 Care Coordination Clinical Reasoning systems model worksheet.

[a] Practice Issues can come from any discipline; nursing, medicine, pharmacy, social work, and so on.

BiPAP, bilevel positive airway pressure; COPD, chronic obstructive pulmonary disease; ICU, intensive care unit.

Once the advanced practice nurse has experience coordinating care for military patients, the cases become part of a clinical reasoning learning history, which become prototypes or schemas for other similar cases. These schemas and experience build on each other over time and result in the development of pattern recognition for future clinical reasoning applications. If the scenario results in a negative judgment or progress is not being made to transition patients from present to desired states, the advanced practice nurse may have to reframe the situation, reconsider the keystone priority, reconsider the care coordination activities, and/or consult with members of the interprofessional team for the problem to be solved and the outcome to be achieved. The key question to ask here is: How will this clinical learning experience impact future reasoning about similar cases?

CARE COORDINATION USING CCCR MODEL WORKSHEETS

The next step in the nursing diagnostic reasoning process is to augment the plan of care to include activities related to interprofessional care planning using the CCCR systems model framework (Exhibit 9.9), which builds on the OPT model of clinical reasoning. The systems dynamics and interactions between and among the patient issues determine the care needed and the services provided. The complexities in this case are the issues related to his lack of social support, veteran's status and comorbidities in his health status. The CCCR systems model web (Figure 9.4) visually represents the complexities in this case along with the essential care coordination practice issues that need attention to organize thinking that focuses on the patient's priority needs.

The CCCR systems model web (Exhibit 9.10) provides a blueprint for consideration of the care coordination practice issues so that clinicians can determine interventions, outcomes, and the value exchange that supports safe, high-quality care. This process involves patient-centered systems thinking, team-centered systems thinking, and organization-centered systems thinking to thoroughly and efficiently manage all aspects of patient cases. The steps to create the web for this case start at the center with the patient description and medical diagnoses (Ralph Wiseman, a 64-year-old male Vietnam veteran with chronic obstructive pulmonary disease, pneumonia, and sepsis), priority nursing domain (elimination and exchange), and ICD-10 codes (acute exacerbation of chronic obstructive pulmonary disease J44.1

EXHIBIT 9.9 CARE COORDINATION CLINICAL REASONING DEFINITION

The authors define *care coordination clinical reasoning* as the application of critical, creative, systems, and complexity thinking to determine the practice issues, interdependencies, and interconnections of role relationships for collaborative work in service of caring for people to address problems, interventions, and outcomes through time and across health care contexts and services.

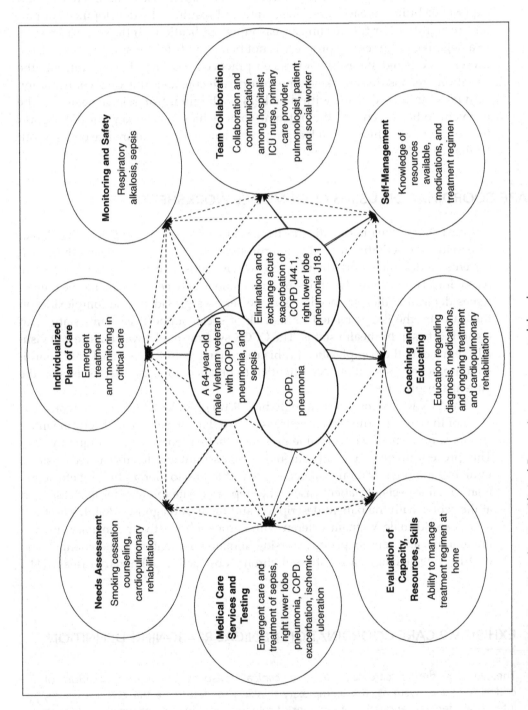

FIGURE 9.4 Care Coordination Clinical Reasoning systems model web.

COPD, chronic obstructive pulmonary disease; ICU, intensive care unit.

EXHIBIT 9.10 CCCR SYSTEMS MODEL WEB DEFINITION

The Care Coordination Clinical Reasoning systems model web enables one to visually represent the complexities and essential care coordination practice issues that need attention so as to organize thinking that focuses on the patient's and/or family's priority needs within the context of services provided within and between health care delivery systems.

and right lower lobe pneumonia J18.1) that show the overlap of patient issues that must be addressed by the advanced practice nurse and the care coordination interprofessional team.

Next, each large circle in this web represents the essential care coordination practice issues with evidence and defining characteristics for this patient story: needs assessment (smoking-cessation counseling and cardiopulmonary rehabilitation); individualized plan of care (emergent treatment and monitoring in critical care); medical care services and testing (emergent care and treatment of sepsis, right lower lobe pneumonia, chronic obstructive pulmonary disease exacerbation, and ischemic ulceration of right foot); evaluation of capacity, resources, and skills (ability to manage treatment regimen at home); monitoring and safety (respiratory alkalosis and sepsis); team collaboration (collaboration and communication among providers—hospitalist, intensive care nurse, primary care provider, pulmonologist, and social worker—and the patient); coaching and educating (education regarding diagnosis, medications, ongoing treatment, and cardiopulmonary rehabilitation); and self-management (knowledge of resources available, medications, and treatment regimen).

The provider then reflects on the total picture on the worksheet and begins to draw lines of relationship, connection, or association among the essential needs. As directional lines are drawn to create the web, functional relationships between and among the needs are recognized. Clinical reasoning and thinking processes are used to explain and justify the reasons for connecting these care coordination needs as central supporting elements in the patient's story based on an analysis and synthesis of possible priorities as represented in the web. The priority care coordination needs that would most efficiently and effectively represent the key issues of the patient are addressed that align with the patient story. A key question to ask is: Does the CCCR systems model web provide a comprehensive consideration of the most pertinent evidence for care coordination practice issues?

The CCCR systems model worksheet (see Figure 9.3) is the next worksheet in the framework designed to provide a graphic representation or visual map of the structure of the CCCR systems model and to help guide team-centered and organization-centered systems thinking. Some key questions to ask here are: What clinical decisions and interventions will help to achieve the outcomes identified on the

OPT model of clinical reasoning (see Figure 9.2)? What specific interventions will the clinicians and members of the team implement? Why are providers considering these activities?

Writing each element on the worksheet shows how parts of the model relate to each other. In Figure 9.3, on the far left-hand side, there is space to write the description of the patient's health care situation that was at the center of the CCCR systems model web. Three essential needs are placed in the first boxes to the right of the description and include basic needs assessment, medical care services and testing, and coaching and education. Each of the care coordination needs identified in this model includes practice issues, interventions, outcomes, and value specification.

From patient-centered systems-thinking processes used to create the OPT clinical reasoning model worksheets for this patient story, the identified basic needs practice issues include airway, breathing, and hydration. Targeted interventions for the team would be to admit to the intensive care unit, BiPAP, intravenous fluids, and intravenous antibiotics. The documented desired outcomes would be hemodynamic stabilization. A key question to ask is: Have the basic needs been identified given the frame of the situation? Consider the value-impact analysis in this case using the questions from Table 9.4.

KNOWLEDGE MANAGEMENT AND VALUE ANALYSIS

The explicit value for role clarity, collaboration, and interaction of the team placed on the needs assessment is explicit knowledge. From Table 9.4, the value-networking reflection question for basic needs is: What knowledge is codified and conveyed to others through dialogue, demonstration, or media? Name three knowledge classification systems that could be used to represent the patient characteristics in this case:

1.
2.
3.

From team-centered systems-thinking processes used for the basic needs assessment, the identified medical care services and testing practice issues include respiratory alkalosis requiring BiPAP and hypotension. Targeted interventions for the team are hydration with intravenous fluids, intravenous broad spectrum antibiotics, and admission to the intensive care unit. The documented desired outcomes are to prevent mechanical ventilation and hemodynamic stabilization. A key question to ask is: Do the testing and interventions sufficiently manage the primary care needs? The explicit value for role clarity, collaboration, and interaction of the team placed on the medical care services and testing is to deliver evidence-based interventions based on the health care provider role. From Table 9.4, the value-networking reflection question for medical care services and testing basic needs is: What is the specific value or object that is conveyed from one role or participant to another role

TABLE 9.4 Value Definitions and Reflection Questions

Deliverable	The specific values or objects that are conveyed from one role or participant to another role or participant.
	What are the deliverables that you offer and expect of others?
Exchange	Two or more transactions between two or more roles or participants that evoke reciprocity. A process in which one role as agent receives resources from another role or agent and provides resources in return.
	What are the resource exchanges between roles or participants on your interprofessional health care team?
Explicit knowledge	The knowledge that is codified and conveyed to others through dialogue, demonstration, or media.
	What is the explicit knowledge shared among members of the team?
Feedback	Feedback is the return of information about the impact of an activity. It can also mean the return of a portion of the output of a process as new input.
	What feedback is returned about activities or outputs in your care coordination activities? How does feedback influence team dynamics and goal attainment?
Human capital/ competence	The knowledge, skills, and competencies that reside in individuals who work in an organization or that are embedded in the organization's internal and external social networks.
	What human capital resources are needed in order for care coordination in your context to be successful?
Impact analysis	An assessment of how an input for a role is handled.
	What are the tangible/intangible costs, gains, or values from the input that generate a response or activity, or increases/decreases tangible assets?
Knowledge management	The degree to which the team facilitates and supports processes for creating, sustaining, sharing, and renewing organizational knowledge in order to generate social or economic gain or improve performance.
	Who is responsible and how is knowledge managed in the care coordination process?
Perceived value	The degree of value participants feel they receive from individual deliverables, which can come from roles, participants, or the network.
	What are the value-added dimensions of individual, collective, team, and organizational networks?
Resilience	The degree to which the network is able to reconfigure to respond to changing conditions and then return to the original form.
	What is the resilience capacity of the team and organization in which you work?
Structural capital	The infrastructure, routines, concepts, models, information systems, work systems, and business processes that support productivity and sustainability.
	To what degree do the structural capital and infrastructure support interprofessional teamwork and care coordination processes?
Systems thinking	An analysis and synthesis of the forces and interrelationships that shape the behavior of systems.
	To what degree do members of the team think about the system dynamics at the patient, group, team, or organizational levels?
Value realization	The degree to which tangible or intangible values turn the input into gains, benefits, capabilities, or assets that contribute to the success of an individual, group, organization, or network (Allee, 2008).
	To what degree do members of the team intentionally negotiate and manage competing values related to collaborating, creating, competing, and or controlling?

Adapted from Allee, Schwabe, and Babb (2015).

or participant? Name three deliverables that are essential for the care coordination success of this case:

1.
2.
3.

Organization-centered systems thinking is used by the team for enhancing coaching and educating the patient. The identified coaching and educating practice issues include educating the patient regarding medications, diagnoses, and available resources. Targeted interventions for the team are to educate and demonstrate the use of respiratory equipment needed at home. The documented desired outcomes are to ensure understanding and agreement on the plan of care. A key question to ask is: Do the content and methods for coaching and teaching match the patient's cognitive abilities and understanding? From Table 9.4, the value-networking reflection question for educating and coaching involves evaluating the transactions between two or more roles or participants when one role as an agent receives resources from another role or agent and provides resources in return. The question would be: What is the exchange of resources and information between the providers and the patient regarding medication and available resources? Name three resources that could be exchanged between the providers and the patient in this case:

1.
2.
3.

The diagram at the center of the worksheet is the activity plan from the interprofessional team (Exhibit 9.11). The team engages in collaborating, creating, competing, and controlling dynamics through communication (Quinn, Bright, Faerman, Thompson, & McGrath, 2014; Quinn, Heynoski, Thomas, & Spreitzer, 2014; Quinn & Quinn, 2015; Quinn & Rohrbough, 1983) to manage essential areas of organizational culture to realize the intangible value exchanges used to develop and manage an activity plan that considers interventions from the individualized plan of care, monitoring processes, evaluation of patient and family capacity with regard to resources and skills, and promotion of self-management. For example, in terms of collaboration, people must understand themselves and communicate honestly and effectively. Individuals mentor and develop others collaboratively and know how to participate and lead teams. Often this knowledge requires encouraging and managing constructive conflict. Competition enhances productivity and profitability. In this domain, vision and goal setting are the path to motivating self and others so that systems can be developed and organized to get results. Creating and promoting the adoption of new ideas or clinical innovations requires attention to judicious use of power and ethics as well as championing new ideas and innovations through negotiating commitments and agreements for implementing and sustaining change. Control contributes to the development of stability and continuity as people work and manage across functions, organize information exchange, measure and monitor performance and quality, and enable compliance.

EXHIBIT 9.11

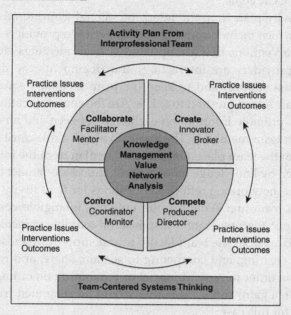

Key questions to consider for the four dimensions of the competing-values framework in the CCCR model are as follows:

- What are the desired outcomes in this case?
- What are the values I expect of myself and others?
- How are the feelings of the patient, family, and team considered in this case?
- What strategies could the team use to coordinate care?

Key ingredients to team-centered systems thinking are that the members must be purpose centered, internally directed, other focused, and externally open to negotiation and communication surrounding competing values (Quinn, 2015; Quinn & Quinn, 2015). The activity plan from the interprofessional team in the CCCR model is guided by these principles and will promote the development of positive organizations and relationships. Each team member should be externally open to challenges, feedback and freedom from labels, higher performance, and the cultivation and development of communities of practice. When this outcome is challenged and false fixed, some team members are valued more than others in the context of competitive versus collaborative goals. Being other influenced cultivates empathy, rapport, energy, and calmness. Together, the team members feel safe and secure enough to take risks and act with trust, integrity, and resilience. Creating such a culture supports a spirit of inquiry, learning, and experimentation resulting in higher performance. Such behavior requires the activation of a reflective self in contrast to automatic self-justification and reactive modes of being and communicating. In order to be a positive influence and bring a state of leadership to the team, each member of the team needs to be vigilant about being purpose centered, choosing goals that create focus, energy, and meaning for the team. A focused, purpose-centered team is likely to attract and create resources related to the reasoning required to communicate across settings to achieve CCCR goals.

The activity plan from the interprofessional team iteratively visits the practice issues, which include communication between providers specific to this case; targeted interventions that are updated at team meetings across the contexts in which the providers are interacting; and documents the desired outcomes to maintain team support and to keep the team members equally informed about patient status. A key question to ask is: Are the communication processes in place and do they promote information exchange between and among the interprofessional health team members? The explicit value for role clarity, collaboration, and interaction of the team placed on the activity plan from the interprofessional team is determined by knowledge management and value-impact analysis. From Table 9.4, the value-networking reflection questions for the activity plan from the interprofessional team are: What are the tangible/intangible costs, gains, or values from the input that generate a response or activity, or increase/decrease tangible assets? How does the team facilitate and support processes for collaborating, controlling, creating, and competing to sustain, share, and renew organizational knowledge in order to generate social or economic gain or improve performance? Name a cost, a gain, and a value that would be generated from the activity plan of the team for this case:

1.
2.
3.

To the far right of the CCCR system model worksheet are four essential care coordination needs that evolve from the activity plan from the interprofessional team stemming from patient-centered systems thinking, team-centered systems thinking, and organization-centered systems thinking. These needs include the individualized plan of care; monitoring safety, needs assessment and plan of care; evaluation of capacity, resources, and skills; and promoting self-management. Each of these care coordination essentials is defined as well by practice issues, interventions, outcomes, and values.

The patient-centered systems-thinking and team-centered systems-thinking activities are used for the individualized plan of care. The identified practice issues revolve around the exacerbation of chronic obstructive pulmonary disease, right lower lobe pneumonia, and respiratory alkalosis. Targeted interventions for the provider and team are to provide intensive care and stabilize the patient hemodynamically. The documented desired outcomes are to treat pneumonia, sepsis, and resolution of respiratory alkalosis. Some key questions to ask are: Does the individualized plan of care include team collaboration? Is there any input that was not yet considered, or are there providers that were overlooked? The explicit value for role clarity, collaboration, and interaction of the provider and team placed on the individualized plan of care is on structural capital. From Table 9.4, the value-networking reflection question for the individualized plan of care is: What are the infrastructure, routines, concepts, models, information systems, work systems, and business processes that support productivity and have sustainability? Name three routines, systems, or processes that support and sustain the productivity of the care coordination in this case:

1.
2.
3.

From the patient-centered systems-thinking and team-centered systems-thinking processes used for monitoring safety, needs assessment, and plan of care, identified practice issues include patient safety. Targeted interventions for the team are to closely monitor the comorbidities. The documented desired outcomes are to prevent complications. A key question to ask is: Does the plan of care promote safety and meet the patient needs? The explicit value for role clarity, collaboration, and interaction of the team placed on monitoring safety, needs assessment, and plan of care is to obtain feedback and assess resilience in the network. From Table 9.4, the value-networking reflection questions for medical care services and testing basic needs are: What feedback is returned about activities or outputs? Was the network able to reconfigure itself to respond to changing conditions and then return to its original form? Name three areas of need and/or safety that were reassessed to determine whether the plan of care needed to be adjusted:

1.
2.
3.

Organization-centered systems-thinking processes, such as coaching and education, are used by the team to evaluate capacity, resources, and skills. The identified practice issues include the identification of the decline in respiratory status functioning. Targeted interventions for the team are to support and empower the patient through resources, education, and monitoring. The documented desired outcomes are to prevent injury and complications from pneumonia and sepsis. A key question to ask is: Do the interventions in the plan of care required skilled help and/or can the patient manage care needs independently? The explicit value for role clarity, collaboration, and interaction of the team placed on evaluating capacity, resources, and skills is identifying human capital and competence. From Table 9.4, the value-networking reflection question for educating and coaching involves evaluating the transactions between two or more roles or participants in which one role as an agent receives resources from another role or agent and provides resources in return. The question would be: What is the exchange of resources and information between the providers and the patient regarding medication and available resources? Name three exchanges of resources, skills, or information with the patient that are essential to the care coordination success of this case:

1.
2.
3.

Organization-centered systems-thinking processes, such as coaching and education, are used by the team to promote self-management. The identified practice issues include knowledge of resources available to the patient. Targeted interventions for the team are to educate and empower the patient. The documented desired outcomes are to have stability of medical conditions and increased functioning for the patient. A key question to ask is: Is the patient able to identify the resources he or she needs and self-manage the health care system? The explicit value for role clarity, collaboration, and interaction of the team placed on promoting self-management is perceived value realization. From Table 9.4, the value-networking reflection question for promoting self-management is: What is the level of value that roles or participants feel they receive from individual deliverables, which can come from roles, participants, or the network? Name three examples of learned self-management that resulted from the care coordination of this case:

1.
2.
3.

With the use of the CCCR systems model, the advanced practice nurse and other providers address practice issues by using and developing evidence-based interventions, implementing measures of adherence, and evaluating processes and outcomes. This requires clinical reasoning at different levels of perspective—the individual patient needs, interprofessional team contributions, and attention to the systems in which people work and provide care. These practice issues, interventions, and outcomes for patient care coordination stem from the National Quality Forum (NQF, 2010a, 2010b) and the Agency for Healthcare Research and Quality (AHRQ, 2014).

As the center of attention for health care needs is managed by webs of relationships between and among providers, each interaction supports a specific value exchange as participant's partner for successful outcomes (Allee, 2003). The dynamic relationships that occurred, for this veteran patient who will return alone to home, among the advanced practice nurse, intensive care nursing staff, physician, social worker, and pulmonologist were collaborative, trusting, dynamic, and interdependent. Application of the competing-value competencies will relate to collaboration, creating, competing, and controlling, and help make explicit knowledge shared and managed to support innovation, coordination, and directing. Through the use of the electronic health record, connectivity impacted the value networking with greater access to knowledge and information. This process provided quick and effective feedback among team members for the complex needs this patient had related to exacerbation of chronic obstructive pulmonary disease and other health problems.

CLINICAL JUDGMENTS AND CCCR

The final phase of the clinical reasoning process is to determine whether outcomes were met and whether care coordination activities were successful. The OPT model of clinical reasoning is revisited for the final phase of care coordination in which judgments are made about achieving outcomes from the interprofessional team activity plan (see Exhibit 9.8). The worksheet (see Figure 9.2) is revisited to make judgments about the care coordination essentials (needs; individualized plan of care; safety; capacity, resources, and skills; and self-management). Shifting to the next level of perspective, using team-centered and organization-centered systems-thinking activities, collaboration, and coordination of the plan of care, reveals ongoing planning and evaluation to provide appropriate patient support during this exacerbation of chronic obstructive pulmonary disease. The goal is to provide a supportive environment with the appropriate resources for this single, male veteran. His sepsis and pneumonia should be treated and discharge planning should include resource personnel to help him manage his chronic illnesses. The patient will need education about smoking, pulmonary medications, ulcer care, coronary artery disease, and the role of rehabilitation. These resources lead to the best possible management and safety for this patient with chronic obstructive pulmonary disease and depression related to life situations. Some remaining questions may arise as the evaluation of outcomes occurs: Can the organizations provide continuing resources and reach care coordination outcomes for this patient? Was communication and the feedback loop effective between the health care providers and the patient? Did the complexity of the system hinder or enhance the achievement of outcomes? How do the competencies of the competing-values framework support the interprofessional dialogue and reasoning about the care coordination of this particular case? How do members of the team share and manage knowledge in service of care coordination? The advanced practice nurse as the care coordinator views all the systems and is the key informant to communicate with the team regarding the efficiency and effectiveness of the processes for care outcomes. Judgments are made about whether the outcomes from case management have been achieved, and the information is recycled back to revise or enhance the plan of care.

The thinking processes used by the advanced practice nurse and other health care providers while implementing the CCCR systems model is promoted through monitoring of thinking, the environment, and behaviors for goal attainment (Zimmerman & Schunk, 2001). The courses of action chosen to manage issues and to ensure that this patient remained safe revolve around behaviors and actions taken, thinking processes used, and environmental structuring. Critical reflective questions that can be used to prompt clinical reasoning to make judgments about the achievement of patient outcomes are listed in Table 9.5. Critical-, creative-, and systems-thinking processes are used for total care coordination, flow from patient-centered (see Table 9.3), team-centered (Table 9.5), and organization-centered systems thinking (Table 9.5) for case management.

TABLE 9.5 Team-Centered and Organization-Centered Systems-Thinking Reflection Questions

SELF-REGULATION ACTIVITIES	REFLECTION QUESTIONS

Monitoring thinking	I. **Reflect on the thinking processes the team used to navigate organizational systems for care coordination of this case.**
	1. The baseline needs identified by the team in this case are.... Adjustments in the plan of care for future successes include.... Difficulties were resolved by...
	2. Team reactions during the care coordination of this case in regard to organizational systems could be described as...and they were handled by...
	3. When the team was dealing with important facts to develop the plan of care, coach, and educate the patient/family about organizational systems, it...
	4. Looking back on meaningful activities, the resources the team could have spent:
	  a. More time on...
	  b. Less time on...

Monitoring the environment	II. **Reflect on the environmental circumstances you encountered in the care coordination of this case.** 5. When the team prepares to carry out coaching and education activities for care coordination, it... 6. When the team considers particular distractions in the organizations that impede medical care services and supports for care coordination, it... 7. When the teamworks and communicates with organizational partners for care coordination of this case, it... 8. If the team had the chance to redo the care coordination activities, it would do...instead of...because ...

Monitoring behavior	III. **Reflect on your behaviors and reactions to the care coordination of this case.**
	9. Impressions of the team performance in evaluating capacity, energy, support, readiness, and skills to organize and manage the plan of care within organizational systems are...
	10. The team ensures that it will update the needs assessment and individualized plan of care by...and if it needs to make changes, it...
	11. The team makes sure it empowers the patient/family to navigate through organizational systems for management of health care needs by...and if it needs to make changes, it...
	12. The team reaction to care coordination of this case...
	  a. Reaction to what it likes about the navigation of organizational systems to facilitate the care coordination of this case...
	  b. Reaction to what it did not like about the navigation of organizational systems to facilitate the care coordination of this case...
	Optional prompt: Other comments about the care coordination of this case...

Adapted from Kuiper, Pesut, and Kautz (2009).

SUMMARY

The clinical reasoning challenge for a veteran's care begins with a description and understanding of the patient's story. The thinking strategies used in this case provided a safe and health-promoting environment for a veteran patient with declining pulmonary health. As the providers practice self-monitoring, self-evaluation, and self-correction, successful strategies are employed, and flaws in thinking are corrected as they collaborate and align interventions for patient success. The OPT clinical reasoning model provides the structure for clinical reasoning and systems thinking within an individual patient situation. The OPT structure and process can be used at several levels for care planning by the provider, by the team, and by the organization to discern alignment and coordination of care activities. The CCCR systems model provides the structure for clinical reasoning for the care coordination essential needs and their related practice issues, interventions, outcomes, and values.

KEY CONCEPTS

1. Clinical reasoning for care coordination with a veteran/military patient with chronic health problems can be promoted with a framework that includes structure, content, and process.
2. A supporting framework for CCCR extends case management using patient-centered systems thinking and the OPT clinical reasoning model across levels of perspective that also include team-centered and organization-centered systems thinking to align care coordination activities.
3. The process of CCCR involves critical reflection for the individual provider and the team.
4. Value-network analysis helps one to define and describe the unique contributions that individual providers make to CCCR efforts supported through knowledge management and value-impact analysis.
5. A supporting framework for CCCR is completed by attending to the organization-centered systems thinking to make judgments about care coordination essentials.

STUDY QUESTIONS AND ACTIVITIES

1. Describe in your own words the benefits and processes of using the CCCR systems model with military care cases.
2. Using the CCCR systems model, identify the care coordination essential needs of cases in military care.
3. To what degree can you explicitly identify and describe the value exchanges associated with care coordination in military care situations?
4. How can an interprofessional team use the competencies of the competing values of collaboration, creating, competing, and controlling to ensure efficiency and effectiveness of care coordination that supports knowledge management

and sharing as well as value-impact analysis and evaluation? How does your team negotiate roles of mentor, broker, director, and coordinator?

5. Identify all the possible standardized health care languages and communication strategies that could be considered in a military care case. Does language impact on communication and the patient outcomes? How does a discipline-specific framework influence the feedback, decisions, and outcomes with military care situations?

6. Identify the relationship between critical reflection and thinking strategies as they are applied to the three levels of system-thinking perspectives that are required—patient centered, team centered, and organization centered. What unique reflections are required to focus on team and organizational function with military care?

REFERENCES

Agency for Healthcare Research and Quality (AHRQ). (2014). *What is care coordination? Care coordination measures atlas update.* Rockville, MD: Author. Retrieved from http://www.ahrq.gov/professionals/prevention-chronic-care/improve/coordination/index.html

Allee, V. (2003). *The future of knowledge: Increasing prosperity through value networks.* Burlington, MA: Butterworth-Heinemann.

Allee, V. (2008). Value network analysis and value conversion of tangible and intangible assets. *Journal of Intellectual Capital, 9*(1), 5–24.

Allee, V., Schwabe, O., & Babb, M. K. (Eds.). (2015). *Value networks and the true nature of collaboration.* Tampa, FL: Megher–Kifer Press ValueNet Works and Verna Allee Associates.

Haas, S. A., Swan, B. A., & Haynes, T. S. (2014). *Care coordination and transition management core curriculum.* Pitman, NJ: American Academy of Ambulatory Care Nursing.

Kuiper, R., Pesut, D., & Kautz, D. (2009). Promoting the self-regulation of clinical reasoning skills in nursing students. *Open Nursing Journal, 3,* 76–85. Retrieved from http://www.ncbi.nlm.nih.gov/pmc/articles/PMC2771264

National Quality Forum (NQF). (2010a). *Preferred practices and performance measures for measuring and reporting care coordination: A consensus report.* Washington, DC: Author.

National Quality Forum (NQF). (2010b). *Quality connections: Care coordination.* Washington, DC: Author.

Pesut, D. J. (2008). Thoughts on thinking with complexity in mind. In C. Lindberg, S. Nash, & C. Lindberg (Eds.), *On the edge: Nursing in the age of complexity* (pp. 211–238). Bordentown, NJ: Plexus Press.

Quinn, R. (2015). *The positive organization: Breaking free from conventional cultures, constraints, and beliefs.* Oakland, CA: Berrett-Koehler.

Quinn, R., & Quinn, R. E. (2015). *Lift: Becoming a positive force in any situation.* San Francisco, CA: Berrett-Koehler.

Quinn, R. E., Bright, D., Faerman, S. R., Thompson, M. P., & McGrath, M. R. (2014). *Becoming a master manager: A competing values approach.* Hoboken, NJ: John Wiley & Sons.

Quinn, R. E., Heynoski, K., Thomas, M., & Spreitzer, G. M. (2014). *The best teacher in you: How to accelerate learning and change lives.* San Francisco, CA: Berrett-Koehler.

Quinn, R. E., & Rohrbough, J. (1983). A spatial model of effectiveness criteria: Towards a competing values approach to organizational analysis. *Management Science, 29,* 363–377.

World Health Organization. (2015). *Manual of the International Classification of Diseases and related health problems* (10th rev. ed.). Geneva, Switzerland: Author. Retrieved from http://www.icd10data.com

Zimmerman, B., & Schunk, D. S. (2001). *Self-regulated learning and academic thought.* Mahwah, NJ: Lawrence Erlbaum.

CHAPTER 10

CARE COORDINATION FOR A PEDIATRIC PATIENT

In this chapter, we use the Care Coordination Clinical Reasoning (CCCR) systems model as described in Part I and explain how the model can be used to reason about a pediatric case. The advanced practice nurse is working with a family that is in need of health and wellness services to promote quality-of-life outcomes in a child who has diabetes. The provider/clinic is the point of access for patients/families. The advanced practice nurse provides care coordination through the application and use of critical-, creative-, systems-, and complexity-thinking processes to manage patient problems with an interprofessional team to design appropriate interventions and establish patient-centered outcomes. Depending on the nature of need involved in the case, referrals to other specialty or primary care providers, community services, and living environments are determined and considered in managing care coordination and transitions (Haas, Swan, & Haynes, 2014).

The CCCR systems model framework begins with the patient story, which is derived from gathering data and evidence from an interview, history, physical examination, and the health record. The advanced practice nurse then develops a patient-centered plan of care using the Outcome-Present State-Test (OPT) model worksheets. In order to do this, one activates the patient-centered systems-thinking skills for complex patient stories and habitually uses key questions to reflect on the specific sections of the model (Pesut, 2008), as well as the dimensions and elements of care coordination.

LEARNING OUTCOMES

After completing this chapter, the reader should be able to:

1. Explain the components of a care coordination framework that are needed to manage the problems, interventions, and outcomes for pediatric patients and their families
2. Describe the different thinking processes that support clinical reasoning skills and strategies for determining priorities in pediatric health care coordination

3. Define the cognitive and metacognitive self-regulatory processes that support individual provider critical reflection related to levels and perspectives associated with clinical reasoning for pediatric care coordination
4. Describe how the communication among interprofessional health care team members is essential for care coordination to address the pediatric patient and family needs
5. Describe the critical meta-reflective processes that support team reflection related to levels and perspectives associated with the care coordination challenges and clinical reasoning required to navigate patient care plans for pediatric patients and their families

THE PATIENT STORY

We begin with the history and story of a 12-year-old White female child, Sally Jones, who presents to the pediatric office with her mother, who states "She seems to be losing weight even though she eats all the time." The mother reports she is concerned about Sally because the teachers at school have been reporting that "she is more irritable and seems to be having a difficult time focusing and asking to go to the restroom frequently." One of the teachers has expressed concern that "she perhaps has attention deficit disorder and may need pharmacological intervention for this." The advanced practice nurse asks the child whether she is sleeping well because she complains of nocturia. Sally's developmental history is described by the mother as "normal" and she has not started menses yet. She is an only child in this family. In school, she is usually on the honor roll and achieves A and B grades for her work. In the past month, this has also changed as she is achieving only Cs and Ds.

During the interview, Sally appears fatigued and has difficulty focusing on the conversation. She is continually drinking water from a bottle and maintains poor eye contact. She is not on any prescribed medications at the time of the interview. Her physical examination reveals her breath has a faint fruity odor and her finger-stick blood sugar is 240 mg/dL. Her vital signs show a heart rate of 100 beats per minute and a respiratory rate of 22 breaths per minute. Her height is 4 feet 11 inches (59 inches), weight is 87 pounds (39.5 kg), and her body mass index (BMI) is 17.5.

The patient is referred to the nearest pediatric intensive care unit and her initial serum laboratory values show glucose 240 mg/dL, sodium 130 mEq/L, chloride 80 mEq/L, and potassium 3.3 mEq/L. Arterial blood gases were drawn and they reveal a pH of 7.19, $PaCO_2$ of 25 mmHg, PaO_2 of 92 mmHg, and an HCO_3 of 10 mEq/L.

PATIENT-CENTERED PLAN OF CARE USING OPT WORKSHEETS

Once the story is obtained from all possible sources, care planning and reasoning proceed using the OPT clinical reasoning web worksheet (Figure 10.1), which helps determine relationships among issues and highlights potential keystone

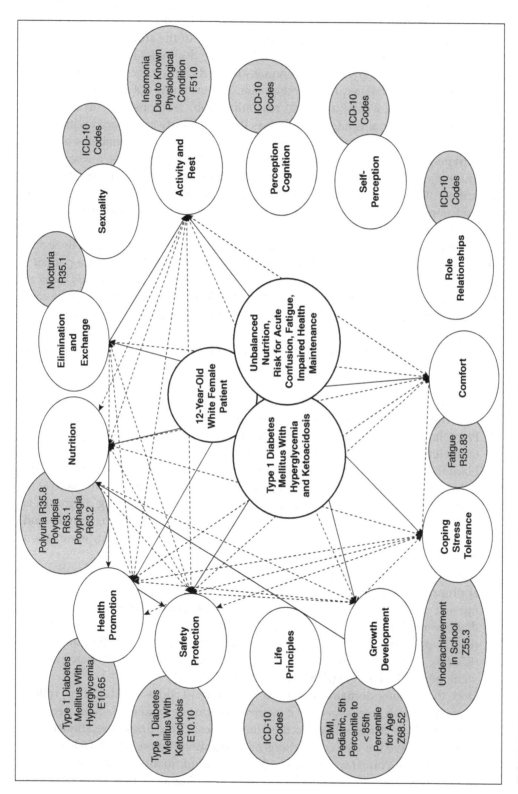

FIGURE 10.1 Outcome-Present State-Test clinical reasoning web worksheet.

BMI, body mass index; ICD-10, International Classification of Diseases, 10th edition.

issues. The OPT clinical reasoning web is a graphic representation of the functional relationships between and among diagnostic hypotheses derived from the analysis and synthesis regarding how each element of the story and issues relate to one another. This activates critical and creative thinking. The visual diagram that results illustrates dynamics among issues and a convergence helps to point out central issues that require nursing care. As one thinks about this case, and begins to spin and weave a clinical reasoning web, relationships are identified among nursing domains and diagnoses as they are jointly considered with medical conditions. The pediatric conditions in this case are type 1 diabetes mellitus with hyperglycemia and ketoacidosis. Once the advanced practice nurse considers these medical diagnoses, the nursing care domains associated with them are identified. The complementary nursing diagnoses most impacted in this case are imbalanced nutrition, risk of acute confusion, fatigue, and ineffective health maintenance.

To spin and weave the web, the provider uses thinking processes to analyze and synthesize relationships among diagnostic hypotheses associated with a patient's health status. The visual representation and mapping of these relationships support the development of patient-centered systems thinking and the ability to make connections between and among the medical and nursing diagnoses under consideration, given the patient story.

The steps to the creation of the OPT clinical reasoning web using the worksheet are as follows:

1. Place a general description of the patient in the respective middle circle—12-year-old White female who is unable to focus on the health interview.
2. Place the major medical diagnoses in the respective middle circle—type 1 diabetes mellitus with hyperglycemia and ketoacidosis.
3. Place the major nursing diagnoses in the respective middle circle—unbalanced nutrition, risk of acute confusion, fatigue, and impaired health maintenance.
4. Choose the nursing domains for which each medical and nursing diagnoses is appropriate—safety and protection, health promotion, nutrition, activity and rest, comfort, coping/stress tolerance, growth and development, elimination and exchange, perception and cognition, and health promotion.
5. Generate all the International Classification of Diseases (ICD)-10 codes that are appropriate for the particular patient and family story that coincide with the nursing domains—type 1 diabetes mellitus with ketoacidosis (E10.10), type 1 diabetes mellitus with hyperglycemia (E10.65), polydipsia (R63.1), polyphagia (R63.2), polyuria (R35.8), insomnia due to physiologic condition (F51.0), fatigue (R53.83), underachievement in school (Z55.3), BMI-pediatric (5th percentile to <85th percentile for age) (Z68.52), and nocturia (R35.1).
6. Once the nursing domains, diagnoses, and ICD-10 codes are identified, reflect on the total web worksheet and concurrently consider and explain how each of the issues is or is not related to the other issues. Draw lines of relationship to spin and weave the web connections or associations among the ICD-10 codes/diagnoses. As you draw the lines, think out loud, justify the reasons for the connections, and explain specifically how the diagnoses may or may not be connected or related.

7. After you have spent some time connecting the relationships, determine which domain/domains have the highest priority for care coordination and most efficiently and effectively represent the keystone nursing care needs of the patient by counting the arrows that connect the medical problems (ICD-10 codes). In this case, counting 11 lines (Table 10.1) pointing to or from the nursing domain of safety protection represents the priority present state keystone issue.

8. Look once again at the sets of relationships and determine the theme or keystone that summarizes the patient-in-context or the patient story—the problems related to type 1 diabetes mellitus and the nursing domains of safety and protection, health promotion, and nutrition are the keystone issues for this case.

The OPT clinical reasoning web worksheet in Figure 10.1 shows a template with the patient health care situation, medical diagnoses, and nursing diagnoses at the center. Around the outer edges of the web are nursing domains with ICD-10 codes derived from history and physical assessment associated with the patient story. The directional arrows that create the web effect represent connections, explanations, and functional relationships between and among the diagnostic possibilities. As one can see, the domains and ICD-10 codes with more connections converging on one of the circles display the priority problem or keystone, in this case safety and protection, health promotion, and nutrition. The keystone issues are one or more central supporting elements of the patient's story that help focus and determine a root cause or center of gravity of the system dynamics and helps guide reasoning and care coordination based on an analysis (breaking things down into discrete parts) and synthesis (putting the parts together in a greater whole) of diagnostic possibilities as represented in the web. A key question to ask here is: How does the clinical reasoning web reveal relationships between and among the identified diagnoses and to what degree do these relationships make practical clinical sense according to the evidence and patient story? Table 10.1 shows a summary of the connections highlighting the priorities with the most connections.

After considering the full picture using the clinical reasoning web worksheet, the next step is to use the OPT clinical reasoning model worksheet to facilitate and structure the patient-centered systems thinking about the care coordination of the identified problems highlighted in Table 10.1. As the advanced practice nurse thinks about the patient, she or he will concurrently consider the frame, outcome state, and present state. Each aspect of the OPT clinical reasoning model contributes to the other. The OPT clinical reasoning model worksheet is a map of the structure designed to provide an illustrative representation and to guide thinking processes about relationships between and among competing issues and problems. Some questions that guide the use of the OPT clinical reasoning model are shown in Table 10.2 (Pesut, 2008).

By writing each element on the worksheet, all the parts of the model become related to each other. As the health care provider moves from right to left, the model structures the plan of care. Critical thinking skills are used to consider the patient story, and creative thinking is used to identify and reason about the keystone issues/themes/cues to determine the most significant evidence in the present state. Complexity thinking helps the provider to consider the outcomes desired and the

TABLE 10.1 Relationships Among Nursing Domains, Medical Diagnoses, and Web Connections

NURSING DOMAINS	MEDICAL DIAGNOSES (ICD-10 CODES)	WEB CONNECTIONS
Safety and protection	Type 1 DM with ketoacidosis E10.10	11
Health promotion	Type 1 DM with hyperglycemia E10.65	10
Nutrition	Polydipsia R63.1 Polyphagia R 63.2 Polyuria R 35.8	10
Activity and rest	Insomnia due to known physiological condition F51.0	8
Comfort	Fatigue R53.83	7
Growth and development	BMI, pediatrics, 5th percentile to < 85th percentile for age Z68.52	7
Coping and stress tolerance	Underachievement in school Z55.3	6
Elimination and exchange	Nocturia R35.1	6

BMI, body mass index; DM, diabetes mellitus.

Source: World Health Organization (2015).

gaps between the present and outcomes states. Once interventions and tests are decided, the plan of care transitions over to a care coordination model and team-centered systems thinking that consider patient and family preferences within the frame of the situation.

The patient-in-context story (Exhibit 10.1) is depicted in Figure 10.2 on the far right-hand side. The advanced practice nurse notes relevant facts of the story, which in this case include the patient demographics and characteristics; sick child brought into the office by her mother for concerns of decline in school function and weight loss. Her teachers report concerns of a possible attention deficit disorder as grades have significantly dropped. The child reports fatigue, nocturia causing insomnia, polyuria, polydipsia, and polyphagia. Menses has not begun. The BMI calculation shows she is below the percentile for her age.

A key point at this juncture is to review and reflect on the patient story for accuracy and thoroughness to be able to proceed with care planning for care coordination.

Moving to the left, there is a place to list the diagnostic cluster cues on the web of medical diagnoses and ICD-10 codes (Exhibit 10.2). At the bottom of this box is placed the designated keystone issues or themes that fall under the most significant nursing domain—type 1 diabetes mellitus with hyperglycemia E10.65 and keto-acidosis E10.10. Remember diagnostic cluster cue web logic is the use of inductive and deductive thinking skills. Some key questions to ask here are: What diagnoses were generated? Is there evidence to support those diagnoses? Is the keystone issue appropriate given this patient story?

TABLE 10.2 Questions That Guide the Use of the OPT Model

Patient-in-context	What is the patient story?
Diagnostic cue/web logic	What diagnoses have you generated?
	What outcomes do you have in mind given the diagnoses?
	What evidence supports those diagnoses?
	How does a reasoning web reveal relationships among the identified problems (diagnoses)?
	What keystone issue(s) emerge?
Framing	How are you framing the situation?
Present state	How is the present state defined?
Outcome state	What are the desired outcomes?
	What are the gaps or complementary pairs (~) of outcomes and present states?
Test	What are the clinical indicators of the desired outcomes?
	On what scales will the desired outcomes be rated?
	How will you know when the desired outcomes are achieved?
	How are you defining your testing in this particular case?
Decision making (interventions)	What clinical decisions or interventions help to achieve the outcomes?
	What specific intervention activities will you implement?
	Why are you considering these activities?
Judgment	Given your testing, what is your clinical judgment?
	Based on your judgment, have you achieved the outcome or do you need to reframe the situation?
	How, specifically, will you take this experience and learning with you into the future as you reason about similar cases?

OPT, Outcome-Present State-Test.
Adapted from Pesut (2008).

EXHIBIT 10.1 PATIENT-IN-CONTEXT STORY

Sally Jones is a 12-year-old White female who comes to the office with her mother for a sick-child visit. There are concerns of a decline in functioning at school and weight loss.

Teachers report concerns of possible attention deficit disorder; grades decreased significantly

Child reports fatigue, nocturia causing insomnia, polyuria, polydipsia, polyphagia. Menses has not begun

Ht: 4' 11" (59 in.), Wt: 87 lb. (39.5 kg), BMI: 17.5

Admitted to the pediatric intensive care unit at the nearby hospital. Initial laboratory tests performed

BMI, body mass index; Ht, height; Wt, weight.

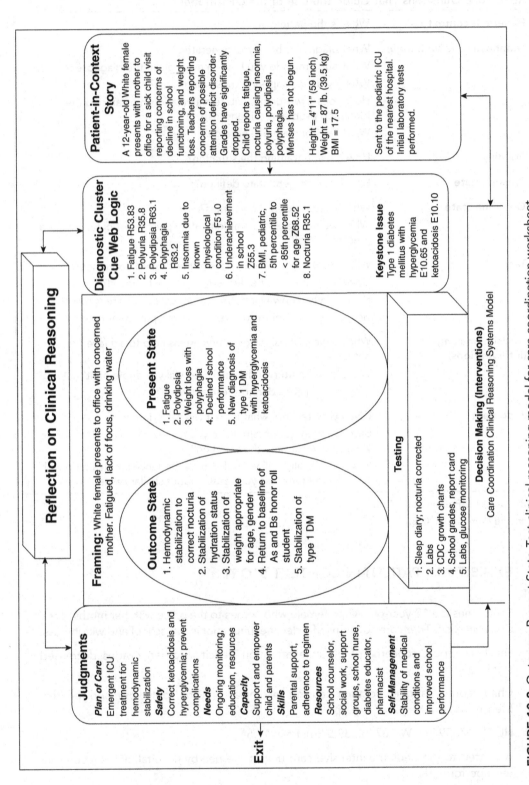

FIGURE 10.2 Outcome-Present State-Test clinical reasoning model for care coordination worksheet.

BMI, body mass index; CDC, Centers for Disease Control and Prevention; DM, diabetes mellitus; ICU, intensive care unit.

EXHIBIT 10.2 DIAGNOSTIC CLUSTER CUE WEB LOGIC

1. Fatigue R53.83
2. Polyuria R35.8
3. Polydipsia R63.1
4. Polyphagia R63.2
5. Insomnia due to known physiologic condition F51.0
6. Underachievement in school Z55.3
7. BMI-pediatric (5th percentile to <85th percentile for age) Z68.52
8. Nocturia R35.1

KEYSTONE ISSUE/THEME

1. Type 1 diabetes mellitus with hyperglycemia E10.65
2. Type 1 diabetes mellitus with ketoacidosis E10.10

EXHIBIT 10.3 FRAMING

White female child presents to the office with a concerned mother. Child is fatigued, unable to focus, and drinks a lot of water.

At the center and background of the worksheet are places to indicate the frame or theme that best represents the background issues regarding thinking about the patient story (Exhibit 10.3). The frame of this case is a White female child who presents to the office with her concerned mother. Child is fatigued, unable to focus, and drinks a lot of water. This frame (White female child with physiologic health and cognitive issues) helps one to organize the present state, outcome state, illustrates the gaps, and provides insights about what tests need to be considered to fill the gap. Decision making and reflection surround the framing as the advanced practice nurse thinks of many things simultaneously. Reflective thinking is used to monitor thinking and behavior. Some key questions to ask here are: How am I framing the situation and does it agree with the patient's view of the situation? Given my disciplinary perspectives, what are the results I want to create for this person?

At the center of the sheet are spaces to place the present state (Exhibit 10.4) and the outcome state (Exhibit 10.5) side by side. The present state in this case shows six primary health care problems related to the keystone issue: fatigue, polydipsia, weight loss with polyphagia, declined school performance, and new diagnosis of diabetes mellitus with hyperglycemia and ketoacidosis. The outcome state shows six matching goals to be achieved through care coordination: hemodynamic stabilization to correct nocturia, stabilization of hydration status, stabilization of weight appropriate for age and gender, return to baseline of As and Bs as honor roll student, and stabilization of type 1 diabetes mellitus. Putting the two

EXHIBIT 10.4 PRESENT STATE

1. Fatigue
2. Polydipsia
3. Weight loss with polyphagia
4. Declined school performance
5. New diagnosis of diabetes mellitus with hyperglycemia and ketoacidosis

EXHIBIT 10.5 OUTCOME STATE

1. Hemodynamic stabilization to correct nocturia
2. Stabilization of hydration status
3. Stabilization of weight appropriate for age and gender
4. Return to baseline of As and Bs as honor roll student
5. Stabilization of type 1 diabetes mellitus

states together creates a gap analysis that naturally shows where the patient is and what the goals are in terms of the patient's care. Some key questions to ask here are: Are the outcomes appropriate given the diagnoses? Are there gaps between the outcomes and present state? Are there clinical indicators of the desired outcome state?

The gap between where the patient is and where the advanced practice nurse wants the patient to be is one way to create a test (Exhibit 10.6). Clinical decisions are choices made about interventions that will help the patient transition from the present state to a desired outcome state. As interventions are tested, the advanced practice nurse evaluates the degree to which outcomes are or are not being achieved. The tests chosen in this case include sleep diary, laboratory data, Centers for Disease Control and Prevention (CDC) growth charts, school grades–report card, and glucose monitoring.

Testing is concurrent and iterative as one gets closer and closer in successive increments toward goal achievement. Some key questions to ask here are: How does the advanced practice nurse define *testing*? On what scales will the desired outcome be rated and how will the advanced practice nurse know when the desired targeted outcomes are achieved?

The reflection box at the top of Figure 10.2 (Exhibit 10.7) reminds the advanced practice nurse of the thinking strategies used for the patient situation. These strategies also help make explicit many of the relationships among ideas and issues associated with the patient problems. Examples of clinical reasoning reflection questions that could be used during patient-centered systems thinking are listed in Table 10.3.

EXHIBIT 10.6 TESTING

1. Sleep diary
2. Laboratory data
3. CDC growth charts
4. School grades, report card
5. Glucose monitoring

EXHIBIT 10.7 REFLECTION ON CLINICAL REASONING

What clinical decisions or interventions help to achieve the outcomes?

What specific intervention activities will you implement?

Why are you considering these activities?

Finally, the judgment space on the far left-hand side of the model (Exhibit 10.8) is the place to write in the results of the conclusions drawn from the CCCR model. Based on the degree of gap or comparison of where the patient is, and where the health care team wants the patient to be, there may or may not be an evidence gap. Once there is evidence that fills that gap, the nurse has to attribute meaning to the data. Making judgments about clinical issues is about the meaning the advanced practice nurse attributes to the evidence derived from the test or gap analysis of present to desired state. Complexity thinking, team-centered systems-thinking and organization-centered systems-thinking skills are used by the care coordination team at this point to evaluate and judge the successes or deficits from the plan of care. Interprofessional team activity requires negotiation of the competing values of collaboration—creating, competing, and controlling— and involves managing shared knowledge; acknowledgment of values impacted; and the brokering, directing, coordinating, and monitoring of practice issues, interventions, and outcomes. The judgments made in this case are made by the team after the care coordination essential-need outcomes are evaluated. Each of the items in the judgment column corresponds to an essential need addressed in the CCCR systems model (Figure 10.3). Some key questions to ask here are: Given the testing, what are the clinical judgments? Have the outcomes been achieved? Does the situation need to be reframed?

Once the advanced practice nurse has experience coordinating care for pediatric patients, the cases become part of a clinical reasoning learning history, which become prototypes or schemas for other similar cases. These schemas and experience build on each other over time and result in the development of pattern recognition for future clinical reasoning applications. If the scenario results in negative judgments, or progress is not being made to transition patients from present to

TABLE 10.3 Patient-Centered Systems-Thinking Reflection Questions

SELF-REGULATION ACTIVITIES	REFLECTION QUESTIONS

Monitoring thinking	I. **Reflect on the thinking processes you used with the care coordination of this case.**
	  1. The baseline needs I identify in this case are.... I think I can identify future adjustments in the plan of care by.... If I have difficulty I...
	  2. When I think about my feelings during the care coordination of this case, I describe them as...and I handle them by...
	  3. When I try to remember or understand important facts to develop the plan of care, coach, and educate the patient/family, I...
	  4. As I look back on meaningful activities, the resources I could have spent:
	    a. More time on...
	    b. Less time on...

Monitoring the environment	II. **Reflect on the environmental circumstances you encountered in the care coordination of this case.**
	  5. When I prepare to carry out coaching and education activities for care coordination, I...
	  6. When I think about particular distractions to facilitating medical care services and supports for care coordination, I...
	  7. When I work and communicate with interprofessional partners for care coordination of this case, I...
	  8. If I had the chance to redo the care coordination activities, I would do...instead of...because ...

Monitoring behavior	III. **Reflect on your behaviors and reactions to the care coordination of this case.**
	  9. My impression of my performance in evaluating capacity, energy, support, readiness, and skills to organize and manage the plan of care, is...
	  10. I make sure I will update the needs assessment and individualized plan of care by...and if I need to make changes, I...
	  11. I make sure I empower the patient/family for self-management of health care needs by...and if I need to make changes, I...
	  12. Reaction to care coordination of this case...
	    a. My reaction to what I like about the care coordination of this case...
	    b. My reaction to what I do not like about the care coordination of this case...
	Optional prompt: Other comments I have about the care coordination of this case...

Adapted from Kuiper, Pesut, and Kautz (2009).

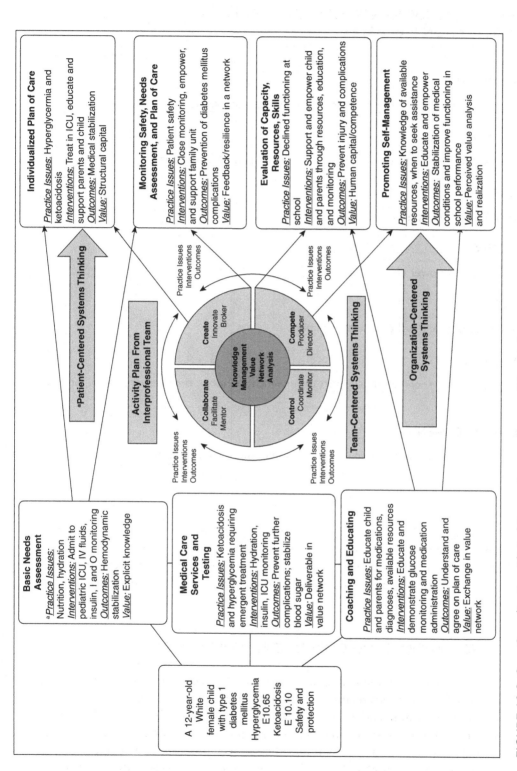

FIGURE 10.3 Care Coordination Clinical Reasoning systems model worksheet.

[a]Practice Issues can be from any discipline; nursing, medicine, pharmacy, social work, and so on.
DM, diabetes mellitus; ICU, intensive care unit; I and O, input and output; IV, intravenous.

EXHIBIT 10.8 JUDGMENTS RELATED TO CARE COORDINATION VARIABLES

PLAN OF CARE

Emergent intensive care treatment for hemodynamic stabilization

SAFETY

Correct ketoacidosis and prevent complications of diabetes mellitus

NEEDS

Ongoing monitoring, education, and resources

CAPACITY

Support and empower child and parents

SKILLS

Parental support and adherence to regimen

RESOURCES

School counselor, social work, support groups, school nurse, diabetes counselor, and pharmacist

SELF-MANAGEMENT

Maintenance of stabilized medical conditions and improved school performance

desired states, the advanced practice nurse may have to reframe the situation, reconsider the keystone priority, and reconsider the care coordination activities for the problem to be solved and the outcome to be achieved. The key question to ask here is how this clinical learning experience will impact future reasoning about similar cases?

CARE COORDINATION USING CCCR MODEL WORKSHEETS

The next step in the nursing diagnostic reasoning process is to augment the plan of care to include activities related to interprofessional care planning using the CCCR systems model framework (Exhibit 10.9), which builds on the OPT model of clinical reasoning. The systems dynamics and interactions between and among the patient issues determine the care needed and the services provided. The complexities in this case are the physical and behavioral issues related to the new diagnosis of diabetes mellitus. The CCCR systems model web (Figure 10.4) visually represents the

EXHIBIT 10.9 CARE COORDINATION CLINICAL REASONING DEFINITION

The authors define *care coordination clinical reasoning* as the application of critical, creative, systems, and complexity thinking to determine the practice issues, interdependencies, and interconnections of role relationships for collaborative work in service of caring for people to address problems, interventions, and outcomes through time and across health care contexts and services.

complexities in this case along with the essential care coordination practice issues that need attention so as to organize thinking that focuses on the patient's and/or family's priority needs.

The CCCR systems model web (Exhibit 10.10) provides a blueprint for consideration of the care coordination practice issues so that clinicians can determine interventions, outcomes, and the value exchange that supports safe, high-quality care. This process involves patient-centered, team-centered, and organization-centered systems thinking to thoroughly and efficiently manage all aspects of patient and family cases. The steps to create the web for this case start at the center with the patient description and medical diagnoses (Sally Jones, a 12-year-old White female child with type 1 diabetes mellitus), priority nursing domain (safety and protection, nutrition, and health promotion), and ICD-10 codes (type 1 diabetes mellitus hyperglycemia E10.65, ketoacidosis E10.10) that show the overlap of patient issues that must be addressed by the advanced practice nurse and the care coordination interprofessional team.

Next, each large circle in this web represents the essential care coordination practice issues with evidence and defining characteristics for this patient story: needs assessment (nutritional and education needs with new diabetes mellitus diagnosis); individualized plan of care (emergent treatment and monitoring of diabetes mellitus); medical care services and testing (emergent care in treatment of type 1 diabetes mellitus ketoacidosis, serum glucose, and hydration); evaluation of capacity, resources, and skills (decreased functioning in school performance); monitoring and safety (ketoacidosis, hyperglycemia, and tachypnea); team collaboration (collaboration and communication among the provider, parents, school nurse, and diabetes educator); coaching and educating (educate child and parents regarding diagnosis, medications, and ongoing treatment); and self-management (knowledge of resources available to child and parents, and diabetes mellitus education and management).

The provider then reflects on the total picture offered by the worksheet, and begins to draw lines of relationship, connection, or association among the essential needs. As directional lines are drawn to create the web, functional relationships between and among the needs are recognized. Clinical reasoning and thinking processes are used to explain and justify the reasons for connecting these care coordination needs as central supporting elements in the patient's story based on an analysis and synthesis of possible priorities, as represented in the web. The priority

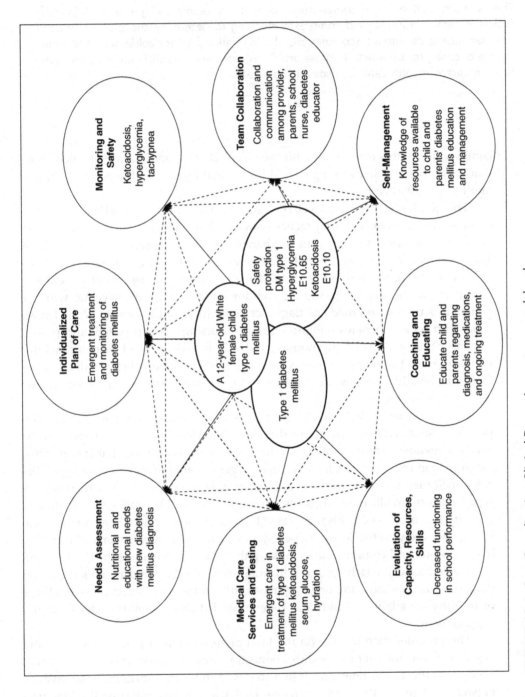

FIGURE 10.4 Care Coordination Clinical Reasoning systems model web.

DM, diabetes mellitus; ICU, intensive care unit; IV, intravenous.

EXHIBIT 10.10 CCCR SYSTEMS MODEL WEB DEFINITION

The Care Coordination Clinical Reasoning systems model web enables one to visually represent the complexities and essential care coordination practice issues that need attention so as to organize thinking that focuses on the patient's and/or family's priority needs within the context of services provided within and between health care delivery systems.

care coordination needs that would most efficiently and effectively represent the key issues of the patient are addressed that align with the patient story. A key question to ask here is whether this CCCR systems model web provides a comprehensive consideration of the most pertinent evidence for care coordination practice issues.

The CCCR systems model worksheet (see Figure 10.3) is the next worksheet in the framework designed to provide a graphic representation or visual map of the structure of the CCCR systems model and to help guide team-centered and organization-centered systems thinking. Some key questions to ask here are: What clinical decisions and interventions will help to achieve the outcomes identified on the OPT model of clinical reasoning (see Figure 10.3)? What specific interventions will the advanced practice nurse and/or the team implement, and are providers considering these activities?

Writing each element on the worksheet shows how parts of the model relate to each other. In Figure 10.3, on the far left-hand side, there is space to write the description of the patient's health care situation that was at the center of the CCCR systems model web. Three essential needs are placed in the first boxes to the right of the description and include basic needs assessment, medical care services and testing, and coaching and education. Each of the care coordination needs identified in this model includes practice issues, interventions, outcomes, and value specification.

From patient-centered systems-thinking processes used to create the OPT clinical reasoning model worksheets for this patient story, the identified basic needs practice issues include nutrition and hydration. Targeted interventions for the team would be to admit to a pediatric intensive care unit, administer intravenous fluids, administer insulin, and monitor intake and output. The documented desired outcomes would be hemodynamic stabilization. A key question to ask is: Have the basic needs been identified given the frame of the situation? Consider the value-impact analysis in this case using the questions from Table 10.4.

KNOWLEDGE MANAGEMENT AND VALUE ANALYSIS

The explicit value for role clarity, collaboration, and interaction of the team placed on the needs assessment is explicit knowledge. From Table 10.4, the value-networking reflection question for basic needs is: What knowledge is codified and conveyed to others through dialogue, demonstration, or media? Name three knowledge

TABLE 10.4 Value Definitions and Reflection Questions

Deliverable	The specific values or objects that are conveyed from one role or participant to another role or participant. What are the deliverables that you offer and expect of others?
Exchange	Two or more transactions between two or more roles or participants that evoke reciprocity. A process in which one role as agent receives resources from another role or agent and provides resources in return. What are the resource exchanges between roles or participants on your interprofessional health care team?
Explicit knowledge	The knowledge that is codified and conveyed to others through dialogue, demonstration, or media. What is the explicit knowledge shared among members of the team?
Feedback	This return of information about the impact of an activity. It can also mean the return of a portion of the output of a process as new input. What feedback is returned about activities or outputs in your care coordination activities? How does feedback influence team dynamics and goal attainment?
Human capital/ competence	The knowledge, skills, and competencies that reside in individuals who work in an organization or that are embedded in the organization's internal and external social networks. What human capital resources are needed in order for care coordination in your context to be successful?
Impact analysis	An assessment of how an input for a role is handled. What are the tangible/intangible costs, gains, or values from the input that generate a response or activity, or increase/decrease tangible assets?
Knowledge management	The degree to which the team facilitates and supports processes for creating, sustaining, sharing, and renewing organizational knowledge in order to generate social or economic gain or improve performance. Who is responsible and how is knowledge managed in the care coordination process?
Perceived value	The degree of value participants feel they receive from individual deliverables, which can come from roles, participants, or the network. What are the value-added dimensions of individual, collective, team, and organizational networks?
Resilience	The degree to which the network is able to reconfigure itself to respond to changing conditions and then return to its original form. What is the resilience capacity of the team and organization in which you work?
Structural capital	The infrastructure, routines, concepts, models, information systems, work systems, and business processes that support productivity and sustainability. To what degree do the structural capital and infrastructure support interprofessional teamwork and care coordination processes?

(continued)

TABLE 10.4 Value Definitions and Reflection Questions *(continued)*

Systems thinking	An analysis and synthesis of the forces and interrelationships that shape the behavior of systems.
	To what degree do members of the team think about the system dynamics at the patient, group, team, or organizational levels?
Value realization	The degree to which tangible or intangible values turn the input into gains, benefits, capabilities, or assets that contribute to the success of an individual, group, organization, or network (Allee, 2008).
	To what degree do members of the team intentionally negotiate and manage competing values related to collaborating, creating, competing, and or controlling?

Adapted from Allee, Schwabe, and Babb (2015).

classification systems that could be used to represent the patient characteristics in this case:

1.
2.
3.

From team-centered systems-thinking processes used for the basic needs assessment, the identified medical care services and testing practice issues include keto-acidosis and hyperglycemia requiring emergent treatment. Targeted interventions for the team are hydration, administration of insulin, and intensive care monitoring. The documented desired outcomes are to prevent further complications and stabilize the blood sugar. A key question to ask is: Do the testing and interventions sufficiently manage the primary care needs? The explicit value for role clarity, collaboration, and interaction of the team placed on the medical care services and testing is to deliver evidence-based interventions based on the health care provider role. From Table 10.4, the value-networking reflection question for medical care services and testing basic needs is: What is the specific value or object that is conveyed from one role or participant to another role or participant? Name three deliverables that are essential for the care coordination success of this case:

1.
2.
3.

Organization-centered systems thinking is used by the team to enhance coaching and educate the patient and family. The identified coaching and education practice issues include education of the child and parents for medications, diagnosis, and available resources. Targeted interventions for the team are to educate patient and family, and demonstrate glucose monitoring and medication administration. The documented desired outcomes are to ensure understanding and agreement on the plan of care. A key question to ask is: Do the content and methods for coaching and teaching match the patient and family cognitive abilities and understanding? From Table 10.4, the value-networking reflection question for educating and coaching involves evaluating the transactions between two or more roles or participants in which one role as an agent receives resources from another role or agents and provides resources in return. The question would be: What is the exchange of resources and information between the providers and the patient and family regarding medication and available resources? Name three resources that could be exchanged between the providers and the patient in this case:

1.

2.

3.

The diagram at the center of the worksheet is the activity plan from the interprofessional team (Exhibit 10.11). The team engages in collaborating, creating, competing, and controlling dynamics through communication (Quinn, Bright, Faerman, Thompson, & McGrath, 2014; Quinn, Heynoski, Thomas, & Spreitzer, 2014; Quinn & Quinn, 2015; Quinn & Rohrbough, 1983) to manage essential areas of organizational culture to realize the intangible value exchanges used to develop and manage an activity plan that considers interventions from the individualized plan of care, monitoring processes, evaluation of patient and family capacity with regard to resources and skills, and promotion of self-management. For example, in terms of collaboration, people must understand themselves and communicate honestly and effectively. Individuals mentor and develop others collaboratively and know how to participate and lead teams. Often this knowledge requires encouraging and managing constructive conflict, and enhances productivity and profitability. In this domain, vision and goal setting are the path to motivating self and others so that systems can be developed and organized to get results. Creating and promoting the adoption of new ideas or clinical innovations requires attention to judicious use of power and ethics as well as championing new ideas and innovations through negotiating commitments and agreements for implementing and sustaining change. Control contributes to the development of stability and continuity as people work and manage across functions, organize information exchange, measure and monitor performance and quality, and enable compliance.

Key ingredients to team-centered systems thinking are that the members must be purpose centered, internally directed, other focused, and externally open to negotiation and communication surrounding competing values (Quinn, 2015; Quinn & Quinn, 2015). The activity plan from the interprofessional team in the CCCR model is guided by these principles and will promote the development of positive organizations and relationships. Each team member should be externally open to challenges, feedback and freedom from labels, higher performance, and the cultivation and development of communities of practice. When this outcome is challenged and false fixed, some team members are valued more than others in the context of competitive versus collaborative goals. Being other influenced cultivates empathy, rapport,

EXHIBIT 10.11

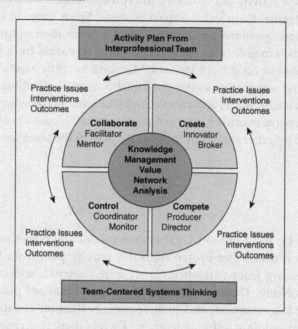

Key questions to consider for the four dimensions of the competing-values framework in the CCCR model are as follows:

- What are the desired outcomes in this case?
- What are the values I expect of myself and others?
- How are the feelings of the patient, family, and team considered in this case?
- What strategies could the team use to coordinate care?

energy, and calmness. Together, the team members feel safe and secure enough to take risks and act with trust, integrity, and resilience. Creating such a culture supports a spirit of inquiry, learning, and experimentation, which results in higher performance. Such behavior requires the activation of a reflective self in contrast to automatic self-justification and reactive modes of being and communicating. In order to be a positive influence and to bring a state of leadership to the team, each member of the team needs to be vigilant about being purpose centered, choosing goals that create focus, energy, and meaning for the team. A focused, purpose-centered team is likely to attract and create resources related to the reasoning required to communicate across settings to achieve CCCR goals.

The activity plan from the interprofessional team iteratively visits the practice issues, which include communication among providers specific to this case; targeted interventions, which are updated at team meetings across the contexts in which the providers are interacting; and documents the desired outcomes to maintain team support and to keep the team equally informed about patient status. A key question to ask is: Are the communication processes in place and do they promote information exchange between and among the interprofessional health team members? The explicit value for role clarity, collaboration, and interaction of the team placed on the activity plan from the interprofessional team is determined by knowledge management and value impact analysis. From Table 10.4, the value-networking reflection questions for the activity plan from the interprofessional team are: What are the tangible/intangible costs, gains, or values from the input that generate a response or activity, or increase/decrease tangible assets? How does the team facilitate and support processes for collaborating, controlling, creating, and competing to sustain, share, and renew organizational knowledge in order to generate social or economic gain or improve performance? Name a cost, a gain, and a value that would be generated from the activity plan of the team for this case:

1.
2.
3.

To the far right of the CCCR system model worksheet are four essential care coordination needs that evolve from the activity plan from the interprofessional team stemming from patient-centered, team-centered, and organization-centered systems thinking. These needs include the individualized plan of care; monitoring safety, needs assessment, and plan of care; evaluation of capacity, resources, and skills; and promoting self-management. Each of these care coordination essentials is defined as well by practice issues, interventions, outcomes, and values.

The patient-centered and team-centered systems-thinking activities are used for the individualized plan of care. The identified practice issues revolve around a female child with hyperglycemia and ketoacidosis from type 1 diabetes mellitus. Targeted interventions for the provider and team are to treat the emergent condition in the intensive care unit, and educate and support the parents and the child. The documented desired outcomes are to provide medical stabilization. Some key questions to ask are: Does the individualized plan of care include team collaboration? Is there any input that was not yet considered? Or are there providers who were overlooked? The explicit value for role clarity, collaboration, and interaction of the provider and team placed on the individualized plan of care is on structural capital. From Table 10.4, the value-networking reflection question for the individualized plan of care is: What are the infrastructure, routines, concepts, models, information systems, work systems, and business processes that support productivity and have sustainability? Name three routines, systems, or processes that support and sustain the productivity of the care coordination in this case.

1.
2.
3.

From the patient-centered and team-centered systems-thinking processes used for monitoring safety, needs assessment, and plan of care, identified practice issues include patient safety. Targeted interventions for the team are close monitoring and empowering the family unit with support. The documented desired outcomes are to prevent diabetes mellitus complications. A key question to ask is: Does the plan of care promote safety and meet the patient and family needs? The explicit value for role clarity, collaboration, and interaction of the team placed on monitoring safety, needs assessment, and plan of care is to obtain feedback and assess resilience in the network. From Table 10.4, the value-networking reflection questions for medical care services and testing basic needs are: What feedback is returned about activities or outputs? Was the network able to reconfigure itself to respond to changing conditions and then return to its original form? Name three areas of need and/or safety that were reassessed to determine if the plan of care needed to be adjusted:

1.
2.
3.

Organization-centered systems-thinking processes such as coaching and education, are used by the team to evaluate capacity, resources, and skills. The identified practice issues include the identification of cognitive decline in functioning at school. Targeted interventions for the team are to support and empower the child and parents through identifying resources, education, and monitoring. The documented desired outcomes are to prevent injury and complications. A key question to ask is: Do the interventions in the plan of care required skilled help and/or can the patient and family manage care needs independently? The explicit value for role clarity, collaboration, and interaction of the team placed on evaluating capacity, resources, and skills is identifying human capital and competence. From Table 10.4, the value-networking reflection question for educating and coaching involves evaluating the transactions between two or more roles or participants in which one role as an agent receives resources from another role or agent and provides resources in return. The question would be: What is the exchange of resources and information between the providers and the patient and family regarding medication and available resources? Name three exchanges of resources, skills, or information with the patient that are essential to the care coordination success of this case:

1.
2.
3.

Organization-centered systems-thinking processes, such as coaching and education, are used by the team to promote self-management. The identified practice issues include knowledge of available resources and when to seek assistance. Targeted interventions for the team are to educate and empower the child and family. The documented desired outcomes are to maintain a stable condition and improve functioning in school performance. A key question to ask is: Are the patient and family able to identify the resources they need to navigate the health care system? The explicit value for role clarity, collaboration, and interaction of the team placed on promoting self-management is perceived value realization. From Table 10.4, the value-networking reflection question for promoting self-management is: What is the level of value that roles or participants feel they receive from individual deliverables, which can come from roles, participants, or the network? Name three examples of learned self-management that resulted from the care coordination of this case:

1.
2.
3.

With the use of the CCCR systems model, the advanced practice nurse and other providers address practice issues by using and developing evidence-based interventions, implementing measures of adherence, and evaluating processes and outcomes. This requires clinical reasoning at different levels of perspective—the individual patient needs, interprofessional team contributions, and attention to the systems in which people work and provide care. These practice issues, interventions, and outcomes for patient and family care coordination stem from the National Quality Forum (NQF, 2010a, 2010b) and the Agency for Healthcare Research and Quality (AHRQ, 2014).

As the center of attention for health care needs is managed by webs of relationships between and among providers, each interaction supports a specific value exchange as participant's partner for successful outcomes (Allee, 2003). The dynamic relationships that occurred for this patient among the advanced practice nurse, nursing staff, physician, pharmacist, school officials, and social worker was collaborative, trusting, dynamic, and interdependent. Application of the competing-value competencies will relate to collaboration, creating, competing, and controlling. Through the use of the electronic health record, connectivity impacted the value networking with greater access to knowledge and information. This process provided quick and effective feedback among team members for the complex needs this patient had related to physical abuse and multiple health problems.

CLINICAL JUDGMENTS AND CCCR

The final phase of the clinical reasoning process is to determine whether outcomes were met and whether care coordination activities were successful. The OPT model of clinical reasoning is revisited for the final phase of care coordination, where judgments are made about achieving outcomes from the interprofessional team activity plan (see Exhibit 10.8). The worksheet (see Figure 10.2) is revisited to make judgments about the care coordination essentials (needs; individualized plan of care; safety; capacity, resources, and skills; and self-management). Shifting to the next level of perspective, using team-centered and organization-centered systems-thinking activities, collaboration, and coordination of the plan of care reveals ongoing planning and evaluation to provide emergent care in the intensive care unit to provide initial hemodynamic stability. The safety concerns are to correct the ketoacidosis and prevent complications. The need for this family unit is ongoing monitoring, education, and identifying available resources. The child and parent capacity will be assessed, supported, and empowered. Their skills to manage diabetes mellitus and adhere to the regimen will also have to be monitored. Appropriate resources for this case are the school counselor, social worker, support groups, school nurse, diabetes educator, and pharmacist. The goal is to promote self-management by the child and parents to stabilize the diabetes mellitus and improve school performance.

Some remaining questions may arise as the evaluation of outcomes occurs: Can the organization provide continuing resources and reach care coordination outcomes for this patient? Were communication and the feedback loop effective between the healthcare providers, and patient and family? Did the complexity of the system hinder or enhance the achievement of outcomes? How do the competencies of the competing-values framework support the interprofessional dialogue and reasoning about the care coordination of this particular case? The advanced practice nurse as the care coordinator views all the systems and is the key informant to communicate with the team regarding the efficiency and effectiveness of the processes for care outcomes. Judgments are made about whether the outcomes from case management have been achieved, and the information is recycled back to revise or enhance the plan of care.

The thinking processes used by the advanced practice nurse and other health care providers while implementing the CCCR systems model is promoted through monitoring of thinking, the environment, and behaviors for goal attainment (Zimmerman & Schunk, 2001). The courses of action chosen to manage issues and ensure that this patient remained safe revolve around behaviors and actions taken, thinking processes used, and environmental structuring. Critical reflective questions that can be used to prompt clinical reasoning to make judgments about the achievement of patient and family outcomes are listed in Table 10.5. Critical-, creative-, and systems-thinking processes are used for total care coordination, flow from patient-centered systems thinking (Table 10.3), team-centered systems thinking (Table 10.5), and organization-centered systems thinking (Table 10.5) for case management.

SUMMARY

The clinical reasoning challenge for pediatric health care begins with a description and understanding of the patient's story. The thinking strategies used in this case provided a safe and health-promoting environment for a child who was newly diagnosed with type 1 diabetes mellitus. As the providers practice self-monitoring, self-evaluation, and self-correction, successful strategies are employed, and flaws in thinking are corrected as they collaborate and align interventions for patient and family success. The OPT clinical reasoning model provides the structure for clinical reasoning and systems thinking within an individual patient and family situation. The OPT structure and process can be used at several levels for care planning by the provider, by the team, and by the organization to discern alignment and coordination of care activities. The CCCR systems model provides the structure for clinical reasoning for the care coordination essential needs and their related practice issues, interventions, outcomes, and values.

KEY CONCEPTS

1. Clinical reasoning for care coordination with psychological/mental health can be promoted with a framework that includes structure, content, and process.

TABLE 10.5 Team-Centered and Organization-Centered Systems-Thinking Reflection Questions

SELF-REGULATION ACTIVITIES	REFLECTION QUESTIONS

Monitoring thinking	**I. Reflect on the thinking processes the team used to navigate organizational systems for care coordination of this case.**
	
	1. The baseline needs identified by the team in this case are.... Adjustments in the plan of care for future successes include.... Difficulties were resolved by...
	
	2. Team reactions during the care coordination of this case in regard to organizational systems could be described as...and they were handled by...
	
	3. When the team was dealing with important facts to develop the plan of care, coach, and educate the patient/family about organizational systems it...
	
	4. Looking back on meaningful activities, the resources the team could have spent:
	  a. More time on...
	  b. Less time on...

Monitoring the environment	**II. Reflect on the environmental circumstances you encountered in the care coordination of this case.** 5. When the team prepares to carry out coaching and education activities for care coordination, it... 6. When the team considers particular distractions in the organizations that impede medical care services and supports for care coordination, it... 7. When the teamworks and communicates with organizational partners for care coordination of this case, it... 8. If the team had the chance to redo the care coordination activities, it would do...instead of...because ...

Monitoring behavior	**III. Reflect on your behaviors and reactions to the care coordination of this case.**
	
	9. Impressions of the team performance in evaluating capacity, energy, support, readiness, and skills to organize and manage the plan of care within organizational systems are...
	
	10. The team assures that it will update the needs assessment and individualized plan of care by...and if it needs to make changes, it...
	
	11. The team makes sure that it empowers the patient/family to navigate through organizational systems for management of health care needs by...and if it needs to make changes, it...
	
	12. The team reaction to care coordination of this case...
	  a. Reaction to what it likes about the navigation of organizational systems to facilitate the care coordination of this case...
	  b. Reaction to what it does not like about the navigation of organizational systems to facilitate the care coordination of this case...
	
	Optional prompt: Other comments about the care coordination of this case...

Adapted from Kuiper, Pesut, and Kautz (2009).

2. A supporting framework for care coordination clinical reasoning extends case management using patient-centered systems thinking and the OPT clinical reasoning model across levels of perspective that also include team-centered systems thinking and organization-centered systems thinking to align care coordination activities.

3. The process of care coordination clinical reasoning involves critical reflection for the individual provider and the team.

4. Value-network analysis helps one to define and describe the unique contributions that individual providers make to CCCR efforts supported through knowledge management and value-impact analysis.

5. A supporting framework for care coordination clinical reasoning is completed by attending to the organizational systems thinking to make judgments about care coordination essentials.

STUDY QUESTIONS AND ACTIVITIES

1. Describe in your own words the benefits and processes of using the CCCR systems model with pediatric health cases.

2. Using the CCCR systems model, identify the care coordination essential needs of cases in pediatric health.

3. To what degree can you explicitly identify and describe the value exchanges associated with care coordination in pediatric health situations.

4. How can an interprofessional team use the competencies of the competing values of collaboration, creating, competing, and controlling to ensure efficiency and effectiveness of care coordination. How does your team negotiate roles of mentor, broker, director, and coordinator?

5. Identify all the possible standardized health care languages and communication strategies that could be considered in a pediatric health case. Does language impact on communication and the patient outcomes? How does a discipline-specific framework influence the feedback, decisions, and outcomes with pediatric health?

6. Identify the relationship between critical reflection and thinking strategies as they are applied to the three levels of system-thinking perspectives that are required— patient, individual provider, team, and organization. What unique reflections are required to focus on team and organizational function with pediatric health?

REFERENCES

Agency for Healthcare Research and Quality (AHRQ). (2014). *What is care coordination? Care coordination measures atlas update*. Rockville, MD: Author. Retrieved from http://www.ahrq.gov/professionals/prevention-chronic-care/improve/coordination/index.html

Allee, V. (2003). *The future of knowledge: Increasing prosperity through value networks*. Burlington, MA: Butterworth-Heinemann.

Allee, V. (2008). Value network analysis and value conversion of tangible and intangible assets. *Journal of Intellectual Capital, 9*(1), 5–24.

Allee, V., Schwabe, O., & Babb, M. K. (Eds.) (2015). *Value networks and the true nature of collaboration*. Tampa, FL: Megher–Kifer Press ValueNet Works and Verna Allee Associates.

Haas, S. A., Swan, B. A., & Haynes, T. S. (2014). *Care coordination and transition management core curriculum*. Pitman, NJ: American Academy of Ambulatory Care Nursing.

Kuiper, R., Pesut, D., & Kautz, D. (2009). Promoting the self-regulation of clinical reasoning skills in nursing students. *Open Nursing Journal, 3*, 76–85. Retrieved from http://www.ncbi.nlm.nih.gov/pmc/articles/PMC2771264

National Quality Forum (NQF). (2010a). *Preferred practices and performance measures for measuring and reporting care coordination: A consensus report*. Washington, DC: Author.

National Quality Forum (NQF). (2010b). *Quality connections: Care coordination*. Washington, DC: Author.

Pesut, D. J. (2008). Thoughts on thinking with complexity in mind. In C. Lindberg, S. Nash, & C. Lindberg (Eds.), *On the edge: Nursing in the age of complexity* (pp. 211–238). Bordentown, NJ: Plexus Press.

Quinn, R. (2015). *The positive organization: Breaking free from conventional cultures, constraints, and beliefs*. Oakland, CA: Berrett-Koehler.

Quinn, R., & Quinn, R. E. (2015). *Lift: Becoming a positive force in any situation*. San Francisco, CA: Berrett-Koehler.

Quinn, R. E., Bright, D., Faerman, S. R., Thompson, M. P., & McGrath, M. R. (2014). *Becoming a master manager: A competing values approach*. Hoboken, NJ: John Wiley & Sons.

Quinn, R. E., Heynoski, K., Thomas, M., & Spreitzer, G. M. (2014). *The best teacher in you: How to accelerate learning and change lives*. San Francisco, CA: Berrett-Koehler.

Quinn, R. E., & Rohrbough, J. (1983). A spatial model of effectiveness criteria: Towards a competing values approach to organizational analysis. *Management Science, 29*, 363–377.

World Health Organization (WHO). (2015). *Manual of the International Classification of Diseases and related health problems* (10th rev. ed.). Geneva, Switzerland: Author. Retrieved from http://www.icd10data.com

Zimmerman, B., & Schunk, D. S. (2001). *Self-regulated learning and academic thought*. Mahwah, NJ: Lawrence Erlbaum.

CHAPTER 11

CARE COORDINATION FOR
A MATERNITY PATIENT

In this chapter, we use the Care Coordination Clinical Reasoning (CCCR) systems model as described in Part I and explain how the model can be used to reason about a case, given the context of a patient in maternity care (labor and delivery). The case presented in this chapter illustrates how an advanced practice nurse works with an obstetrician coordinating the care for a patient who is in need of interventions for complications during pregnancy. The patient was admitted to a hospital labor and delivery unit for abdominal pain, vaginal bleeding, and decreased fetal movement. The advanced practice nurse provides care coordination through the application and use of critical-, creative-, systems-, and complexity-thinking processes to manage patient problems with an interprofessional team to design appropriate interventions and establish patient-centered outcomes. Depending on the nature of need involved in the case, referrals to other specialty or primary care providers are determined and considered in managing care coordination and transitions (Haas, Swan, & Haynes, 2014).

The CCCR systems model framework begins with the patient story, which is derived from gathering data and evidence from an interview, history, physical examination, and the health record. The advanced practice nurse then develops a patient-centered plan of care using the Outcome-Present State-Test (OPT) model worksheets. In order to do this, one activates patient-centered systems-thinking skills for complex patient stories and consistently uses key questions to reflect on the specific sections of the model (Pesut, 2008), as well as the dimensions and elements of care coordination processes.

LEARNING OUTCOMES

After completing this chapter, the reader should be able to:

1. Explain the components of a care coordination framework that are needed to manage the problems, interventions, and outcomes of maternity patients managing health care issues
2. Describe the different thinking processes that support clinical reasoning skills and strategies for determining priorities and desired outcomes for the maternity patient

3. Define the cognitive and metacognitive self-regulatory processes that support individual provider critical reflection related to levels and perspectives associated with clinical reasoning for the maternity patient and care coordination
4. Describe how the communication and knowledge management between interprofessional health care team members is essential for care coordination to address maternity patient needs
5. Describe the critical meta-reflective processes that support team reflection, communication, and value-added impact related to levels and perspectives associated with the care coordination challenges and clinical reasoning required to navigate maternity patient care plans

THE PATIENT STORY

We begin with the history and story of a 19-year-old English-speaking, Asian female, Sarah Chinn, who presents to the labor and delivery unit because of abdominal cramping. She is at 36 weeks gestation and for the past 3 hours rated her pain a 10 on a 1-to-10 scale. She is a gravida 2, para 0 (G2P0), and the electronic health record shows no prenatal care since week 22 of gestation and a net loss of 10 pounds at that visit.

Social assessment reveals that Sarah was "kicked out" of her parent's home and has been staying with different friends. The father of the baby is no longer involved with her. She was waiting to "settle down" before resuming prenatal care. Sarah does not know where she will live after the baby is born. She denies taking childbirth classes or being prepared to take the baby home from the hospital. Ms. Chinn has no significant past medical history and she denies illicit drug use. She does not take any medications currently and denies taking prenatal vitamins.

The physical examination reveals a highly agitated young woman who is inappropriately dressed for cold weather. She is uncooperative with the application of the fetal monitor. The staff notes a moderate amount of bright red vaginal bleeding and no obvious leakage of fluid. Vaginal examination reveals a 1-cm dilated and 30% effaced cervix. The vertex is ballotable. Contractions are moderate to strong, lasting 40 to 60 seconds every 2 to 3 minutes. Sarah's height is 5′ 7″ (67 in.), her weight is 115 pounds at 22 weeks gestation, and her body mass index (BMI) is 18.01.

Admission laboratory results show a positive drug screen for cocaine and a urinalysis positive for ketones. The complete blood count reveals a hemoglobin of 10.2 g/dL, hematocrit of 30.8%, and platelet count of 98,000/mm^3.

PATIENT-CENTERED PLAN OF CARE USING OPT WORKSHEETS

Once the story is obtained from all possible sources, care planning and reasoning proceed using the OPT clinical reasoning web worksheet (Figure 11.1), which helps determine relationships among issues and highlights potential keystone issues. The OPT clinical reasoning web is a graphic representation of the functional relationships between and among diagnostic hypotheses derived from the analysis and synthesis regarding how each element of the story and issues relate to one another. This activates critical and creative thinking. The visual diagram that results illustrates

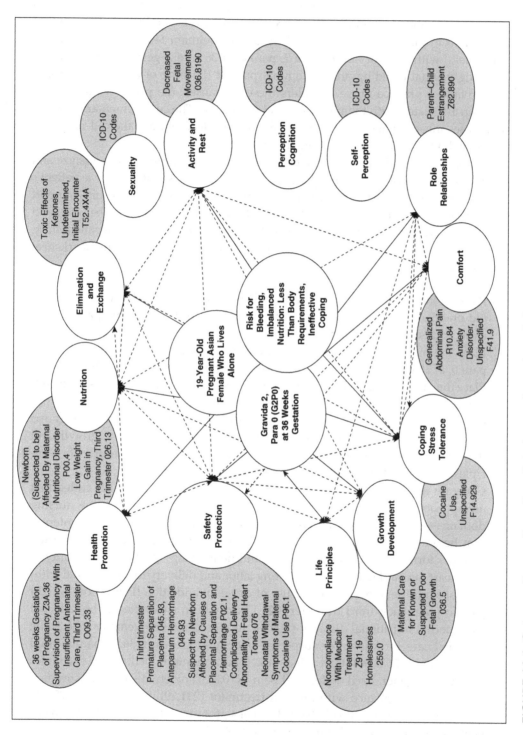

FIGURE 11.1 Outcome-Present State-Test clinical reasoning web worksheet.

ICD-10, International Classification of Diseases, 10th edition.

dynamics among issues and a convergence helps to point out central issues that require nursing care. As one thinks about this case, and begins to spin and weave a clinical reasoning web, relationships are identified among nursing domains and diagnoses as they are jointly considered with medical conditions. The medical conditions in this case are those of a 19-year-old pregnant female who lives alone (homeless) with a history of gravida 2, para 0, at 36 weeks gestation. She is experiencing vaginal bleeding and abdominal pain at the time of examination. Once the advanced practice nurse considers these diagnoses, the priority nursing care domain associated with them is safety and protection. The complementary nursing diagnoses most impacted in this case are risk for bleeding, imbalanced nutrition: less than body requirements, and ineffective coping.

To spin and weave the web, the provider uses thinking processes to analyze and synthesize relationships among diagnostic hypotheses associated with a patient's health status. The visual representation and mapping of these relationships support the development of patient-centered systems thinking and connections between and among the medical and nursing diagnoses under consideration, given the patient story.

The steps to the creation of the OPT clinical reasoning web using the worksheet are as follows:

1. Place a general description of the patient in the respective middle circle—19-year-old pregnant Asian female presents to the labor and delivery unit; patient lives alone and is essentially homeless.
2. Place the major medical diagnoses in the respective middle circle—gravida 2, para 0, at 36 weeks gestation with abdominal pain and vaginal bleeding.
3. Place the major nursing diagnoses in the respective middle circle—risk for bleeding, imbalanced nutrition: less than body requirements, and ineffective coping.
4. Choose the nursing domains for which each medical and nursing diagnosis is appropriate—safety and protection, nutrition, activity and rest, growth and development, role relationships, elimination and exchange, comfort, life principles, coping and stress tolerance, and health promotion.
5. Generate all the International Classification of Diseases (ICD-10) codes that are appropriate for the particular patient story that coincide with the nursing domains—premature separation of placenta, third trimester (045.93); antepartum hemorrhage, third trimester (046.93); newborn (suspected to be) affected by other forms of placental separation and hemorrhage (P02.1); abnormality in fetal heart rate and rhythm complicating labor and delivery (076): neonatal withdrawal symptoms from maternal use of drugs of addiction (P96.1); low weight gain in pregnancy, third trimester (026.13); newborn (suspected to be) affected by maternal nutritional disorder (P00.4): decreased fetal movements (036.8190); maternal care for known or suspected poor fetal growth (036.5); parent–child estrangement (262.890); toxic effect of ketones, undetermined, initial encounter (T52.4X4A); generalized abdominal pain (R10.84); anxiety disorder, unspecified (F41.9); noncompliance with medical treatment (291.19); homelessness (259.0); cocaine use, unspecified (F14,929); 36 weeks gestation of pregnancy with insufficient antenatal care, and third trimester (009.33).
6. Once the nursing domains, diagnoses, and ICD-10 codes are identified, reflect on the total web worksheet and concurrently consider and explain how each of the

TABLE 11.1 Relationships Among Nursing Domains, Medical Diagnoses, and Web Connections

NURSING DOMAINS	MEDICAL DIAGNOSES (ICD-10 CODES)	WEB CONNECTIONS
Safety protection	Premature separation of placenta, third trimester O45.93	10
	Antepartum hemorrhage, third trimester O46.93	
	Newborn (suspected to be) affected by other forms of placental separation and hemorrhage P02.1	
	Abnormality in fetal heart rate and rhythm complicating labor and delivery O76	
	Neonatal withdrawal symptoms from maternal use of drugs of addiction P96.1	
Coping stress tolerance	Cocaine use, unspecified F14.929	8
Nutrition	Low weight gain in pregnancy, third trimester O26.13	7
	Newborn (suspected to be) affected by maternal nutritional disorder P00.4	
Activity and rest	Decreased fetal movements O36.8190	7
Role relationships	Parent–child estrangement 262.890	6
Elimination and Exchange	Toxic effects of ketones, undetermined, initial encounter T52.4X4A	6
Comfort	Generalized abdominal pain R10.84	6
	Anxiety disorder, unspecified F41.9	
Growth development	Maternal care for known or suspected poor fetal growth O36.5	5
Life principles	Noncompliance with medical treatment 291.19	4
	Homelessness 259.0	
Health promotion	36 weeks gestation of pregnancy with insufficient antenatal care, third trimester O09.33	4

Source: World Health Organization (2015).

issues is or is not related to the other issues. Draw lines of relationship to spin and weave the web connections or associations among the ICD-10 codes/diagnoses. As you draw the lines, think out loud, justify the reasons for the connections, and explain specifically how the diagnoses may or may not be connected or related.

7. After the advanced practice nurse has spent some time connecting the relationships, determine which domain/domains have the highest priority for care coordination and most efficiently and effectively represent the keystone nursing care needs of the patient by counting the arrows that connect the medical problems (ICD-10 codes). In this case, counting 10 lines (Table 11.1) pointing to or from the nursing domain of safety/protection represents the priority present-state keystone issues.

8. Look once again at the sets of relationships and determine the theme or keystone that summarizes the patient-in-context or the patient story—safety/protection for a pregnant 19-year-old at 36 weeks gestation.

An OPT clinical reasoning web worksheet, as seen in Figure 11.1, shows a template with the patient health care situation, medical diagnoses, and nursing diagnoses in the center. Around the outer edges of the web are nursing domains with ICD-10 codes derived from history and physical assessment associated with the patient story. The arrows create the web effect and represent connections, explanations, and functional relationships between and among the diagnostic possibilities. As one can see, the domains and ICD-10 codes with more connections converging on the circles display the priority problem or keystone, in this case, safety and protection. A keystone issue is one or more of the central supporting elements of the patient's story that help focus and determine a root cause or center of gravity of the system dynamics and help guide reasoning and care coordination based on an analysis (breaking things down into discrete parts) and synthesis (putting the parts together in a greater whole) of diagnostic possibilities as represented in the web. A key question to ask here is: How does the clinical reasoning web reveal relationships between and among the identified diagnoses and to what degree do these relationships make practical clinical sense according to the evidence and patient story? Table 11.1 shows a summary of the connections highlighting the priority with the most connections.

After considering the full picture using the clinical reasoning web worksheet, the next step is to use an OPT clinical reasoning model worksheet to facilitate and structure the patient-centered systems thinking about the care coordination of the identified problems highlighted in Table 11.1. As the advanced practice nurse thinks about the patient, he or she will concurrently consider the frame, outcome state, and present state. Each aspect of the OPT clinical reasoning model contributes to the other. The OPT clinical reasoning model worksheet is a map of the structure designed to provide an illustrative representation and guide thinking processes about relationships between and among competing issues and problems. Some questions that guide the use of the OPT clinical reasoning model are shown in Table 11.2 (Pesut, 2008).

By writing each element on the worksheet, all the parts of the model become related to each other. As the health care provider moves from right to left, the model structures the plan of care. Critical thinking skills are used to consider the patient story and creative thinking is used to identify and reason about the keystone issues/themes/cues to determine the most significant evidence in the present state. Complexity thinking helps the provider to consider the outcomes desired and the gaps between the present and outcome states. Once interventions and tests are decided, the plan of care transitions over to a care coordination model and team-centered systems thinking that considers patient preferences within the frame of the situation.

The patient-in-context story (Exhibit 11.1) is on the far right-hand side, as depicted in Figure 11.2. The advanced practice nurse notes relevant facts of the story, which in this case include the patient demographics and characteristics; 19-year-old pregnant Asian female who lacks any social support and is homeless. Sarah has a diagnosis of pregnancy at 36 weeks gestation with complications. She is very agitated and uncooperative with the application of a fetal monitor. She has abdominal pain, vaginal bleeding, symptoms of fetal distress, and the cervix is 1-cm dilated.

TABLE 11.2 Questions That Guide the Use of the OPT Model

Patient-in-context	What is the patient story?
Diagnostic cue/ web logic	What diagnoses have you generated?
	What outcomes do you have in mind given the diagnoses?
	What evidence supports those diagnoses?
	How does a reasoning web reveal relationships among the identified problems (diagnoses)?
	What keystone issue(s) emerge?
Framing	How are you framing the situation?
Present state	How is the present state defined?
Outcome state	What are the desired outcomes?
	What are the gaps or complementary pairs (~) of outcomes and present states?
Test	What are the clinical indicators of the desired outcomes?
	On what scales will the desired outcomes be rated?
	How will you know when the desired outcomes are achieved?
	How are you defining your testing in this particular case?
Decision making (interventions)	What clinical decisions or interventions help to achieve the outcomes?
	What specific intervention activities will you implement?
	Why are you considering these activities?
Judgment	Given your testing, what is your clinical judgment?
	Based on your judgment, have you achieved the outcome or do you need to reframe the situation?
	How, specifically, will you take this experience and learning with you into the future as you reason about similar cases?

OPT, Outcome-Present State-Test.

Adapted from Pesut (2008).

She is underweight with a BMI of 18.01 at 22 weeks. She has not received any prenatal care since 22 weeks gestation. She has not had any prenatal classes and is not prepared to take the baby home from the hospital. Significant laboratory data show anemia, thrombocytopenia, and urinalysis positive for ketones and cocaine. A key point at this juncture is to review and reflect on the patient story for accuracy and thoroughness to before proceeding with care planning for care coordination.

Moving to the left of the worksheet, there is a place to list the diagnostic cluster cues on the web of medical diagnoses and ICD-10 codes (Exhibit 11.2). At the bottom of this box are placed the designated keystone issues or themes that fall under the most significant nursing domain—safety/protection: premature separation of placenta, third trimester 045.93; antepartum hemorrhage, third trimester 046.93; newborn (suspected to be) affected by other forms of placental separation and hemorrhage P02.1; abnormality in fetal heart rate and rhythm complicating labor and delivery 076; and neonatal withdrawal symptoms from maternal use of drugs P96.1. Remember diagnostic cluster cues web logic is the use of inductive and deductive

EXHIBIT 11.1 PATIENT-IN-CONTEXT STORY

Sarah Chinn is a 19-year-old Asian female who is at 36 weeks gestation and presents to the emergency department and labor and delivery unit with abdominal pain and vaginal bleeding. Social history is that she lives with friends, but is homeless without a support system. She has had no prenatal care since 22 weeks and has not been taking vitamins. She denies illicit drug use.

Significant laboratory data: anemia, thrombocytopenia, and urinary drug screen positive for cocaine; urinalysis is positive for ketones

thinking skills. Some key questions to ask here are: What diagnoses were generated? Is there evidence to support those diagnoses? Is the keystone issue appropriate, given this patient story?

In the center and background of the worksheet are places to indicate the frame or theme that best represents the background issues regarding thinking about the patient story (Exhibit 11.3). The frame of this case is a 19-year-old adolescent female who is at 36 weeks gestation with high levels of anxiety and agitation, restlessness, and is uncooperative. The frame helps to organize the present state, outcome state, illustrates the gaps, and provides insights about what tests need to be considered to fill the gap. Decision making and reflection surround the framing as the advanced practice nurse thinks of many things simultaneously. Reflective thinking is used to monitor thinking and behavior. Some key questions to ask here are: How am I framing the situation and does it agree with the patient view of the situation? Given my disciplinary perspectives, what are the results I want to create for this person?

At the center of the sheet are spaces to place the present state (Exhibit 11.4) and outcome state (Exhibit 11.5) side by side. The present state in this case shows six primary health care problems related to the keystone issue: generalized abdominal pain for 3 hours; moderate amount of bright-red vaginal bleeding; gravida 2, para 0; fetal heart rate of 170 with repetitive late decelerations; 1-cm dilated 30% effaced cervix with vertex ballotable; and positive urine drug screen for cocaine.

The outcome state shows six matching goals to be achieved through care coordination: control of pain, hemodynamic stability, delivery of healthy newborn, fetal viability and maternal stability, emergent C-section with positive course of recovery, and substance use control. Putting the two states together creates a gap analysis that naturally shows where the patient is and what the goals are in terms of the patient's care. Some key questions to ask here are: Are the outcomes appropriate given the diagnose? Are there gaps between the outcomes and present state? Are there clinical indicators of the desired outcome state?

The gap between where the patient is and where the advanced practice nurse wants the patient to be is one way to create a test (Exhibit 11.6). Clinical decisions are choices made about interventions that will help the patient transition from present state to a desired outcome state. As interventions are tested, the advanced practice nurse evaluates the degree to which outcomes are being achieved or not. The tests chosen in this case include: pain scale rating, feminine napkin pad count, Apgar score, fetal

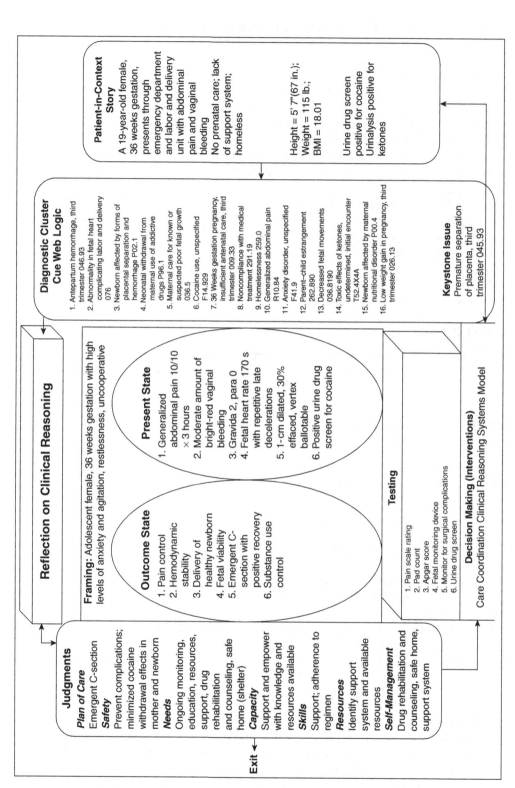

FIGURE 11.2 Outcome–Present State–Test clinical reasoning model for care coordination worksheet.

BMI, body mass index.

EXHIBIT 11.2 DIAGNOSTIC CLUSTER CUE WEB LOGIC

1. Antepartum hemorrhage, third trimester O46.93
2. Abnormality in fetal heart rate complicating labor and delivery O76
3. Newborn affected by forms of placental separation and hemorrhage P02.1
4. Neonatal withdrawal from maternal use of addictive drugs P96.1
5. Maternal care for known or suspected poor fetal growth O36.5
6. Cocaine use, unspecified F14.929
7. 36 weeks gestation pregnancy, insufficient antenatal care, third trimester O09.33
8. Noncompliance with medical treatment 291.19
9. Homelessness 259.0
10. Generalized abdominal pain R10.84
11. Anxiety disorder, unspecified F41.9
12. Parent–child estrangement 262.890
13. Decreased fetal movements O36.8190
14. Toxic effects of ketones, undetermined, initial encounter T52.4X4A
15. Newborn affected by maternal nutritional disorder P00.4
16. Low weight gain in pregnancy, third trimester O26.13

KEYSTONE ISSUE

1. Premature separation of placenta, third trimester O45.93

EXHIBIT 11.3 FRAMING

An adolescent female at 36 weeks gestation with high levels of anxiety, agitation, restlessness who is uncooperative

EXHIBIT 11.4 PRESENT STATE

1. Generalized abdominal pain 10/10 × 3 hours
2. Moderate amount of bright red vaginal bleeding
3. Gravida 2, para 0
4. Fetal heart rate of 170 beats per minute with repetitive late decelerations
5. 1-cm dilated, 30% effaced, and vertex ballotable
6. Positive urine drug screen for cocaine

monitoring device, no postsurgical complications, and urine drug screen. Testing is concurrent and iterative as one gets closer and closer in successive increments toward goal achievement. Some key questions to ask here are: How is the advanced practice nurse defining *testing*? On what scales will the desired outcome be rated? How will the advanced practice nurse know when the desired targeted outcomes are achieved?

EXHIBIT 11.5 OUTCOME STATE

1. Pain control
2. Hemodynamic stability
3. Delivery of healthy newborn
4. Fetal viability
5. Emergent C-section with positive recovery
6. Substance use control

EXHIBIT 11.6 TESTING

1. Pain scale rating
2. Pad count
3. Apgar score
4. Fetal monitoring device
5. Monitor for surgical complications
6. Urine drug screen

EXHIBIT 11.7 REFLECTION ON CLINICAL REASONING

What clinical decisions or interventions help to achieve the outcomes?

What specific intervention activities will you implement?

Why are you considering these activities?

The reflection box at the top of Figure 11.2 (Exhibit 11.7) reminds the advanced practice nurse of the thinking strategies used for the patient situation. These strategies also help make explicit many of the relationships among ideas and issues associated with the patient problems. Examples of reflection questions that support and engage patient-centered systems thinking are listed in Table 11.3.

Finally, the judgment space on the far left-hand side of the model (Exhibit 11.8) offers the place to write in the results of the conclusions drawn from the CCCR model. Based on the degree of gap or comparison of where the patient is, and where the health care team wants the patient to be, there may or may not be an evidence gap. Once there is evidence that fills that gap, the nurse has to attribute meaning to the data. Making judgments about clinical issues is about the meaning the advanced practice nurse attributes to the evidence derived from the test or gap analysis of present to desired state. Complexity thinking, team-centered systems-thinking and organization-centered systems-thinking skills are used by the care coordination team at this point to evaluate and judge the successes or deficits from the plan of care. Interprofessional team activity requires negotiation of the competing values of collaborating, creating, competing, and controlling, and involves managing shared

TABLE 11.3 Patient-Centered Systems-Thinking Reflection Questions

SELF-REGULATION ACTIVITIES	REFLECTION QUESTIONS

Monitoring thinking	I. **Reflect on the thinking processes you used with the care coordination of this case.**
	1. The baseline needs I identify in this case are.... I think I can identify future adjustments in the plan of care by.... If I have difficulty I...
	2. When I think about my feelings during the care coordination of this case, I describe them as...and I handle them by...
	3. When I try to remember or understand important facts to develop the plan of care, coach, and educate the patient/family I...
	4. As I look back on meaningful activities, the resources I could have spent:
	  a. More time on...
	  b. Less time on...

Monitoring the environmental	II. **Reflect on the environmental circumstances you encountered in the care coordination of this case.** 5. When I prepare to carry out coaching and education activities for care coordination, I... 6. When I think about particular distractions to facilitating medical care services and supports for care coordination, I... 7. When I work and communicate with interprofessional partners for care coordination of this case, I... 8. If I had the chance to redo the care coordination activities, I would do... instead of... because...

Monitoring behavioral	III. **Reflect on your behaviors and reactions to the care coordination of this case.**
	9. My impression of my performance in evaluating capacity, energy, support, readiness, and skills to organize and manage the plan of care, I...
	10. I make sure I will update the needs assessment and individualized plan of care by... and if I need to make changes, I...
	11. I make sure I empower the patient/family for self-management of health care needs by...and if I need to make changes, I...
	12. Reaction to care coordination of this case...
	  a. My reaction to what I like about the care coordination of this case...
	  b. My reaction to what I do not like about the care coordination of this case...
	Optional prompt: Other comments I have about the care coordination of this case...

Adapted from Kuiper, Pesut, and Kautz (2009).

knowledge; acknowledgment of values impacted; and the brokering, directing, coordinating, and monitoring of practice issues, interventions, and outcomes. The judgments made in this case are made by the team after the care coordination essential needs outcomes are evaluated. Each of the items in the judgment column corresponds to an essential need addressed in the CCCR systems model (Figure 11.3). Some key questions to ask are: Given the testing, what are the clinical judgments? Have the outcomes been achieved? Does the situation need to be reframed?

EXHIBIT 11.8 JUDGMENTS RELATED TO CARE COORDINATION VARIABLES

PLAN OF CARE

Emergent C-section

SAFETY

Prevent complications; minimize cocaine withdrawal effects in mother and newborn

NEEDS

Ongoing monitoring, education, resources, support, drug rehabilitation and counseling, and safe home (shelter)

CAPACITY

Support and empower with knowledge and resources available

SKILLS

Support, adherence to regimen

RESOURCES

Identify support systems and available resources

SELF-MANAGEMENT

Drug rehabilitation and counseling, safe home, and support system

Once the advanced practice nurse has experience coordinating care for acute care patients, the cases become part of a clinical reasoning learning history, which become prototypes or schemas for other similar cases. These schemas and experience build on each other over time and result in the development of pattern recognition for future clinical reasoning applications. If the situation results in a negative judgment, or progress is not being made to transition patients from present to desired states, the advanced practice nurse may have to reframe the situation, reconsider the keystone priority, reconsider the care coordination activities, and/or consult with members of the interprofessional team for the problem to be solved and the outcome to be achieved. The key question to ask here is: How will this clinical learning experience impact future reasoning about similar cases?

CARE COORDINATION USING CCCR MODEL WORKSHEETS

The next step in the nursing diagnostic reasoning process is to augment the plan of care to include activities related to interprofessional care planning using the CCCR model framework (Exhibit 11.9) that builds on the OPT model of clinical reasoning.

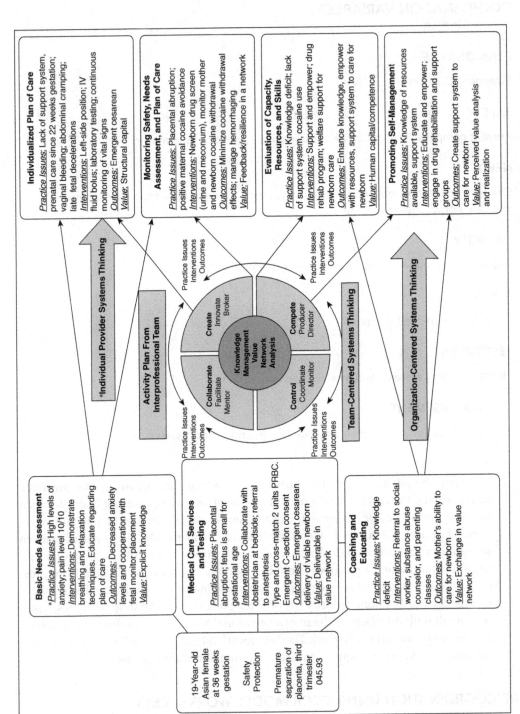

FIGURE 11.3 Care Coordination Clinical Reasoning systems model worksheet.

[a] Practice Issues can come from any discipline: nursing, medicine, pharmacy, social work, and so on.

IV, intravenous; PRBC, packed red blood cells.

EXHIBIT 11.9 CARE COORDINATION CLINICAL REASONING DEFINITION

The authors define *care coordination clinical reasoning* as the application of critical, creative, systems, and complexity thinking to determine the practice issues, interdependencies, and interconnections of role relationships for collaborative work in service of caring for people to address problems, interventions, and outcomes through time and across health care contexts and services.

The systems dynamics and interactions between and among the patient issues determine the care needed and the services provided. The complexities in this case are the issues related to Sarah's lack of social support, substance abuse, noncompliance with taking prenatal vitamins, and adhering to prenatal care. The CCCR systems model web (Figure 11.4) visually represents the complexities in this case along with the essential care coordination practice issues that need attention to organize thinking that focuses on the patient's priority needs.

The CCCR systems model web (Exhibit 11.10) provides a blueprint for consideration of the care coordination practice issues so clinicians can determine interventions, outcomes, and the value exchange that supports safe, high-quality care. This process involves patient-centered systems thinking, team-centered systems thinking, and organization-centered systems thinking to thoroughly and efficiently manage all aspects of patient cases. The steps to create the web for this case start in the center, with the patient description and medical diagnoses (Sarah Chinn is a 19-year-old pregnant Asian female who lives alone), priority nursing domain (safety protection), and ICD-10 code (premature separation of placenta, third trimester 045.93), which show the overlap of patient issues that must be addressed by the advanced practice nurse, obstetrician, and the care coordination interprofessional team.

Next, each large circle in this web represents the essential care coordination practice issues with evidence and defining characteristics for this patient story: needs assessment (decrease anxiety level, explanation of procedures with possible reasons for presenting symptoms, manage pain level); individualized plan of care (lack of support system; offer to call support person); medical care services and testing (intravenous fluids, bedside ultrasound to rule out placental abruption, laboratory testing, oxygen at 10 L nonrebreather mask); evaluation of capacity, resources, and skills (lack of support system); monitoring and safety (continuous electronic fetal monitoring, maternal vital signs, pad count, and intake and output); team collaboration (collaboration and communication among family, nurse practitioner, obstetrician, staff nurse); coaching and educating (coaching with relaxation and breathing methods); and self-management (knowledge of resources available, illicit drug-use cessation).

The provider then reflects on the total picture on the worksheet and begins to draw lines of relationship, connection, or association among the essential needs. As directional lines are drawn to create the web, functional relationships between and among the needs are recognized. Clinical reasoning and thinking processes are used to explain and justify the reasons for connecting these care coordination needs as central supporting elements in the patient's story based on an analysis and synthesis of possible priorities, as represented in the web. The priority care coordination

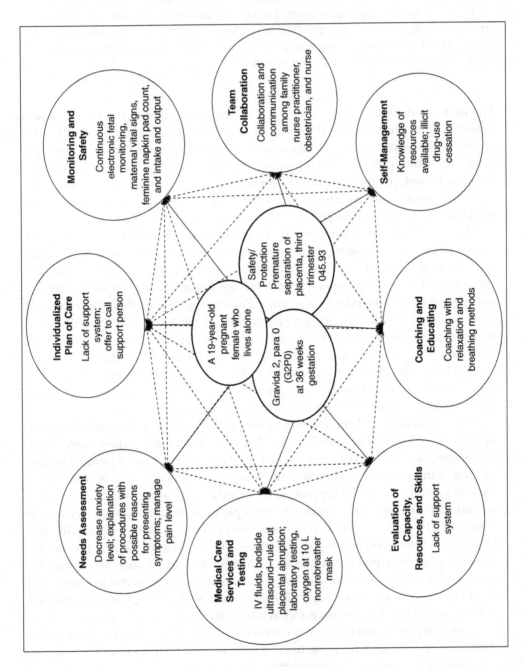

FIGURE 11.4 Care Coordination Clinical Reasoning systems model web.

IV, intravenous.

EXHIBIT 11.10 CCCR SYSTEMS MODEL WEB DEFINITION

The Care Coordination Clinical Reasoning systems model web enables one to visually represent the complexities and essential care coordination practice issues that need attention so as to organize thinking that focuses on the patient's and/or family's priority needs within the context of services provided within and between health care delivery systems.

needs that would most efficiently and effectively represent the key issues of the patient are addressed that align with the patient story. A key question to ask is: Does the CCCR systems model web provide a comprehensive consideration of the most pertinent evidence for care coordination practice issues?

The CCCR systems model worksheet (see Figure 11.3) is the next worksheet in the framework designed to provide a graphic representation or visual map of the structure of the CCCR systems model and help guide team-centered and organization-centered systems thinking. Some key questions to ask are: What clinical decisions and interventions will help to achieve the outcomes identified on the OPT model of clinical reasoning (see Figure 11.2)? What specific interventions will the clinicians and members of the team implement? Why are providers considering these activities?

Writing each element on the worksheet shows how parts of the model relate to each other. In Figure 11.3, on the far left-hand side, there is space to write the description of the patient's health care situation that was at the center of the CCCR systems model web. Three essential needs are placed in the first boxes to the right of the description and include basic needs assessment, medical care services and testing, and coaching and education. Each of the care coordination needs identified in this model includes practice issues, interventions, outcomes, and value specification.

From patient-centered systems-thinking processes used to create the OPT clinical reasoning model worksheets for this patient story, the identified basic needs practice issues include high levels of anxiety and pain (10/10). Targeted interventions for the team would be to demonstrate breathing and relaxation techniques and educate regarding the plan of care. The documented desired outcomes would be anxiety control and cooperation with fetal monitor placement. A key question to ask is: Have the basic needs been identified, given the frame of the situation? Consider the value-impact analysis in this case using the questions from Table 11.4.

KNOWLEDGE MANAGEMENT AND VALUE ANALYSIS

The explicit value for role clarity, collaboration, and interaction of the team placed on the needs assessment is explicit knowledge. From Table 11.4, the value-networking reflection question for basic needs is: What knowledge is codified and conveyed to others through dialogue, demonstration, or media? Name three knowledge classification systems that could be used to represent the patient characteristics in this case:

1.
2.
3.

TABLE 11.4 Value Definitions and Reflection Questions

Deliverable	The specific values or objects that are conveyed from one role or participant to another role or participant. What are the deliverables that you offer and expect of others?
Exchange	Two or more transactions between two or more roles or participants that evoke reciprocity. A process in which one role as agent receives resources from another role or agent and provides resources in return. What are the resource exchanges between roles or participants on your interprofessional health care team?
Explicit knowledge	The knowledge that is codified and conveyed to others through dialogue, demonstration, or media. What is the explicit knowledge shared among members of the team?
Feedback	The return of information about the impact of an activity. It can also mean the return of a portion of the output of a process as new input. What feedback is returned about activities or outputs in your care coordination activities? How does feedback influence team dynamics and goal attainment?
Human capital/ competence	The knowledge, skills, and competencies that reside in individuals who work in an organization or that are embedded in the organization's internal and external social networks. What human capital resources are needed in order for care coordination in your context to be successful?
Impact analysis	An assessment of how an input for a role is handled. What are the tangible/intangible costs, gains, or values from the input that generate a response or activity, or increases/decreases tangible assets?
Knowledge management	The degree to which the team facilitates and support processes for creating, sustaining, sharing, and renewing organizational knowledge in order to generate social or economic gain or improve performance. Who is responsible and how is knowledge managed in the care coordination process?
Perceived value	The degree of value participants feel they receive from individual deliverables that can come from roles, participants, or the network. What are the value-added dimensions of individual, collective, team, and organizational networks?
Resilience	The degree to which the network is able to reconfigure to respond to changing conditions and then return to original form. What is the resilience capacity of the team and organization in which you work?
Structural capital	The infrastructure, routines, concepts, models, information systems, work systems, and business processes that support productivity and sustainability. To what degree do the structural capital and infrastructure support interprofessional team work and care coordination processes?
Systems thinking	An analysis and synthesis of the forces and interrelationships that shape the behavior of systems? To what degree do members of the team think about the system dynamics at the patient, group, team, or organizational levels?
Value realization	The degree to which tangible or intangible values, turn the input into gains, benefits, capabilities, or assets that contribute to the success of an individual, group, organization, or network (Allee, 2008). To what degree do members of the team intentionally negotiate and manage competing values related to collaborating, creating, competing, and or controlling?

Adapted from Allee, Schwabe, and Babb (2015).

From team-centered systems-thinking processes used for the basic needs assessment, the identified medical care services and testing practice issues include placental abruption and fetus that is small for gestational age. Targeted interventions for the team are collaboration with the obstetrician at the bedside, referral to anesthesia, type and cross match for two units of blood, and emergent C-section consent. The documented desired outcomes are to emergent cesarean delivery of viable newborn. A key question to ask is: Does the testing and interventions sufficiently manage the primary care needs? The explicit value for role clarity, collaboration, and interaction of the team placed on the medical care services and testing is to deliver evidence-based interventions based on the health care provider role. From Table 11.4, the value-networking reflection question for medical care services and testing basic needs is: What is the specific value or object that is conveyed from one role or participant to another role or participant? Name three deliverables that are essential for the care coordination success of this case:

1.
2.
3.

Organization-centered systems thinking is used by the team for enhancing coaching and educating the patient. The identified coaching and educating practice issues include knowledge deficit of current health status. Targeted interventions for the team are referral to a social worker, referral to a substance abuse counselor, and parenting classes. The documented desired outcomes are to have the mother be able to care for the newborn. A key question to ask is: Does the content and methods for coaching and teaching match the patient cognitive abilities and understanding? From Table 11.4, the value-networking reflection question for educating and coaching involves evaluating the transactions between two or more roles or participants where one role as an agent receives resources from another role or agents and provides resources in return. The question would be: What is the exchange of resources and information between the providers and the patient regarding medication and available resources? Name three resources that could be exchanged between the providers and patient in this case:

1.
2.
3.

The diagram in the center of the worksheet is the activity plan from the interprofessional team (Exhibit 11.11). The team engages in collaborating, creating, competing, and controlling dynamics through communication (Quinn, Bright, Faerman, Thompson, & McGrath, 2014; Quinn, Heynoski, Thomas, & Spreitzer, 2014; Quinn & Quinn, 2015; Quinn & Rohrbough, 1983) to manage essential areas of organizational culture to realize the intangible value exchanges used to develop and manage an activity plan that considers interventions from the individualized plan of care, monitoring processes, evaluation of patient and family capacity with regard to resources and skills, and promotion of self-management. For example, in terms of collaboration, people must understand themselves and communicate honestly and effectively. Individuals mentor and develop

EXHIBIT 11.11

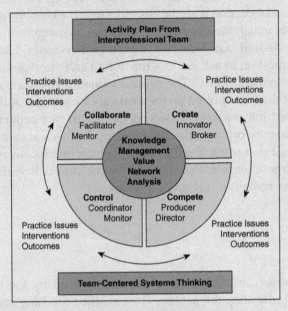

Key questions to consider for the four dimensions of the competing-values framework in the CCCR model.

- What are the desired outcomes in this case?
- What are the values I expect of myself and others?
- How are the feelings of the patient, family, and team considered in this case?
- What strategies could the team use to coordinate care?

others collaboratively and know how to participate and lead teams. Often this knowledge requires encouraging and managing constructive conflict. Competition enhances productivity and profitability. In this domain, vision and goal setting are a path to motivating self and others so that systems can be developed and organized to get results. Creating and promoting the adoption of new ideas or clinical innovations requires attention to judicious use of power and ethics as well as championing new ideas and innovations through negotiating commitments and agreements for implementing and sustaining change. Control contributes to the development of stability and continuity as people work and manage across functions, organize information exchange, measure and monitor performance and quality, and enable compliance.

Key ingredients to team-centered systems thinking are that the members must be purpose centered, internally directed, other focused, and externally open to negotiation and communication surrounding competing values (Quinn, 2015; Quinn & Quinn, 2015). The activity plan from the interprofessional team in the CCCR model is guided by these principles and will promote the development of positive organizations and relationships. Each team member should be externally open to challenges, feedback and freedom from labels, higher performance, and the cultivation and development of communities of practice. When this outcome is challenged and false fixed, some team members are valued more than others in the context of competitive versus collaborative goals. Being other influenced cultivates empathy, rapport, energy, and calmness. Together, the team members feel safe and secure enough to take risks and act with trust, integrity, and resilience. Creating such a culture supports a spirit of inquiry, learning, and experimentation, which results in higher performance. Such behavior requires the activation of a reflective self in contrast to automatic self-justification and reactive modes of being and communicating. In order to be a positive influence and bring a state of leadership to the team, each member of the team needs to be vigilant about being purpose centered, choosing goals that create focus, energy, and meaning for the team. A focused purpose-centered team is likely to attract and create resources related to the reasoning required to communicate across settings to achieve CCCR goals.

The activity plan from the interprofessional team iteratively visits the practice issues, which include communication among providers specific to this case; targeted interventions that are updated at team meetings across the contexts in which the providers are interacting; and documents the desired outcomes to maintain team support and to keep the team equally informed about patient status. A key question to ask is: Are the communication processes in place and do they promote information exchange between and among the interprofessional health team members? The explicit value for role clarity, collaboration, and interaction of the team placed on the activity plan from the interprofessional team is determined by knowledge management and value impact analysis. From Table 11.4, the value-networking reflection questions for the activity plan from the interprofessional team are: What are the tangible/intangible costs, gains, or values from the input that generate a response or activity, or increases/decreases tangible assets? How does the team facilitate and support processes for collaborating, controlling, creating, and competing to sustain, share, and renew organizational knowledge in order to generate social or economic gain or improve performance? Name a cost, gain, and value that would be generated from the activity plan of the team for this case:

1.
2.
3.

To the far right of the CCCR system model worksheet are four essential care coordination needs that evolve from the activity plan from the interprofessional team stemming from patient-centered systems thinking, team-centered systems thinking, and organizational-centered systems thinking. These needs include the individualized plan of care; monitoring safety, needs assessment, and plan of care; evaluating capacity, resources, and skills; and promoting self-management. Each of these care coordination essentials is defined as well by practice issues, interventions, outcomes, and values.

The patient-centered systems-thinking and team-centered systems-thinking activities are used for the individualized plan of care. The identified practice issues revolve around the lack of support system, lack of prenatal care since 22 weeks gestation, vaginal bleeding, abdominal cramping, and late fetal decelerations. Targeted interventions for the provider and team are left-side positioning, administering intravenous fluids, laboratory testing, and continuous monitoring of vital signs.

The documented desired outcomes are to carry out an emergent cesarean. Some key questions to ask are: Does the individualized plan of care include team collaboration? Is there any input that was not yet considered? Are there providers who were overlooked? The explicit value for role clarity, collaboration, and interaction of the provider and team placed on the individualized plan of care is on structural capital. From Table 11.4, the value-networking reflection question for the individualized plan of care is: What are the infrastructure, routines, concepts, models, information systems, work systems, and business processes that support productivity and have sustainability? Name three routines, systems, or processes that support and sustain the productivity of the care coordination in this case:

1.
2.
3.

From the patient-centered systems-thinking and team-centered systems-thinking processes used for monitoring safety, needs assessment, and plan of care, identified practice issues include placental abruption and positive maternal cocaine avoidance. Targeted interventions for the team are to carry out a screen for newborn urine and meconium, and monitor mother and newborn for cocaine withdrawal. The documented desired outcomes are to minimize cocaine withdrawal effects and manage hemorrhage in the mother. A key question to ask is: Does the plan of care promote safety and meet the patient needs? The explicit value for role clarity, collaboration, and interaction of the team placed on monitoring safety, needs assessment, and plan of care is to obtain feedback and assess resilience in the network. From Table 11.4, the value-networking reflection questions for medical care services and testing basic needs are: What feedback is returned about activities or outputs? Was the network able to reconfigure itself to respond to changing conditions and then return to its original form? Name three areas of need and/or safety that were reassessed to determine whether the plan of care needed to be adjusted:

1.
2.
3.

Organization-centered systems-thinking processes, such as coaching and education, are used by the team from to evaluate capacity, resources, and skills. The identified practice issues include knowledge deficit, lack of support systems, and cocaine use. Targeted interventions for the team are to support and empower, enrollment in a drug rehabilitation program, and welfare support for newborn care. The documented desired outcomes are to enhance knowledge and empower with resources and support systems to care for the newborn. A key question to ask is: Do the interventions in the plan of care require skilled help and/or can the patient manage care needs independently? The explicit value for role clarity, collaboration, and interaction of the team placed on evaluating capacity, resources, and skills is identifying human capital and competence. From Table 11.4, the value-networking reflection question for educating and coaching involves evaluating the transactions between two or more roles or participants in which one role as an agent receives resources from another role or agent and provides resources in return. The question would be: What is the exchange of resources and information between the providers and the patient regarding available resources? Name three exchanges of resources, skills, or information with the patient that are essential to the care coordination success of this case:

1.

2.

3.

Organization-centered systems-thinking processes, such as coaching and education, are used by the team to promote self-management. The identified practice issues include knowledge of resources available to the patient and support systems. Targeted interventions for the team are to educate and empower the patient, engage the patient in drug rehabilitation, and make the patient aware of support groups. The documented desired outcomes are to create a support system to care for the newborn. A key question to ask is: Is the patient able to identify the resources he or she needs and navigate the health care system? The explicit value for role clarity, collaboration, and interaction of the team placed on promoting self-management is perceived-value realization. From Table 11.4, the value-networking reflection question for promoting self-management is: What is the level of value that roles or participants feel they receive from individual deliverables, which can come from roles, participants, or the network? Name three examples of learned self-management that resulted from the care coordination of this case:

1.

2.

3.

With the use of the CCCR systems model, the advanced practice nurse and other providers address practice issues by using and developing evidence-based interventions, implementing measures of adherence, and evaluating processes and outcomes. This requires clinical reasoning at different levels of perspective—the individual patient needs, interprofessional team contributions, and attention to the systems in which people work and provide care. These practice issues, interventions, and outcomes for patient care coordination stem from the National Quality Forum (NQF, 2010a, 2010b) and the Agency for Healthcare Research and Quality (AHRQ, 2014).

As the center of attention for health care needs is managed by webs of relationships between and among providers, each interaction supports a specific value exchange as the participant's partner for successful outcomes (Allee, 2003). The dynamic relationships that occurred, for this acute care patient who will return home alone, with the advanced practice nurse, labor and delivery staff, obstetrician, social worker, substance abuse counselor, and support groups for the homeless were collaborative, trusting, dynamic, and interdependent. Application of the competing-value competencies will relate to collaboration, creating, competing, and controlling, and help make explicit knowledge shared and managed to support innovation, coordination, and directing care. Through the use of the electronic health record, connectivity impacted the value networking with greater access to knowledge and information. This process provided quick and effective feedback among team members for the complex needs this patient had related to complications from a high-risk pregnancy.

CLINICAL JUDGMENTS AND CCCR

The final phase of the clinical reasoning process is to determine whether outcomes were met and if care coordination activities were successful. The CCCR model of clinical reasoning is revisited for the final phase of care coordination, when judgments are made about achieving outcomes from the interprofessional team activity plan (see Exhibit 11.8). The worksheet (see Figure 11.2) is revisited to make judgments about the care coordination essentials (needs, individualized plan of care; safety; capacity, resources, skills, and self-management). Shifting to the next level of perspective, using team-centered systems and organization-centered systems-thinking activities, collaboration, and coordination of the plan of care, reveals ongoing planning and evaluation to provide appropriate patient support. The goal is to provide a supportive environment with the appropriate resources for this homeless 19-year-old Asian adolescent female. Her pregnancy, delivery, and drug abuse should be managed initially on entry into the health care system. Discharge planning from the hospital should include resource personnel to help her manage postnatal and newborn care. The patient will need education about abstaining from illicit cocaine use and be empowered to use resources to maintain a healthy and safe environment for herself and the baby. These resources lead to the best possible management and safety for this homeless patient.

Some remaining questions may arise as the evaluation of outcomes occurs, such as: Can the organization provide continuing resources and reach care coordination outcomes for this patient? Were communication and the feedback loop effective between the health care providers and the patient? Did the complexity of the system hinder or enhance the achievement of outcomes? How do the competencies of the competing-values framework support the interprofessional dialogue and reasoning about the care coordination of this particular case? How do members of the team share and manage knowledge in service of care coordination? The advanced practice nurse as care coordinator views all the systems and is the key informant to communicate with the team regarding the efficiency and effectiveness of the processes for care outcomes. Judgments are made about whether the outcomes from case management have been achieved, and the information is recycled back to revise or enhance the plan of care.

The thinking processes used by the advanced practice nurse and other health care providers while implementing the CCCR systems model are promoted through monitoring of thinking, the environment, and behaviors for goal attainment (Zimmerman & Schunk, 2001). The courses of action chosen to manage issues and ensure that this patient remained safe revolve around behaviors and actions taken, thinking processes used, and environmental structuring. Critical reflective questions that can be used to prompt clinical reasoning to make judgments about the achievement of patient outcomes are listed in Table 11.5. Critical-, creative-, and systems-thinking processes are used for total care coordination, flow from

TABLE 11.5 Team-Centered and Organization-Centered Systems-Thinking Reflection Questions

SELF-REGULATION ACTIVITIES	REFLECTION QUESTIONS

Monitoring thinking	**I. Reflect on the thinking processes the team used to navigate organizational systems for care coordination of this case.**
	1. The baseline needs identified by the team in this case are…. Adjustments in the plan of care for future successes include…. Difficulties were resolved by…
	2. Team reactions during the care coordination of this case in regard to organizational systems could be described as… and they were handled by…
	3. When the team was dealing with important facts to develop the plan of care, coach, and educate the patient/family about organizational systems it …
	4. Looking back on meaningful activities, the resources the team could have spent:
	   a. More time on…
	   b. Less time on…

Monitoring the environmental	**II. Reflect on the environmental circumstances you encountered in the care coordination of this case.** 5. When the team prepares to carry out coaching and education activities for care coordination, it… 6. When the team considers particular distractions in the organization that impede medical care services and supports for care coordination, it… 7. When the team works and communicates with organizational partners for care coordination of this case, it… 8. If the team had the chance to redo the care coordination activities, it would do… instead of… because …

Monitoring behavioral	**III. Reflect on your behaviors and reactions to the care coordination of this case.**
	9. Impressions of the team performance in evaluating capacity, energy, support, readiness, and skills to organize and manage the plan of care within organizational systems are…
	10. The team ensures that it will update the needs assessment and individualized plan of care by… and if it needs to make changes, it…
	11. The team makes sure it empowers the patient/family to navigate through organizational systems for management of health care needs by… and if it needs to make changes, it…
	12. The team reaction to care coordination of this case…
	   a. Reaction to what it likes about the navigation of organizational systems to facilitate the care coordination of this case…
	   b. Reaction to what it did not like about the navigation of organizational systems to facilitate the care coordination of this case…
	Optional prompt: Other comments about the care coordination of this case…

Adapted from Kuiper, Pesut, and Kautz (2009).

patient-centered systems (Table 11.3), team-centered systems thinking (Table 11.5), and organization-centered systems thinking (Table 11.5) for case management.

SUMMARY

The clinical reasoning challenge for acute care begins with a description and understanding of the patient's story. The thinking strategies used in this case attempt to provide a safe and health-promoting environment for a young single mother and her baby. As the providers practice self-monitoring, self-evaluation, and self-correction, successful strategies are employed, and flaws in thinking are corrected as they collaborate and align interventions for patient success. The OPT clinical reasoning model provides the foundation and structure for clinical reasoning and systems thinking within an individual patient situation. The OPT structure and process can be used at several levels for care planning by the provider, by the team, and by the organization to discern alignment and coordination of care activities. The CCCR systems model provides the structure for clinical reasoning for the care coordination essential needs and their related practice issues, interventions, outcomes, and values.

KEY CONCEPTS

1. Clinical reasoning for care coordination with a maternity patient with a high-risk pregnancy can be promoted with a framework that includes structure, content, and process.
2. A supporting framework for CCCR extends case management using patient-centered systems thinking and the OPT clinical reasoning model across levels of perspective that also includes team-centered systems thinking and organization-centered systems thinking to align care coordination activities.
3. The process of CCCR involves critical reflection for the individual provider and team.
4. Value-network analysis helps to define and describe the unique contributions that individual providers make to CCCR efforts supported through knowledge management and value-impact analysis.
5. A supporting framework for CCCR is completed by attending to the organization-centered systems thinking to make judgments about care coordination essentials.

STUDY QUESTIONS AND ACTIVITIES

1. Describe in your own words the benefits and processes of using the CCCR systems model with a maternity patient.
2. Using the CCCR systems model, identify the care coordination essential needs of maternity cases.

3. To what degree can you explicitly identify and describe the value exchanges associated with care coordination in obstetric situations?

4. How can an interprofessional team use the competencies of the competing values of collaboration, creating, competing, and controlling to ensure efficiency and effectiveness of care coordination? How does your team negotiate roles of mentor, broker, director, and coordinator?

5. Identify all the possible standardized health care languages and communication strategies that could be considered in an acute care case. Does language impact on communication and the patient outcomes? How does a discipline-specific framework influence the feedback, decisions, and outcomes with maternity care?

6. Identify the relationship between critical reflection and thinking strategies as they are applied to the three levels of system-thinking perspectives that are required—patient, individual provider, team, and organization. What unique reflections are required to focus on team and organizational function with maternity patients?

REFERENCES

Agency for Healthcare Research and Quality (AHRQ). (2014). *What is care coordination? Care coordination measures atlas update*. Rockville, MD: Author. Retrieved from http://www.ahrq.gov/professionals/prevention-chronic-care/improve/coordination/index.html

Allee, V. (2003). *The future of knowledge: Increasing prosperity through value networks*. Burlington, MA: Butterworth-Heinemann.

Allee, V. (2008). Value network analysis and value conversion of tangible and intangible assets. *Journal of Intellectual Capital, 9*(1), 5–24.

Allee, V., Schwabe, O., & Babb, M. K. (Eds.). (2015). *Value networks and the true nature of collaboration*. Tampa, FL: Megher–Kifer Press ValueNet Works and Verna Allee Associates.

Haas, S. A., Swan, B. A., & Haynes, T. S. (2014). *Care coordination and transition management core curriculum*. Pitman, NJ: American Academy of Ambulatory Care Nursing. ICD10Data.com. Retrieved from http://www.icd10data.com/ICD10CM/Codes

Kuiper, R., Pesut, D., & Kautz, D. (2009). Promoting the self-regulation of clinical reasoning skills in nursing students. *Open Nursing Journal, 3*, 76–85. Retrieved from http://www.ncbi.nlm.nih.gov/pmc/articles/PMC2771264

National Quality Forum. (2010a). *Preferred practices and performance measures for measuring and reporting care coordination: A consensus report*. Washington, DC: Author.

National Quality Forum. (2010b). *Quality connections: Care coordination*. Washington, DC: Author.

Pesut, D. J. (2008). Thoughts on thinking with complexity in mind. In C. Lindberg, S. Nash, & C. Lindberg (Eds.), *On the edge: Nursing in the age of complexity* (pp. 211–238). Bordentown, NJ: Plexus Press.

Quinn, R. (2015). *The positive organization: Breaking free from conventional cultures, constraints, and beliefs*. Oakland, CA: Berrett-Koehler.

Quinn, R. E., Bright, D., Faerman, S. R., Thompson, M. P., & McGrath, M. R. (2014). *Becoming a master manager: A competing values approach*. Hoboken, NJ: John Wiley & Sons.

Quinn, R. E., Heynoski, K., Thomas, M., & Spreitzer, G. M. (2014). *The best teacher in you: How to accelerate learning and change lives*. San Francisco, CA: Berrett-Koehler.

Quinn, R., & Quinn, R. E. (2015). *Lift: Becoming a positive force in any situation*. San Francisco, CA: Berrett-Koehler.

Quinn, R. E., & Rohrbough, J. (1983). A spatial model of effectiveness criteria: Towards a competing values approach to organizational analysis. *Management Science, 29,* 363–377.

World Health Organization. (2015). *Manual of the International Classification of Diseases and related health problems* (10th rev. ed.). Geneva, Switzerland: Author. Retrieved from http://www.icd10data.com/

Zimmerman, B., & Schunk, D. S. (2001). *Self-regulated learning and academic thought.* Mahwah, NJ: Lawrence Erlbaum.

CHAPTER 12

CARE COORDINATION FOR A NEONATAL PATIENT

In this chapter, we use the Care Coordination Clinical Reasoning (CCCR) systems model as described in Part I and explain how the model can be used to reason about a primary care neonatal case. The advanced practice nurse is working with a mother who is in need of support services and education to promote quality outcomes for a preterm newborn. The provider–clinic is the point of access for patients–families. The advanced practice nurse provides care coordination through the application and use of critical-, creative-, systems-, and complexity-thinking processes to manage patient problems with an interprofessional team to design appropriate interventions and establish patient-centered outcomes. Depending on the nature of need involved in the case, referrals to other specialty or primary care providers, community services, and living environments are determined and considered in managing care coordination and transitions (Haas, Swan, & Haynes, 2014).

The CCCR systems model framework begins with the patient story, which is derived from gathering data and evidence from an interview, history, physical examination, and the health record. The advanced practice nurse then develops an individual plan of care using the Outcome-Present State-Test (OPT) model worksheets. In order to do this, one activates the patient-centered systems-thinking skills for complex patient stories and habitually uses key questions to reflect on the specific sections of the model (Pesut, 2008), as well as the dimensions of the care coordination processes.

LEARNING OUTCOMES

After completing this chapter, the reader should be able to:

1. Explain the components of a care coordination framework that are needed to manage the problems, interventions, and outcomes of neonatal patients
2. Describe the different thinking processes that support clinical reasoning skills and strategies for determining priorities for neonatal patient care coordination

3. Define the cognitive and metacognitive self-regulatory processes that support individual provider critical reflection related to levels and perspectives associated with clinical reasoning for neonatal patient care coordination

4. Describe how the communication between interprofessional health care team members is essential for care coordination to address neonatal patient and family needs

5. Describe the critical meta-reflective processes that support team reflection related to levels and perspectives associated with the care coordination challenges and clinical reasoning required to navigate neonatal patient care plans

THE PATIENT STORY

We begin with the history and story of a 5-day-old White female baby, Ashley Ford, who was born at 36 weeks and is in the pediatric office for a weight check at 72 hours after hospital discharge. She was delivered at 2,021 g, placing her in the 10th percentile. Ashley's occipital frontal circumference (OFC) was 32.5 cm (50th percentile) and her length was 45.4 cm (25th percentile). After delivery, Ashley remained with her mother on the postpartum unit where there were no problems with blood sugar or temperature. Her weight on the day of discharge was 1,947 g (decreased 5%), and her bilirubin was 8.9 mg/dL.

The physical examination in the pediatrician's office reveals a temperature of 96.2°F rectally, heart rate of 168 beats per minute, respiratory rate of 36 breaths per minute, and oxygen saturation of 98%. Ashley's weight is 1,798 g, which is decreased by 11% from her birthweight. The rest of the examination is unremarkable except that she has jaundiced-appearing skin and a slightly depressed anterior fontanelle. Her muscle tone is normal and her neurological responses are normal. Her mother states that she breastfeeds every 4 hours during the day and every 5 hours during the night, however, she often has to wake the infant up for feedings. Ashley has had four wet diapers and one stool in the past 24 hours. Her bilirubin level in the office is 18.5 mg/dL. The mother was advised to take Ashley to the pediatric unit in the hospital for further assessment and treatment.

Laboratory values on admission to the hospital are as follows—white blood count: 8.2/mm^3 with an unremarkable differential, hemoglobin: 18.5 g/dL, hematocrit: 56%, platelets: 298,000/mcL, reticulocytes: 2.1%, blood urea nitrogen: 22 mg/dL, creatinine: 0.5 gm/dL, glucose: 78 gm/dL, potassium: 4.8 mEq/L, calcium: 8.9 mEq/L, chloride: 112 mEq/L, sodium: 151 mEq/L, aspartate aminotransferase (AST): 52 U/L, alanine aminotransferase (ALT): 24 U/L, bilirubin-total: 18.7 mg/dL (high), and bilirubin-direct: 0.3 mg/dL. Arterial blood gas analysis reveals pH: 7.34, PaO$_2$: 80 mmHg, PaCO$_2$: 39 mmHg, and HCO$_3$: 21 mEq/L. Blood cultures were also drawn and sent to the laboratory.

PATIENT-CENTERED PLAN OF CARE USING OPT WORKSHEETS

Once the story is obtained from all possible sources, care planning and clinical reasoning proceed using the OPT clinical reasoning web worksheet (Figure 12.1)

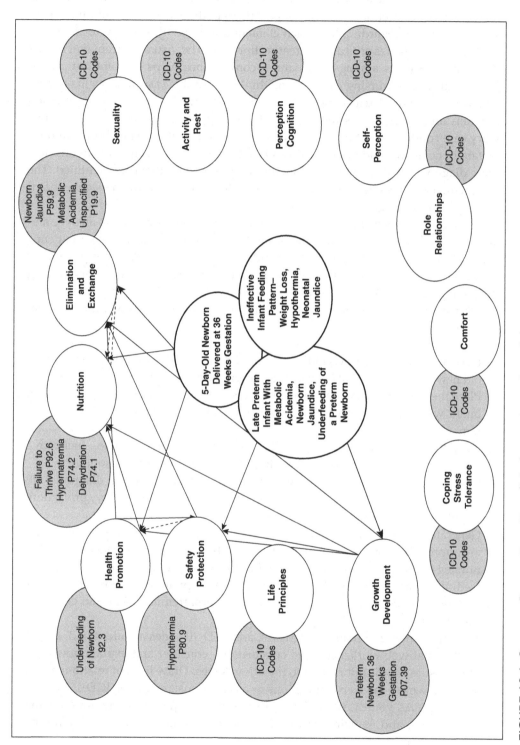

FIGURE 12.1 Outcome-Present State-Test clinical reasoning web worksheet.

ICD-10, International Classification of Diseases, 10th edition.

to help determine relationships among issues and highlight potential keystone issues. The OPT clinical reasoning web is a graphic representation of the functional relationships between and among diagnostic hypotheses derived from the analysis and synthesis regarding how each element and issue of the story relate to one another. This activates critical and creative thinking. The visual diagram that results illustrates dynamics among issues and a convergence helps to point out central issues that require nursing care. As one thinks about this case, and begins to spin and weave a clinical reasoning web, relationships are identified among nursing domains and diagnoses as they are combined with medical conditions. The primary care conditions in this case are a late-preterm infant with newborn jaundice, metabolic acidemia, and underfeeding. Once the advanced practice nurse considers these diagnoses, the nursing care domains associated with them are identified. The complementary nursing diagnoses most impacted in this case are ineffective infant feeding pattern–weight loss, hypothermia, and neonatal jaundice.

To spin and weave the web, the provider uses thinking processes to analyze and synthesize relationships among diagnostic hypotheses associated with a patient's health status. The visual representation and mapping of these relationships support the development of systems thinking and making connections between and among the medical and nursing diagnoses under consideration, given the patient story.

The steps to the creation of the OPT clinical reasoning web using the worksheet are as follows:

1. Place a general description of the patient in the respective middle circle—5-day-old newborn delivered at 36 weeks gestation (Ashley Ford).
2. Place the major medical diagnoses in the respective middle circle—Late-preterm infant with metabolic acidemia, newborn jaundice, and underfeeding of a preterm infant.
3. Place the major nursing diagnoses in the respective middle circle—ineffective infant feeding pattern—weight loss, hypothermia, and neonatal jaundice.
4. Choose the nursing domains for which each medical and nursing diagnoses are appropriate—elimination and exchange, health promotion, safety/protection, growth and development, and nutrition.
5. Generate all the International Classification of Diseases-10 (ICD-10) codes that are appropriate for the particular patient and family story that coincide with the nursing domains—newborn jaundice (P59.9), metabolic acidemia (P19.9), underfeeding of a newborn (P92.3), hypothermia (P80.9), preterm newborn at 36 weeks gestation (P07.39), failure to thrive (P92.6), hypernatremia (P74.2), and dehydration (P74.1).
6. Once the nursing domains, diagnoses, and ICD-10 codes are identified, reflect on the total web worksheet, and concurrently consider and explain how each of the issues is or is not related to the other issues. Draw lines of relationship to spin and weave the web connections or associations among the ICD-10 codes/diagnoses. As you draw the lines, think out loud, justify the reasons for the connections, and explain specifically how the diagnoses may or may not be connected or related.
7. After you have spent some time connecting the relationships, determine which domain/domains have the highest priority for care coordination and most

efficiently and effectively represent the keystone nursing care needs of the patient by counting the arrows that connect the medical problems (ICD-10 codes). In this case, counting six lines (Table 12.1) pointing to or from the nursing domains of elimination and exchange and health promotion represents the priority present-state keystone issue, which result from a late-preterm infant with metabolic acidemia, newborn jaundice, and underfeeding.

8. Look once again at the sets of relationships and determine the theme or keystone that summarizes the patient-in-context or the patient story—the problems related to elimination and exchange and health promotion are the keystone issues for this case.

The OPT clinical reasoning web worksheet offered in Figure 12.1 shows a template with the patient health care situation, medical diagnoses, and nursing diagnoses in the center. Around the outer edges of the web are nursing domains with ICD-10 codes derived from history and physical assessment associated with the patient story. The directional arrows that create the web effect represent connections, explanations, and functional relationships between and among the diagnostic possibilities. As one can see, the domains and ICD-10 codes with more connections converging on one of the circles display the priority problem or keystones, in this case elimination and exchange and health promotion. A keystone issue is one or more central supporting elements of the patient's story that help focus and determine a root cause or center of gravity of the system dynamics and helps guide reasoning and care coordination based on an analysis (breaking things down into discrete parts) and synthesis (putting the parts together in a greater whole) of diagnostic possibilities as represented in the web. A key question to ask here is: How does the clinical reasoning web reveal relationships between and among the identified diagnoses and to what degree do these relationships make practical clinical sense according to the evidence and patient story? Table 12.1 shows a summary of the connections highlighting the priority with the most connections.

TABLE 12.1 Relationships Among Nursing Domains, Medical Diagnoses, and Web Connections

NURSING DOMAINS	MEDICAL DIAGNOSES (ICD-10 CODES)	WEB CONNECTIONS
Elimination and exchange	Newborn jaundice P59.9 Metabolic acidemia P19.9	6
Health promotion	Underfeeding of newborn P92.3	6
Safety/protection	Hypothermia P80.9	5
Growth and development	Preterm newborn 36 weeks gestation P07.39	5
Nutrition	Failure to thrive P92.6 Hypernatremia P74.2 Dehydration P74.1	5

Source: World Health Organization (2015).

TABLE 12.2 Questions That Guide the Use of the OPT Model

Patient-in-context	What is the patient story?
Diagnostic cue/web logic	What diagnoses have you generated?
	What outcomes do you have in mind, given the diagnoses?
	What evidence supports those diagnoses?
	How does a reasoning web reveal relationships among the identified problems (diagnoses)?
	What keystone issue(s) emerge?
Framing	How are you framing the situation?
Present state	How is the present state defined?
Outcome state	What are the desired outcomes?
	What are the gaps or complementary pairs (~) of outcomes and present states?
Test	What are the clinical indicators of the desired outcomes?
	On what scales will the desired outcomes be rated?
	How will you know when the desired outcomes are achieved?
	How are you defining your testing in this particular case?
Decision making (interventions)	What clinical decisions or interventions help to achieve the outcomes?
	What specific intervention activities will you implement?
	Why are you considering these activities?
Judgment	Given your testing, what is your clinical judgment?
	Based on your judgment, have you achieved the outcome or do you need to reframe the situation?
	How, specifically, will you take this experience and learning with you into the future as you reason about similar cases?

OPT, Outcome-Present State-Test.

Adapted from Pesut (2008).

After considering the full picture using the clinical reasoning web worksheet, the next step is to use the OPT clinical reasoning model worksheet to facilitate and structure the patient-centered systems thinking about the care coordination of the identified problems highlighted in Table 12.1. As the advanced practice nurse thinks about the patient, he or she will concurrently consider the frame, outcome state, and present state. Each aspect of the OPT clinical reasoning model contributes to the other. The OPT clinical reasoning model worksheet is a map of the structure designed to provide an illustrative representation and guide thinking processes about relationships between and among competing issues and problems. Some questions that guide the use of the OPT clinical reasoning model are shown in Table 12.2 (Pesut, 2008).

By writing each element on the worksheet, all the parts of the model become related to each other. As the health care provider moves from right to left, the model structures the plan of care. Critical thinking skills are used to consider the

EXHIBIT 12.1 PATIENT-IN-CONTEXT STORY

A 5-year-old White preterm female infant (Ashley Ford) with a diagnosis of weight loss, newborn jaundice, and metabolic acidemia. She shows an 11% weight loss since discharge from the hospital and she has signs and symptoms of dehydration at the 72-hour postdischarge checkup in the pediatrician's office. She has only had four to five wet diapers and one stool in the past 24 hours. Her skin appears jaundiced and she has a depressed anterior fontanelle. She is admitted to an acute care pediatric unit in the hospital for further assessment and treatment of dehydration.

Significant laboratory data—bilirubin: 18.5 mg/dL, weight: 1,798 g, pH: 7.34

patient story and creative thinking is used to identify and reason about the keystone issues/themes/cues to determine the most significant evidence in the present state. Complexity thinking helps the provider to consider the outcomes desired and the gaps between the present and outcomes states. Once interventions and tests are decided, the plan of care transitions over to a care coordination model and team-centered systems thinking that considers patient and family preferences within the frame of the situation.

The patient-in-context story (Exhibit 12.1) is on the far right-hand side, as depicted in Figure 12.2. The advanced practice nurse notes relevant facts of the story, which, in this case, include the patient demographics and characteristics; 5-year-old female late-preterm infant presenting to the pediatrician's office for a routine 72-hour posthospital discharge. She has a diagnosis of weight loss, newborn jaundice, and metabolic acidemia. Her failure to thrive has placed her in the case load of a pediatric nurse practitioner who is to assist the mother in making some primary care decisions about admitting her to the hospital for further assessment and treatment. Significant laboratory data show a total bilirubin of 18.5 mg/dL, pH of 7.34, and sodium of 151 mEq/L. The mother has been breastfeeding every 4 to 5 hours, but the baby has only had four wet diapers and one stool in the past 24 hours. The skin appears jaundiced and there is a depressed anterior fontanelle. Assessment and treatment of Ashley's fluid status need acute care attention at this time. A key point at this juncture is to review and reflect on the patient story for accuracy and thoroughness to proceed appropriately with care planning for care coordination.

Moving to the left of the worksheet, there is a place to list the diagnostic cluster cue on the web of medical diagnoses and ICD-10 codes (Exhibit 12.2). At the bottom of this box are placed the designated keystone issues or themes that fall under the most significant nursing domain—weight loss P92.3, newborn jaundice P59.9, and metabolic acidemia P19.9. Remember diagnostic cluster cue web logic is the use of inductive and deductive thinking skills. Some key questions to ask here are: What diagnoses were generated? Is there evidence to support those diagnoses? Is the keystone issue appropriate, given this patient story?

In the center and background of the worksheet are places to indicate the frame or theme that best represents the background issues regarding thinking about the patient story (Exhibit 12.3). The frame of this case is a 5-day-old female preterm

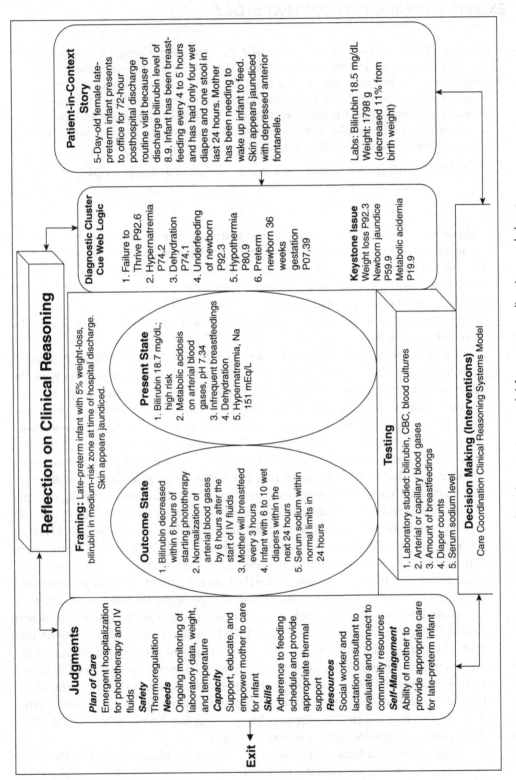

FIGURE 12.2 Outcome–Present State-Test clinical reasoning model for care coordination worksheet.

CBC, complete blood count; IV, intravenous.

EXHIBIT 12.2 DIAGNOSTIC CLUSTER CUE WEB LOGIC

1. Failure to thrive P92.6
2. Hypernatremia P74.2
3. Dehydration P74.1
4. Underfeeding of newborn P92.3
5. Hypothermia P80.9
6. Preterm newborn 36 weeks gestation P07.39

KEYSTONE ISSUE/THEME

1. Weight loss P92.3
2. Newborn jaundice P59.9
3. Metabolic acidemia P19.9

EXHIBIT 12.3 FRAMING

A 5-day-old preterm infant presents with a 5% weight loss, bilirubin in the medium-risk zone at the time of hospital discharge, and jaundiced skin.

infant with a 5% weight loss and bilirubin level in the medium-risk zone at the time of hospital discharge. Her skin appears jaundiced. This helps to organize the present state and outcome state, illustrates the gaps, and provides insights about what tests need to be considered to fill the gap. Decision making and reflection surround the framing as the advanced practice nurse thinks of many things simultaneously. Reflective thinking is used to monitor thinking and behavior. A key question to ask here is: How do I frame the situation and does it agree with the patient–family view of the situation?

At the center of the sheet are spaces to place the present state (Exhibit 12.4) and outcome state (Exhibit 12.5) side by side. The present state in this case shows five primary health care problems related to keystone issue—bilirubin: 18.7 mg/dL, metabolic acidosis pH: 7.34, infrequent breastfeedings, dehydration, and hypernatremia—sodium 151 mEq/L. The outcome state (Exhibit 12.5) shows five matching goals to be achieved through care coordination: bilirubin decreased within 6 hours of starting phototherapy, normalization of arterial blood gases by 6 hours after the start of intravenous fluids, mother breastfeeding every 3 hours, 6 to 10 wet diapers within the next 24 hours, and serum sodium within normal limits within 24 hours. Putting the two states together creates a gap analysis that naturally shows where the patient is and what the goals are in terms of the patient's care. Some key questions to ask here are: Are the outcomes appropriate given the diagnoses? Are there gaps between the outcomes and present state? Are there clinical indicators of the desired outcome state?

EXHIBIT 12.4 PRESENT STATE

1. Bilirubin: 18.7 mg/dL (high risk)
2. Metabolic acidosis pH: 7.34
3. Infrequent breastfeedings
4. Dehydration
5. Hypernatremia—sodium: 151 mEq/L

EXHIBIT 12.5 OUTCOME STATE

1. Bilirubin decreased within 6 hours of phototherapy
2. Normalization of arterial blood gases
3. Mother breastfeeds every 3 hours
4. Infant has 6 to 10 wet diapers within the next 24 hours
5. Serum sodium within normal limits within 24 hours

EXHIBIT 12.6 TESTING

1. Laboratory studies: bilirubin, complete blood count (CBC), blood cultures
2. Arterial blood gases
3. Number of breastfeedings in 24 hours
4. Diaper counts
5. Serum sodium level

The gap between where the patient is and where the advanced practice nurse wants the patient to be is one way to create a test (Exhibit 12.6). Clinical decisions are choices made about interventions that will help the patient transition from present state to a desired outcome state. As interventions are tested, the advanced practice nurse evaluates the degree to which outcomes are or are not being achieved. The tests chosen in this case include bilirubin levels, CBC, blood cultures, arterial blood gases, hourly spacing of breastfeedings, diaper counts, and serum sodium levels.

Testing is concurrent and iterative as one gets closer and closer with successive increments toward goal achievement. Some key questions to ask here are: How is the advanced practice nurse defining *testing*? On what scales will the desired outcome be rated? How will the advanced practice nurse know when the desired targeted outcomes are achieved?

The reflection box at the top of Figure 12.2 (Exhibit 12.7) reminds the advanced practice nurse of the thinking strategies used for the patient situation. These strategies also help make explicit many of the relationships among ideas and issues associated with the patient problems. Examples of clinical reasoning reflection questions that could be used during patient-centered systems thinking are listed in Table 12.3.

EXHIBIT 12.7 REFLECTION ON CLINICAL REASONING

What clinical decisions or interventions help to achieve the outcomes?

What specific intervention activities will you implement?

Why are you considering these activities?

TABLE 12.3 Patient-Centered Systems-Thinking Reflection Questions

SELF-REGULATION ACTIVITIES	REFLECTION QUESTIONS

Monitoring thinking	I. **Reflect on the thinking processes you used with the care coordination of this case.**
	 1. The baseline needs I identify in this case are.... I think I can identify future adjustments in the plan of care by.... If I have difficulty I...
	 2. When I think about my feelings during the care coordination of this case, I describe them as...and I handle them by...
	 3. When I try to remember or understand important facts to develop the plan of care, coach, and educate the patient/family I....
	 4. As I look back on meaningful activities, the resources I could have spent:
	    a. More time on....
	    b. Less time on....

Monitoring the environment	II. **Reflect on the environmental circumstances you encountered in the care coordination of this case.** 5. When I prepare to carry out coaching and education activities for care coordination, I... 6. When I think about particular distractions to facilitating medical care services and supports for care coordination, I... 7. When I work and communicate with interprofessional partners for care coordination of this case, I... 8. If I had the chance to redo the care coordination activities, I would do... instead of... because ...

Monitoring behavior	III. **Reflect on your behaviors and reactions to the care coordination of this case.**
	 9. My impression of my performance in evaluating capacity, energy, support, readiness, and skills to organize and manage the plan of care, is...
	 10. I make sure I will update the needs assessment and individualized plan of care by... and if I need to make changes, I....
	 11. I make sure I empower the patient–family for self-management of health care needs by...and if I need to make changes, I...
	 12. Reaction to care coordination of this case...
	    a. My reaction to what I like about the care coordination of this case...
	    b. My reaction to what I do not like about the care coordination of this case...
	 Optional prompt: Other comments I have about the care coordination of this case...

Adapted from Kuiper, Pesut, and Kautz (2009).

EXHIBIT 12.8 JUDGMENTS RELATED TO CARE COORDINATION VARIABLES

PLAN OF CARE

Emergent hospitalization for phototherapy and intravenous fluids

SAFETY

Thermoregulation

NEEDS

Ongoing monitoring of laboratory data, weight, and temperature

CAPACITY

Support, educate, and empower the mother to care for her infant

SKILLS

Adhere to feeding schedule and provide thermal support

RESOURCES

Social worker, lactation consultant, and community resources

SELF-MANAGEMENT

Mother able to provide appropriate care for late-preterm infant

Finally, the judgment space on the far left-hand side of the worksheet (Exhibit 12.8) is the place to write in the results of the conclusions drawn from the CCCR model. The degree of gap or comparison of where the patient is, and where the health care team wants the patient to be, determines whether there is a gap in the evidence. Once there is evidence that fills that gap, the nurse has to attribute meaning to the data. Making judgments about clinical issues is about the meaning the advanced practice nurse attributes to the evidence derived from the test or gap analysis of the present to he desired state. Complexity thinking, team-centered systems-thinking, and organization-centered systems-thinking skills are used by the care coordination team at this point to evaluate and judge the successes or deficits from the plan of care. Interprofessional team activity requires negotiation and communication about competing values of collaboration—creating, competing, and controlling—and involves managing shared knowledge; acknowledgment of values impacted; and the brokering, directing, coordinating, and monitoring of practice issues, interventions, and outcomes. The judgments in this case are made by the team after the care coordination essential needs outcomes are evaluated. Each of the items in the judgment column corresponds to an essential need addressed in the CCCR systems model (Figure 12.3). Some key questions to ask here are: Given the

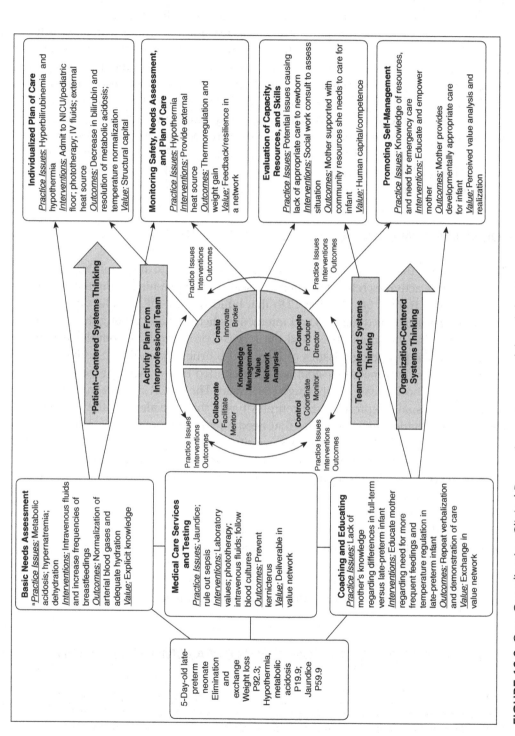

FIGURE 12.3 Care Coordination Clinical Reasoning systems model worksheet.

[a] Practice Issues can be from any discipline: nursing, medicine, pharmacy, social work, and so on.

IV, intravenous; NICU, neonatal intensive care unit.

testing, what are the clinical judgments? Have the outcomes been achieved? Does the situation need to be reframed?

Once the advanced practice nurse has experience coordinating care for neonatal patients, the cases become part of a clinical reasoning learning history, which become prototypes or schemas for other, similar cases. These schemas and experience build on each other over time and result in the development of pattern recognition for future clinical reasoning applications. If the scenario results in negative judgments, or progress is not being made to transition patients from present to desired states, the advanced practice nurse may have to reframe the situation, reconsider the keystone priority, reconsider the care coordination activities for the problem to be solved, and the outcome to be achieved. The key question to ask here is: How will the advanced practice nurse specifically take this clinical-learning experience into the future to reason about similar cases?

CARE COORDINATION USING CCCR MODEL WORKSHEETS

The next step in the nursing diagnostic reasoning process is to augment the plan of care to include activities related to interprofessional care planning using the CCCR systems model framework (Exhibit 12.9) that builds on the OPT model of clinical reasoning. The systems dynamics and interactions between and among the patient issues determine the care needed and the services provided. The complexities in this care are the physiologic issues of increased bilirubin, jaundice, possible sepsis, dehydration, and metabolic acidosis compounded by the fact that the mother does not know how to care for this high-risk infant. The CCCR systems model web (Figure 12.4) visually represents the complexities in this case along with the essential care coordination practice issues that need attention to organize thinking that focuses on the patients' and/or family's priority needs.

The CCCR systems model web (Exhibit 12.10) provides a blueprint for consideration of the care coordination practice issues so that clinicians can determine interventions, outcomes, and the value exchange that supports safe, high-quality care. This process involves patient-centered systems thinking, team-centered systems thinking, and organizational-centered systems thinking to thoroughly and efficiently manage all aspects of patient and family cases. The steps to create the web for this case start in the center with the patient description and medical diagnoses (5-day-old late-preterm female infant, Ashley Ford, with newborn jaundice, metabolic acidemia, and underfeeding), priority nursing domains (elimination and exchange and

EXHIBIT 12.9 CARE COORDINATION CLINICAL REASONING DEFINITION

The authors define *care coordination clinical reasoning* as the application of critical, creative, systems, and complexity thinking to determine the practice issues, interdependencies, and interconnections of role relationships for collaborative work in service of caring for people to address problems, interventions, and outcomes through time and across health care contexts and services.

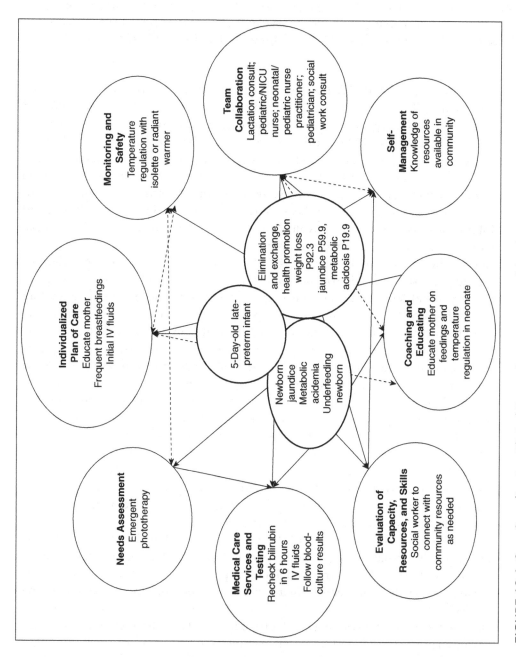

FIGURE 12.4 Care Coordination Clinical Reasoning systems model web.

IV, intravenous; NICU, neonatal intensive care unit.

EXHIBIT 12.10 CCCR SYSTEMS MODEL WEB DEFINITION

The Care Coordination Clinical Reasoning systems model web enables one to visually represent the complexities and essential care coordination practice issues that need attention so as to organize thinking that focuses on the patient's and/or family's priority needs within the context of services provided within and between health care delivery systems.

health promotion), and ICD-10 codes (weight loss P92.3, jaundice P59.9, and metabolic acidosis P19.9) that show the overlap of patient issues that must be addressed by the advanced practice nurse and the care coordination interprofessional team.

Next, each large circle in this web represents the essential care coordination practice issues with evidence and defining characteristics for this patient story: needs assessment (emergent phototherapy); individualized plan of care (education to mother for frequent breastfeedings, initial treatment intravenous fluids); medical care services and testing (recheck bilirubin in 6 hours, intravenous fluids, and follow blood-culture results); evaluation of capacity, resources, and skills (social worker to connect mother with community resources as needed); monitoring and safety (temperature regulation with isolette or radiant warmer); team collaboration (lactation consultant, pediatric/neonatal intensive care nurse, pediatric nurse practitioner, pediatrician, and social worker); coaching and educating (educate mother on feeding schedule and temperature regulation in the neonate); and self-management (knowledge of resources available to the mother in the community).

The provider then reflects on the total picture on the worksheet and begins to draw lines of relationship, connection, or association among the essential needs. As directional lines are drawn to create the web, functional relationships between and among the needs are recognized. Clinical reasoning and thinking processes are used to explain and justify the reasons for connecting these care coordination needs as central supporting elements in the patient's story based on an analysis and synthesis of possible priorities as represented in the web. The priority care coordination needs that would most efficiently and effectively represent the key issues of the patient are addressed that align with the patient story. A key question to ask is: Does this CCCR systems model web provide a comprehensive consideration of the most pertinent evidence for care coordination practice issues?

The CCCR systems model worksheet (see Figure 12.3) is the next worksheet in the framework designed to provide a graphic representation or visual map of the structure of the CCCR systems model and helps guide team-centered systems and organization-centered systems thinking. Some key questions to ask are: What clinical decisions and interventions will help to achieve the outcomes identified on the OPT model of clinical reasoning (see Figure 12.2) What specific interventions will the advanced practice nurse and/or the team implement? Why consider these activities?

Writing each element on the worksheet shows how parts of the model relate to each other. In Figure 12.3, on the far left-hand side, there is space to write the description of the patient's health care situation that was at the center of the CCCR systems model web. Three essential needs are placed in the first boxes to the right of the description and include basic needs assessment, medical care services and testing, and coaching and education. Each of the care coordination needs identified in this model includes practice issues, interventions, outcomes, and value specification.

From patient-centered systems-thinking processes used to create the OPT clinical reasoning model worksheets for this patient story the identified basic needs practice issues include metabolic acidosis, hypernatremia, and dehydration. Targeted interventions for the team would be to administer intravenous fluids and increase the frequency of breastfeedings. The documented desired outcomes would be normalization of arterial blood gases and adequate hydration. A key question to ask is: Have the basic needs been identified, given the frame of the situation? Consider the value-impact analysis in this case, using the questions from Table 12.4.

KNOWLEDGE MANAGEMENT AND VALUE ANALYSIS

The explicit value for role clarity, collaboration, and interaction of the team placed on the needs assessment is explicit knowledge. From Table 12.4, the value-networking reflection question for basic needs is: What knowledge is codified and conveyed to others through dialogue, demonstration, or media? Name three knowledge classification systems that could be used to represent the patient characteristics in this case:

1.
2.
3.

From team-centered systems-thinking processes used for the basic needs assessment, the identified medical care services and testing practice issues include suspicion of jaundice and need to rule out sepsis. Targeted interventions for the team are monitoring laboratory values, phototherapy, intravenous fluids, and to follow blood cultures. The documented desired outcomes are to prevent kernicterus. A key question to ask is: Do the testing and interventions sufficiently manage the primary care needs? The explicit value for role clarity, collaboration, and interaction of the team placed on the medical care services and testing is to deliver evidence-based interventions based on the health care provider role. From Table 12.4, the value-networking reflection question for medical care services and testing basic needs is: What is the specific value or object that is conveyed from one role or participant to another role or participant? Name three deliverables that are essential for the care coordination success of this case:

1.
2.
3.

Organization-centered systems thinking is used by the team to enhance coaching and education of the patient and family. The identified coaching and educating practice issues include inform the mother regarding differences in full- versus late-preterm infant care. Targeted interventions for the team are to educate the mother regarding need for more frequent breastfeedings and temperature regulation in the

TABLE 12.4 Value Definitions and Reflection Questions

Deliverable	The specific values or objects that are conveyed from one role or participant to another role or participant. What are the deliverables that you offer and expect of others?
Exchange	Two or more transactions between two or more roles or participants that evoke reciprocity. A process in which one role as agent receives resources from another role or agent and provides resources in return. What are the resource exchanges between roles or participants on your interprofessional health care team?
Explicit knowledge	The knowledge that is codified and conveyed to others through dialogue, demonstration, or media. What is the explicit knowledge shared among members of the team?
Feedback	This is the return of information about the impact of an activity. It can also mean the return of a portion of the output of a process as new input. What feedback is returned about activities or outputs in your care coordination activities? How does feedback influence team dynamics and goal attainment?
Human capital/ competence	The knowledge, skills, and competencies that reside in individuals who work in an organization or that are embedded in the organization's internal and external social networks. What human capital resources are needed in order for care coordination in your context to be successful?
Impact analysis	An assessment of how an input for a role is handled. What are the tangible/intangible costs, gains, or values from the input that generate a response or activity, or increase/decrease tangible assets?
Knowledge management	The degree to which the team facilitates and supports processes for creating, sustaining, sharing, and renewing organizational knowledge in order to generate social or economic gain or improve performance. Who is responsible and how is knowledge managed in the care coordination process?
Perceived value	The degree of value participants feel they receive from individual deliverables that can come from roles, participants, or the network. What are the value-added dimensions of individual, collective, team, and organizational networks?
Resilience	The degree to which the network is able to reconfigure to respond to changing conditions and then return to original form. What is the resilience capacity of the team and organization in which you work?
Structural capital	The infrastructure, routines, concepts, models, information systems, work systems, and business processes that support productivity and sustainability. To what degree does the structural capital and infrastructure support interprofessional teamwork and care coordination processes?
Systems thinking	An analysis and synthesis of the forces and interrelationships that shape the behavior of systems? To what degree do members of the team think about the system dynamics at the patient, group, team, or organizational levels?
Value realization	The degree to which tangible or intangible values turn the input into gains, benefits, capabilities, or assets that contribute to the success of an individual, group, organization, or network (Allee, 2008). To what degree do members of the team intentionally negotiate and manage competing values related to collaborating, creating, competing, and or controlling?

Adapted from Allee, Schwabe, and Babb (2015).

late-preterm infant. The documented desired outcomes are to repeat verbalization from the mother regarding the teaching and demonstration of appropriate care. A key question to ask is: Do the content and methods for coaching and teaching match the patient and family cognitive abilities and understanding? From Table 12.4, the value-networking reflection question for educating and coaching involves evaluating the transactions between two or more roles or participants in which one role as an agent receives resources from another role or agent and provides resources in return. The question would be: What is the exchange of resources and information between the providers and the patient and family regarding medication and available resources? Name three resources that could be exchanged between the providers and family and patient in this case:

1.
2.
3.

The diagram in the center of the worksheet is the activity plan from the interprofessional team (Exhibit 12.11). The team engages in collaborating, creating, competing, and controlling dynamics through communication (Quinn, Bright, Faerman, Thompson, & McGrath, 2014; Quinn, Heynoski, Thomas, & Spreitzer, 2014; Quinn & Quinn, 2015; Quinn & Rohrbough, 1983) to manage essential areas of organizational culture to realize the intangible value exchanges used to develop and manage an activity plan that considers interventions from the individualized plan of care, monitoring processes, evaluation of patient and family capacity with regard to resources and skills, and promotion of self-management. For example, in terms of collaboration, people must understand themselves and communicate honestly and effectively. Individuals mentor and develop others collaboratively and know how to participate and lead teams. Often this knowledge requires encouraging and managing constructive conflict. Competition enhances productivity and profitability. In this domain, vision and goal setting are a path to motivating self and others so that systems can be developed and organized to get results. Creating and promoting the adoption of new ideas or clinical innovations require attention to judicious use of power and ethics as well as championing new ideas and innovations through negotiating commitments and agreements for implementing and sustaining change. Control contributes to the development of stability and continuity as people work and manage across functions, organize information exchange, measure and monitor performance and quality, and enable compliance.

Key ingredients to team-centered systems thinking are that the members must be purpose centered, internally directed, other focused, and externally open to negotiation and communication surrounding competing values (Quinn, 2015; Quinn & Quinn, 2015). The activity plan from the interprofessional team in the CCCR model is guided by these principles and will promote the development of positive organizations and relationships. Each team member should be externally open to challenges, feedback, and freedom from labels, higher performance, and the cultivation and development of communities of practice. When this outcome is challenged and false fixed, some team members are valued more than others in the context of competitive versus collaborative goals. Being other influenced cultivates

EXHIBIT 12.11

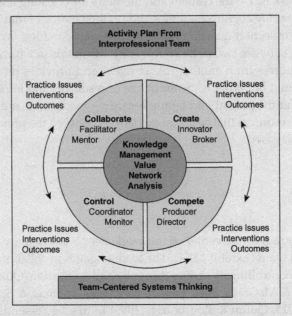

Key questions to consider for the four dimensions of the competing-values framework in the CCCR model.

- What are the desired outcomes in this case?
- What are the values I expect of myself and others?
- How are the feelings of the patient, family, and team considered in this case?
- What strategies could the team use to coordinate care?

empathy, rapport, energy, and calmness. Together, the team members feel safe and secure enough to take risks and act with trust, integrity, and resilience. Creating such a culture supports a spirit of inquiry, learning, and experimentation, which results in higher performance. Such behavior requires the activation of a reflective self in contrast to automatic self-justification and reactive modes of being and communicating. In order to be a positive influence and bring a state of leadership to the team, each member of the team needs to be vigilant about being purpose centered, choosing goals that create focus, energy, and meaning for the team. A focused purpose-centered team is likely to attract and create resources related to the reasoning required to communicate across settings to achieve CCCR goals.

The activity plan from the interprofessional team iteratively visits the practice issues that include communication between providers specific to this case, targeted interventions that are updated at team meetings across the contexts in which the providers are interacting, and documents the desired outcomes to maintain team support and keep the team equally informed about patient status. A key question to ask is: Are the communication processes in place and do they promote information exchange between and among the interprofessional health team members? The explicit value for role clarity, collaboration, and interaction of the team placed on the activity plan from the interprofessional team is determined by knowledge management and value impact analysis. From Table 12.4, the value-networking reflection questions for the activity plan from the interprofessional team are: What are the tangible/intangible costs, gains, or values from the input that generate a response or activity, or increase/decrease tangible assets? How does the team facilitate and support processes for collaborating, controlling, creating, and competing to sustain, share, and renew organizational knowledge in order to generate social or economic gain or improve performance? Name a cost, gain, and value that would be generated from the activity plan of the team for this case:

1.
2.
3.

To the far right of the CCCR system model worksheet are four essential care coordination needs that evolve from the activity plan from the interprofessional team stemming from patient-centered systems thinking, team-centered systems thinking, and organization-centered systems thinking. These needs include the individualized plan of care; monitoring safety, needs assessment, and plan of care; evaluating capacity, resources, and skills; and promoting self-management. Each of these care coordination essentials is defined as well by practice issues, interventions, outcomes, and values.

The patient-centered systems-thinking and team-centered systems-thinking activities are used for the individualized plan of care. The identified practice issues revolve around hyperbilirubinemia and hypothermia. Targeted interventions for the provider and team are to admit to an acute care pediatric unit, phototherapy, intravenous fluids, and use of an external heat source. The documented desired outcomes are to decrease the bilirubin levels, resolve the metabolic acidosis, and normalize thermoregulation. Some key questions to ask are: Does the individualized plan of care include team collaboration? Is there any input that was not yet considered? Are there providers who were overlooked? The explicit value for role clarity, collaboration, and interaction of the provider and team placed on the individualized plan of care is on structural capital. From Table 12.4, the value-networking reflection question for the individualized plan of care is: What are the infrastructure, routines, concepts, models, information systems, work systems, and business processes that support productivity and have sustainability? Name three routines, systems, or processes that support and sustain the productivity of the care coordination in this case:

1.
2.
3.

From the patient-centered systems-thinking and team-centered systems-thinking processes used for monitoring safety, needs assessment, and plan of care, identified practice issues include hypothermia. Targeted interventions for the team are to provide an external heat source. The documented desired outcomes are for thermoregulation and weight gain. A key question to ask is: Does the plan of care promote safety and meet patient and family needs? The explicit value for role clarity, collaboration, and interaction of the team placed on monitoring safety, needs assessment, and plan of care is to obtain feedback and assess resilience in the network. From Table 12.4, the value-networking reflection questions for medical care services and testing basic needs are: What feedback is returned about activities or outputs? Was the network able to reconfigure itself to respond to changing conditions and then return to its original form? Name three areas of need and/or safety that were reassessed to determine whether the plan of care needed to be adjusted:

1.
2.
3.

Organization-centered systems-thinking processes, such as coaching and education, are used by the team to evaluate capacity, resources, and skills. The identified practice issues include the identification of potential issues causing lack of appropriate care to the preterm newborn. Targeted interventions for the team are to consult with social work to assess the environment in which the mother and infant reside. The documented desired outcomes are to support the mother with community resources needed to care for the infant. A key question to ask is: Do the interventions in the plan of care require skilled help and/or can the patient and family manage care needs independently? The explicit value for role clarity, collaboration, and interaction of the team placed on evaluating capacity, resources, and skills is identifying human capital and competence. From Table 12.4, the value-networking reflection question for educating and coaching involves evaluating the transactions between two or more roles or participants in which one role as an agent receives resources from another role or agent and provides resources in return. The question would be: What is the exchange of resources and information between the providers and the patient and family regarding medication and available resources? Name three exchanges of resources, skills, or information with the patient and family that are essential to the care coordination success of this case.

1.
2.
3.

Organization-centered systems-thinking processes, such as coaching and education, are used by the team to promote self-management. The identified practice issues include knowledge of resources and the need for emergency care. Targeted interventions for the team are to educate and empower the mother. The documented desired outcomes are to have the mother provide developmentally appropriate care for the infant. A key question to ask is: Are the patient and family able to identify the resources they need and navigate the health care system? The explicit value for role clarity, collaboration, and interaction of the team placed on promoting self-management is perceived value realization. From Table 12.4, the value-networking reflection question for promoting self-management is: What is the level of value that roles or participants feel they receive from individual deliverables, which can come from roles, participants, or the network? Name three examples of learned self-management that resulted from the care coordination of this case:

1.
2.
3.

With the use of the CCCR systems model, the advanced practice nurse and other providers address practice issues by using and developing evidence-based interventions, implementing measures of adherence, and evaluating processes and outcomes. This requires clinical reasoning at different levels of perspective—the individual patient needs, interprofessional team contributions, and attention to the systems in which people work and provide care. These practice issues, interventions, and outcomes for patient and family care coordination stem from the National Quality Forum (NQF, 2010a, 2010b) and the Agency for Healthcare Research and Quality (AHRQ, 2014).

As the center of attention for health care needs is managed by webs of relationships between and among providers, each interaction supports a specific value exchange as the participant's partner for successful outcomes (Allee, 2003). The dynamic relationships that occurred for this neonatal patient in the acute care facility with the pediatric nurse practitioner, pediatric/neonatal intensive care nurse, pediatrician, social worker, lactation consultant, and mother were collaborative, trusting, dynamic, and interdependent. Application of the competing-value competencies will relate to collaboration, creating, competing, and controlling, and help make explicit knowledge shared and managed to support innovation, coordination, and directing. Through the use of the electronic health record, connectivity impacted the value networking with greater access to knowledge and information. This process provided quick and effective feedback among team members for the complex needs this patient had related to neonatal failure to thrive.

CLINICAL JUDGMENTS AND CCCR

The final phase of the clinical reasoning process is to determine whether outcomes were met and whether care coordination activities were successful. The OPT model of clinical reasoning is revisited for the final phase of care coordination during which judgments are made about achieving outcomes from the interprofessional team activity plan (see Exhibit 12.8). The worksheet (see Figure 12.2) is revisited to make judgments about the care coordination essentials (needs, individualized plan of care; safety; capacity, resources, skills, self-management). Shifting to the next level of perspective, using team-centered systems and organization-centered systems-thinking activities, collaboration and coordination of the plan of care reveal ongoing planning and evaluation to provide appropriate patient and family support during this emergent situation with a preterm infant. The goal is to provide normalization of fluid status, acid–base balance, thermoregulation, and education of the mother. The appropriate community resources need to be identified and the home environment for the family should be assessed. Family support is needed to educate about appropriate care of the preterm newborn. Resources identified for this case would be the pediatric nurse practitioner, pediatrician, social worker, lactation consultant, and community resources. These resources lead to the best possible management of this emergent situation for this infant patient and self-management by the mother delivering appropriate care.

Some remaining questions may arise as the evaluation of outcomes occurs, such as: Can the organizations provide continuing resources and reach care coordination outcomes for this patient? Were communication and feedback loops effective between the health care providers and the mother? Did the complexity of the system hinder or enhance the achievement of outcomes? How do the competencies of the competing-values framework support interprofessional dialogue and reasoning about the care coordination of this particular case? The advanced practice nurse as care coordinator views all the systems and is the key informant to communicate with the team regarding the efficiency and effectiveness of the processes for care outcomes. Judgments are made about whether the outcomes from case management have been achieved, and the information is recycled back to revise or enhance the plan of care.

The thinking processes used by the advanced practice nurse and other health care providers while implementing the CCCR systems model are promoted through monitoring of thinking, the environment, and behaviors for goal attainment (Zimmerman & Schunk, 2001). The courses of action chosen to manage issues and ensure that this patient remained safe revolve around behaviors and actions taken, thinking processes used, and environmental structuring. Critical reflective questions that can be used to prompt clinical reasoning to make judgments about the achievement of patient and family outcomes are listed in Table 12.5. Critical-, creative-, and systems-thinking processes are used for total care coordination, flow from patient-centered systems thinking (Table 12.3), team-centered systems thinking (Table 12.5), and organization-centered systems thinking (Table 12.5) for case management.

SUMMARY

The clinical reasoning challenge for neonatal care begins with a description and understanding of the patient's story. The thinking strategies used in this case provided a safe and health-promoting environment for an infant patient who was declining in health and exhibiting a failure to thrive. As the providers practice self-monitoring, self-evaluation, and self-correction, successful strategies are employed, and flaws in thinking are corrected as they collaborate and align interventions for patient and family success. The OPT clinical reasoning model provides the structure for clinical reasoning and systems thinking within an individual patient and family situation. The OPT structure and process can be used at several levels for care planning by the provider, by the team, and by the organization to discern alignment and coordination of care activities. The CCCR systems model provides the structure for clinical reasoning for the care coordination essential needs and their related practice issues, interventions, outcomes, and values.

TABLE 12.5 Team-Centered and Organization-Centered Systems-Thinking Reflection Questions

SELF-REGULATION ACTIVITIES	REFLECTION QUESTIONS
Monitoring thinking	I. **Reflect on the thinking processes the team used to navigate organizational systems for care coordination of this case.** 1. The baseline needs identified by the team in this case are.... Adjustments in the plan of care for future successes include.... Difficulties were resolved by... 2. Team reactions during the care coordination of this case in regard to organizational systems could be described as...and they were handled by... 3. When the team was dealing with important facts to develop the plan of care, coach, and educate the patient/family about organizational systems it... 4. Looking back on meaningful activities, the resources the team could have spent: a. More time on... b. Less time on...
Monitoring the environment	II. **Reflect on the environmental circumstances you encountered in the care coordination of this case.** 5. When the team prepares to carry out coaching and education activities for care coordination, it... 6. When the team considers particular distractions in the organizations that impede medical care services and supports for care coordination, it... 7. When the team works and communicates with organizational partners for care coordination of this case, it... 8. If the team had the chance to redo the care coordination activities, it would do... instead of... because...
Monitoring behavior	III. **Reflect on your behaviors and reactions to the care coordination of this case.** 9. Impressions of the team performance in evaluating capacity, energy, support, readiness, and skills to organize and manage the plan of care within organizational systems are.... 10. The team assures that it updates the needs assessment and individualized plan of care by...and if it needs to make changes, it... 11. The team makes sure it empowers the patient–family to navigate through organizational systems for management of health care needs by...and if the team needs to make changes, it... 12. The team reaction to care coordination of this case... a. Reaction to what it likes about the navigation of organizational systems to facilitate the care coordination of this case... b. Reaction to what it did not like about the navigation of organizational systems to facilitate the care coordination of this case... Optional prompt: Other comments about the care coordination of this case...

Adapted from Kuiper, Pesut, and Kautz (2009).

KEY CONCEPTS

1. Clinical reasoning for care coordination with neonatal patient issues can be promoted with a framework that includes structure, content, and process.
2. A supporting framework for CCCR extends case management using patient-centered systems thinking and the OPT clinical reasoning model across levels of perspective that also includes team-centered systems thinking and organization-centered systems thinking to align care coordination activities.
3. The process of CCCR involves critical reflection for the individual provider and team.
4. Value-network analysis helps to define and describe the unique contributions that individual providers make to CCCR efforts supported through knowledge management and value-impact analysis.
5. A supporting framework for CCCR is completed by attending to the organization-centered systems thinking to make judgments about care coordination essentials.

STUDY QUESTIONS AND ACTIVITIES

1. Describe in your own words the benefits and processes of using the CCCR systems model with neonatal cases.
2. Using the CCCR systems model, identify the care coordination essential needs of cases in neonatal care.
3. To what degree can you explicitly identify and describe the value exchanges associated with care coordination in preterm infant care situations. How does your team negotiate roles of mentor, broker, director, and coordinator?
4. How can an interprofessional team use the competencies of the competing values of collaboration, creating, competing, and controlling to ensure efficiency and effectiveness of care coordination? How does your team negotiate roles of mentor, broker, director, and coordinator?
5. Identify all the possible standardized health care languages and communication strategies that could be considered in a preterm infant case. Does language impact on communication and the patient outcomes?
6. Identify the relationship between critical reflection and thinking strategies as they are applied to the three levels of system-thinking perspectives that are required—individual provider, team, and organization. What unique reflections are required to focus on team and organizational function with neonatal care?

REFERENCES

Agency for Healthcare Research and Quality (AHRQ). (2014). *What is care coordination? Care coordination measures atlas update.* Rockville, MD: Author. Retrieved from http://www.ahrq.gov/professionals/prevention-chronic-care/improve/coordination/index.html

Allee, V. (2003). *The future of knowledge: Increasing prosperity through value networks.* Burlington, MA: Butterworth-Heinemann.

Allee, V. (2008). Value network analysis and value conversion of tangible and intangible assets. *Journal of Intellectual Capital, 9*(1), 5–24.

Allee, V., Schwabe, O., & Babb, M. K. (Eds.). (2015). *Value networks and the true nature of collaboration.* Tampa, FL: Megher–Kifer Press ValueNet Works and Verna Allee Associates.

Haas, S. A., Swan, B. A., & Haynes, T. S. (2014). *Care coordination and transition management core curriculum.* Pitman, NJ: American Academy of Ambulatory Care Nursing.

Kuiper, R., Pesut, D., & Kautz, D. (2009). Promoting the self-regulation of clinical reasoning skills in nursing students. *Open Nursing Journal, 3,* 76–85. Retrieved from http://www .ncbi.nlm.nih.gov/pmc/articles/PMC2771264

National Quality Forum. (2010a). *Preferred practices and performance measures for measuring and reporting care coordination: A consensus report.* Washington, DC: Author.

National Quality Forum. (2010b). *Quality connections: Care coordination.* Washington, DC: Author.

Pesut, D. J. (2008). Thoughts on thinking with complexity in mind. In C. Lindberg, S. Nash, & C. Lindberg (Eds.), *On the edge: Nursing in the age of complexity* (pp. 211–238). Bordentown, NJ: Plexus Press.

Quinn, R. (2015). *The positive organization: Breaking free from conventional cultures, constraints, and beliefs.* Oakland, CA: Berrett-Koehler.

Quinn, R., & Quinn, R. E. (2015). *Lift: Becoming a positive force in any situation.* San Francisco, CA: Berrett-Koehler.

Quinn, R. E., Bright, D., Faerman, S. R., Thompson, M. P., & McGrath, M. R. (2014). *Becoming a master manager: A competing values approach.* Hoboken, NJ: John Wiley & Sons.

Quinn, R. E., Heynoski, K., Thomas, M., & Spreitzer, G. M. (2014). *The best teacher in you: How to accelerate learning and change lives.* San Francisco, CA: Berrett-Koehler.

Quinn, R. E., & Rohrbough, J. (1983). A spatial model of effectiveness criteria: Towards a competing values approach to organizational analysis. *Management Science, 29,* 363–377.

World Health Organization. (2015). *Manual of the International Classification of Diseases and related health problems* (10th rev. ed.). Geneva, Switzerland: Author. Retrieved from http://www.icd10data.com

Zimmerman, B., & Schunk, D. S. (2001). *Self-regulated learning and academic thought.* Mahwah, NJ: Lawrence Erlbaum.

CHAPTER 13

CARE COORDINATION FOR
A PATIENT IN REHABILITATION

In this chapter, we use the Care Coordination Clinical Reasoning (CCCR) systems model as described in Part I and explain how the model can be used to reason about a case given the context of a patient in rehabilitation. The case presented in this chapter illustrates how an advanced practice nurse works with a patient who is in need of interventions during a cardiac rehabilitation process. The rehabilitation unit was prescribed for this patient after a hospital admission for chest pain and a percutaneous transluminal coronary angioplasty (PTCA) and stent placement into the left anterior descending (LAD) and circumflex (CMX) arteries. The advanced practice nurse provides care coordination through the application and use of critical-, creative-, systems-, and complexity-thinking processes to manage patient problems with an interprofessional team to design appropriate interventions and establish patient-centered outcomes. Depending on the nature of need involved in the case, referrals to other specialty or primary care providers, community services, and living environments are determined and considered in managing care coordination and transitions (Haas, Swan, & Haynes, 2014).

The CCCR systems model framework begins with the patient story, which is derived from gathering data and evidence from an interview, history, physical examination, and the health record. The advanced practice nurse then develops a patient-centered plan of care using the Outcome-Present State-Test (OPT) model worksheets. In order to do this, one activates patient-centered systems-thinking skills for complex patient stories and consistently uses key questions to reflect on the specific sections of the model (Pesut, 2008), as well as the dimensions and elements of care coordination processes.

LEARNING OUTCOMES

After completing this chapter, the reader should be able to:

1. Explain the components of a care coordination framework that are needed to manage the problems, interventions, and outcomes of rehabilitation patients managing health care issues

2. Describe the different thinking processes that support clinical reasoning skills and strategies for determining priorities and desired outcomes for the rehabilitation patient
3. Define the cognitive and metacognitive self-regulatory processes that support individual provider critical reflection related to levels and perspectives associated with clinical reasoning for the rehabilitation patient and care coordination
4. Describe how the communication and knowledge management between interprofessional health care team members are essential for care coordination to address rehabilitation patient needs
5. Describe the critical meta-reflective processes that support team reflection and value-added impact related to levels and perspectives associated with the care coordination challenges and clinical reasoning required to navigate rehabilitation patient care plans

THE PATIENT STORY

We begin with the history and story of a 45-year-old male, Derek Roberts, who presents to the cardiac rehabilitation unit after a percutaneous transluminal coronary angioplasty (PTCA) procedure with stent placement in two arteries. He was having some chest pain at work, his coworkers called 911, and he was brought to the emergency department for evaluation. He subsequently was taken to the cardiac catheterization laboratory for definitive care. After recovery in the coronary care unit, he was referred to the rehabilitation unit for cardiac conditioning and education regarding diet, exercise, medications, and lifestyle guidance to prevent further cardiovascular disease progression.

During admission to the rehabilitation unit, Derek appears tired and unmotivated to begin the rehabilitation process. His motivation is advice from his physician and encouragement from his wife "nagging him to take better care of himself." He denies being angry about his heart condition and does not understand the regimen he needs to follow to prevent further cardiac events. He reports a lot of pain at the catheter puncture site in the right groin. He is limping and having difficulty walking on the treadmill.

Mr. Roberts's past medical history includes the comorbidities of hypertension, type 2 diabetes mellitus, and sleep apnea. He is a nonsmoker at this time since quitting 5 years ago. He drinks approximately six beers per week. His social history includes that he is married and lives with a teenage son. He works full time as an auto mechanic, has returned to work, but takes the time to come to continue with cardiac rehabilitation. Current medications include Plavix 75 mg daily, aspirin 325 mg daily, Lipitor 20 mg at bedtime, lisinopril 10 mg daily, and Glucophage 500 mg three times daily.

The physical examination reveals a height of 5′ 11″, weight of 197 pounds (89.5 kg), and a body mass index (BMI) of 27.5. His lungs are clear, there are no abnormal heart sounds, and the telemetry monitor during exercise shows sinus rhythm with occasional unifocal premature ventricular contractions (PVCs). During exercise, his heart rate ranges 70 to 100 beats per minute, respiratory rate is 22 breaths per minute, and his oxygen saturation is 97%. Finger-stick blood sugar pre-exercise is 242 mg/dL, and post-exercise it is 100 mg/dL. His right groin has a large hematoma at the catheter puncture site.

Other laboratory values are as follows—nonfasting blood glucose: 240 mg/dL, sodium: 137 mEq/L, potassium: 3.9 mEq/L, total cholesterol: 179 mg/dL, low-density lipoprotein (LDL): 85 mg/dL, triglycerides: 189 mg/dL, and high-density lipoprotein (HDL):LDL ratio: 0.5.

PATIENT-CENTERED PLAN OF CARE USING OPT WORKSHEETS

Once the story is obtained from all possible sources, care planning and reasoning proceed using the OPT clinical reasoning web worksheet (Figure 13.1), which helps determine relationships among issues and highlights potential keystone issues. The OPT clinical reasoning web is a graphic representation of the functional relationships between and among diagnostic hypotheses derived from the analysis and synthesis regarding how each element of the story and issues relate to one another. This activates critical and creative thinking. The visual diagram that results illustrates dynamics among issues and a convergence helps to point out central issues that require nursing care. As one thinks about this case, and begins to spin and weave a clinical reasoning web, relationships are identified among nursing domains and diagnoses as they are jointly considered with medical conditions. The medical conditions in this case are history of hypertension, coronary artery disease, nicotine dependence in remission, type 2 diabetes mellitus, hyperglycemia, hypertriglyceridemia, difficulty walking, reaction to severe stress—unspecified, alcohol abuse, fatigue, pain in right leg, nontraumatic hematoma of soft tissue, problems in relationship with spouse, adjustment disorder with depressed mood, and sleep apnea. Once the advanced practice nurse considers these diagnoses, the nursing care domains associated with them are identified. The complementary nursing diagnoses most impacted in this case are fatigue, knowledge deficit, and ineffective self-help management.

To spin and weave the web, the provider uses thinking processes to analyze and synthesize relationships among diagnostic hypotheses associated with a patient's health status. The visual representation and mapping of these relationships support the development of patient-centered systems thinking and connections between and among the medical and nursing diagnoses under consideration, given the patient story.

The steps to the creation of the OPT clinical reasoning web using the worksheet are as follows:

1. Place a general description of the patient in the respective middle circle—45-year-old White male presenting to the cardiac rehabilitation unit who is unmotivated to progress through the program.
2. Place the major medical diagnoses in the respective middle circle—coronary artery disease with stent placement.
3. Place the major nursing diagnoses in the respective middle circle—fatigue, knowledge deficit, and ineffective self-help management.
4. Choose the nursing domains for which each medical and nursing diagnosis is appropriate—health promotion, self-perception, nutrition, safety/protection, life principles, coping/stress tolerance, comfort, role relationships, and activity/rest.

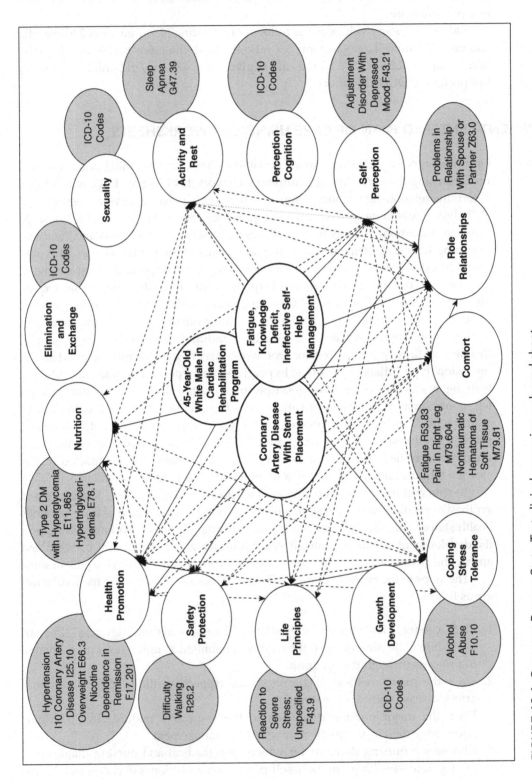

FIGURE 13.1 Outcome-Present State-Test clinical reasoning web worksheet.

DM, diabetes mellitus; ICD-10, International Classification of Diseases, 10th edition.

5. Generate all the International Classification of Diseases (ICD)-10 codes that are appropriate for the particular patient story that coincide with the nursing domains—hypertension (I10), coronary artery disease (I25.10), overweight (E66.3), nicotine dependence in remission (F17.201), difficulty walking (R26.2), reaction to severe stress unspecified (F43.9), sleep apnea (G47.39), adjustment disorder with depressed mood (F43.21), problems in relationship with spouse (Z63.0), fatigue (R53.83), pain in right leg (M79. 604), and alcohol abuse (F10.1).

6. Once the nursing domains, diagnoses, and ICD-10 codes are identified, reflect on the total web worksheet and concurrently consider and explain how each of the issues is or is not related to the other issues. Draw lines of relationship to spin and weave the web connections or associations among the ICD-10 codes/diagnoses. As you draw the lines, think out loud, and justify the reasons for the connections and explain specifically how the diagnoses may or may not be connected or related.

7. After the advanced practice nurse has spent some time connecting the relationships, determine which domain/domains have the highest priority for care coordination and most efficiently and effectively represent the keystone nursing care needs of the patient by counting the arrows that connect the medical problems (ICD-10 codes). In this case, counting 15 lines (Table 13.1) pointing to or from the nursing domain of health promotion represents the priority present-state keystone issues.

8. Look once again at the sets of relationships and determine the theme or keystone that summarizes the patient-in-context or the patient story—health promotion with coronary artery disease.

An OPT clinical reasoning web worksheet, depicted in Figure 13.1, shows a template with the patient health care situation, medical diagnoses, and nursing diagnoses at the center. Around the outer edges of the web are nursing domains with ICD-10 codes derived from history and physical assessment associated with the patient story. The directional arrows create the web effect and represent connections, explanations, and functional relationships between and among the diagnostic possibilities. As one can see, the domains and ICD-10 codes with more connections converging on the circles display the priority problem or keystone, in this case, health promotion. A keystone issue is one or more central supporting elements of the patient's story that help focus and determine a root cause or center of gravity of the system dynamics and helps guide reasoning and care coordination based on an analysis (breaking things down into discrete parts) and synthesis (putting the parts together in a greater whole) of diagnostic possibilities as represented in the web. Some key questions to ask here are: How does the clinical reasoning web reveal relationships between and among the identified diagnoses? To what degree do these relationships make practical clinical sense according to the evidence and patient story? Table 13.1 shows a summary of the connections highlighting the priority with the most connections.

After considering the full picture using the clinical reasoning web worksheet, the next step is to use an OPT clinical reasoning model worksheet to facilitate and structure the patient-centered systems thinking about the care coordination of the identified problems highlighted in Table 13.1. As the advanced practice nurse thinks about the patient, she or he will concurrently consider the frame, outcome state, and present state. Each aspect of the OPT clinical reasoning model contributes to

TABLE 13.1 Relationships Among Nursing Domains, Medical Diagnoses, and Web Connections

NURSING DOMAINS	MEDICAL DIAGNOSES (ICD-10 CODES)	WEB CONNECTIONS
Health promotion	Hypertension I10 Coronary artery disease I25.10 Overweight E66.3 Nicotine dependence, in remission F17.201	15
Self-perception	Adjustment disorder with depressed mood F43.21	13
Coping stress intolerance	Alcohol abuse F10.10	11
Role relationships	Problems in relationship with spouse or partner Z63.0	11
Nutrition	Type 2 diabetes mellitus with hyperglycemia E11.865 Hypertriglyceridemia E78.1	10
Activity and rest	Sleep apnea G47.39	10
Life principles	Reaction to severe stress; unspecified F43.9	9
Comfort	Fatigue R53.83 Pain in right leg M79.604 Nontraumatic hematoma of soft tissue M79.81	8
Safety protection	Difficulty walking R26.2	7

Source: World Health Organization (2015).

the other. The OPT clinical reasoning model worksheet is a map of the structure designed to provide an illustrative representation and guide thinking processes about relationships between and among competing issues and problems. Some questions that guide the use of the OPT clinical reasoning model are shown in Table 13.2 (Pesut, 2008).

By writing each element on the worksheet, all the parts of the model become related to each other. As the health care provider moves from right to left, the model structures the plan of care. Critical thinking skills are used to consider the patient story and creative thinking is used to identify and reason about the keystone issues/themes/cues to determine the most significant evidence in the present state. Complexity thinking helps the provider to consider the outcomes desired and the gaps between the present and outcomes states. Once interventions and tests are decided, the plan of care transitions over to a care coordination model and team-centered systems thinking that considers patient preferences within the frame of the situation.

The patient-in-context story (Exhibit 13.1) is depicted on the far right-hand side in Figure 13.2. The advanced practice nurse notes relevant facts of the story, which in this case include the patient demographics and characteristics: 45-year-old White male who lives with his wife and teenage son. He has diagnoses of coronary

TABLE 13.2 Questions That Guide the Use of the OPT Model

Patient-in-context	What is the patient story?
Diagnostic cue/web logic	What diagnoses have you generated?
	What outcomes do you have in mind given the diagnoses?
	What evidence supports those diagnoses?
	How does a reasoning web reveal relationships among the identified problems (diagnoses)?
	What keystone issue(s) emerge?
Framing	How are you framing the situation?
Present state	How is the present state defined?
Outcome state	What are the desired outcomes?
	What are the gaps or complementary pairs (~) of outcomes and present states?
Test	What are the clinical indicators of the desired outcomes?
	On what scales will the desired outcomes be rated?
	How will you know when the desired outcomes are achieved?
	How are you defining your testing in this particular case?
Decision making (interventions)	What clinical decisions or interventions help to achieve the outcomes?
	What specific intervention activities will you implement?
	Why are you considering these activities?
Judgment	Given your testing, what is your clinical judgment?
	Based on your judgment, have you achieved the outcome or do you need to reframe the situation?
	How, specifically, will you take this experience and learning with you into the future as you reason about similar cases?

OPT, Outcome-Present State-Test.
Adapted from Pesut (2008).

artery disease, hypertension, obesity, type 2 diabetes mellitus, hypertriglyceridemia, sleep apnea, alcohol abuse, fatigue, stress, depression, problems in relationship with spouse, difficulty walking, and pain in right leg from hematoma of soft tissue. He is post–PTCA and stent placement for occlusions in two cardiac arteries. He has returned to work as a mechanic and comes to the cardiac rehabilitation unit for education, exercise training, and lifestyle guidance. He abuses alcohol and stopped smoking 5 years ago. He also has some financial difficulties at home. The acute care nurse practitioner will pull the acute care team together to promote his health and manage his chronic comorbidities while working with him in the rehabilitation program. Significant laboratory data show hyperglycemia, hypertriglyceridemia, and a BMI of 27.5. A key point at this juncture is to review and reflect on the patient story for accuracy and thoroughness to proceed with care planning for care coordination.

Moving to the left, there is a place to list the diagnostic cluster cues on the web of medical diagnoses and ICD-10 codes (Exhibit 13.2). At the bottom of this box is placed the designated keystone issues or themes that fall under the most significant nursing domain—health promotion and coronary artery disease I25.10. Remember diagnostic

EXHIBIT 13.1 PATIENT-IN-CONTEXT STORY

Derek Roberts is a 45-year-old White male who presents to cardiac rehabilitation post–stent placement to left anterior descending (LAD) and circumflex (CFX). He is walking with a limp on the treadmill and reports pain in the right groin. He is unsure as to what he can do to improve his health. Social history is that he works full time as an auto mechanic, he is married, and has a teenage son. He drinks a 6 pack of beer weekly and quit smoking 5 years ago.

Prescribed medications include: Plavix, aspirin, Lipitor, lisinopril, and Glucophage.

Ht: 5′ 11″ (71 in.)

Wt: 197 lb., BMI: 27.5

Blood glucose: 240 mg/dL

Triglycerides: 189 mg/dL

BMI, body mass index; Ht, height; Wt, weight.

cluster cue web logic is the use of inductive and deductive /thinking skills. The key question to ask here is: What diagnoses were generated, is there evidence to support those diagnoses, and is the keystone issue appropriate given this patient story?

In the center and background of the worksheet are places to indicate the frame or theme that best represents the background issues regarding thinking about the patient story (Exhibit 13.3). The frame of this case is a 45-year-old White male who presents to the rehabilitation unit post–PTCA and stent placement. He is fatigued and unmotivated to proceed with the cardiac rehabilitation program. He has a limp from soft tissue injury to the right groin. This frame helps to organize the present state and outcome state, illustrates the gaps, and provides insights about what tests need to be considered to fill the gap. Decision making and reflection surround the framing as the advanced practice nurse thinks of many things simultaneously. Reflective thinking is used to monitor thinking and behavior. Some key questions to ask here are: How am I framing the situation and does the frame agree with the patient view of the situation? Given my disciplinary perspectives, what are the results I want to create for this person?

At the center of the sheet are spaces to place the present state (Exhibit 13.4) and outcome state (Exhibit 13.5) side by side. The present state in this case shows five primary health care problems related to the keystone issue: fatigue, sleep apnea, several combined chronic disease conditions, uncontrolled type 2 diabetes mellitus, and knowledge deficit of his medical conditions.

The outcome state shows five matching goals to be achieved through care coordination: hemodynamic stabilization to correct nocturia, proper-fitting continuous positive airway pressure (CPAP) mask and compliance with that therapy, stabilization of disease conditions, regulation and stabilization of glucose levels, and knowledgeable and compliant with medical regimen. Putting the two states together creates a gap analysis that naturally shows where the patient is and what the goals are in terms of the patient's care. Some key questions to ask here are: Are the outcomes appropriate given the diagnoses? Are there gaps between the outcomes and present state? Are there clinical indicators of the desired outcome state?

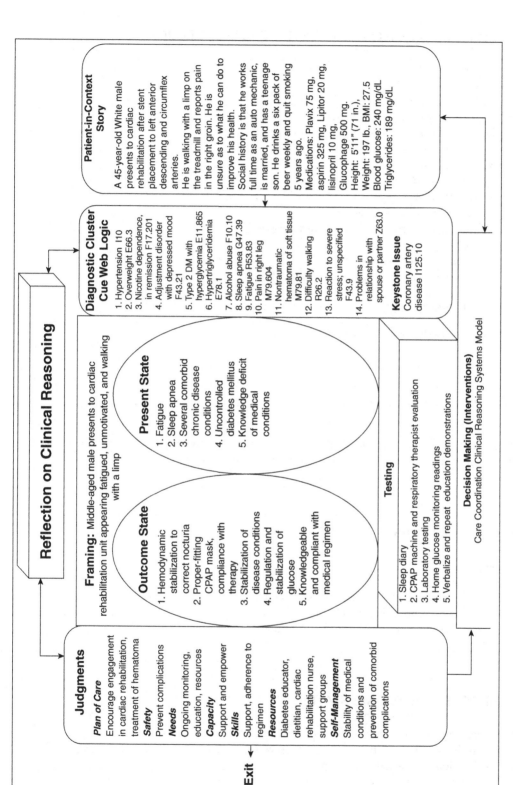

FIGURE 13.2 Outcome-Present State-Test clinical reasoning model for care coordination worksheet.

BMI, body mass index; CPAP, continuous positive airway pressure; DM, diabetes mellitus.

EXHIBIT 13.2 DIAGNOSTIC CLUSTER CUE WEB LOGIC

1. Hypertension I10
2. Overweight E 66.3
3. Nicotine dependence remission F17.210
4. Adjustment disorder; depressed mood F43.21
5. Type 2 diabetes mellitus with hyperglycemia E11.865
6. Hypertriglyceridemia E78.1
7. Alcohol abuse F10.10
8. Sleep apnea G47.39
9. Fatigue R53.83
10. Pain in right leg M79.604
11. Nontraumatic hematoma of soft tissue M79.81
12. Difficulty walking R26.2
13. Reaction to severe stress F43.9
14. Problems in relationship with spouse Z63.0

KEYSTONE ISSUE/THEME

Coronary artery disease I25.10

EXHIBIT 13.3 FRAMING

Derek Roberts, a 45-year-old White male, presents to the rehabilitation unit for a cardiac program. He is fatigued, unmotivated, and walks with a limp.

EXHIBIT 13.4 PRESENT STATE

1. Fatigue
2. Sleep apnea
3. Several combined chronic disease conditions
4. Uncontrolled type 2 diabetes mellitus
5. Knowledge deficit of his medical conditions

EXHIBIT 13.5 OUTCOME STATE

1. Emergency management and health restoration
2. Proper fitting of CPAP mask, compliance with therapy
3. Stabilization of disease conditions
4. Regulation and stabilization of glucose
5. Knowledgeable and compliant with medical regimen

EXHIBIT 13.6 TESTING

1. Sleep diary
2. CPAP machine and respiratory therapist evaluation
3. Laboratory testing
4. Home glucose monitoring readings
5. Verbalize and repeat education demonstration

EXHIBIT 13.7 REFLECTION ON CLINICAL REASONING

What clinical decisions or interventions help to achieve the outcomes?

What specific intervention activities will you implement?

Why are you considering these activities?

The gap between where the patient is and where the advanced practice nurse wants the patient to be is one way to create a test (Exhibit 13.6). Clinical decisions are choices made about interventions that will help the patient's transition from present state to a desired outcome state. As interventions are tested, the advanced practice nurse evaluates the degree to which outcomes are or are not being achieved. The tests chosen in this case include sleep diary, CPAP machine and respiratory therapist evaluation, laboratory testing, home glucose monitoring readings, and verbalize and repeat education demonstration. Testing is concurrent and iterative as one gets closer and closer with successive increments toward goal achievement. Some key questions to ask here are: How is the advanced practice nurse defining *testing*? On what scales will the desired outcome be rated? How will the advanced practice nurse know when the desired targeted outcomes are achieved?

The reflection box at the top of Figure 13.2 (Exhibit 13.7) reminds the advanced practice nurse of the thinking strategies used for the patient situation. These strategies also help make explicit many of the relationships among ideas and issues associated with the patient problems. Examples of reflection questions that support and engage patient-centered systems thinking are listed in Table 13.3.

Finally, the judgment space on the far left-hand side of the model (Exhibit 13.8) provides the place to write in the results of the conclusions drawn from the CCCR model. Based on the degree of gap or comparison of where the patient is, and where the health care team wants the patient to be, there may or may not be an evidence gap. Once there is evidence that fills that gap, the nurse has to attribute meaning to the data. Making judgments about clinical issues is about the meaning the advanced practice nurse attributes to the evidence derived from the test or gap analysis of present to desired state. Complexity thinking, team-centered systems thinking, and organization-centered systems-thinking skills are used by the care coordination team at this point to evaluate and judge the successes or deficits from the plan of care. Interprofessional team activity requires negotiation of the competing values of

TABLE 13.3 Patient-Centered Systems-Thinking Reflection Questions

SELF-REGULATION ACTIVITIES	REFLECTION QUESTIONS

Monitoring thinking	**I. Reflect on the thinking processes you used with the care coordination of this case.**
	1. The baseline needs I identify in this case are.... I think I can identify future adjustments in the plan of care by.... If I have difficulty I...
	2. When I think about my feelings during the care coordination of this case, I describe them as...and I handle them by...
	3. When I try to remember or understand important facts to develop the plan of care, coach, and educate the patient/family, I...
	4. As I look back on meaningful activities, the resources I could have spent:
	   a. More time on...
	   b. Less time on...

Monitoring the environment	**II. Reflect on the environmental circumstances you encountered in the care coordination of this case.** 5. When I prepare to carry out coaching and education activities for care coordination, I... 6. When I think about particular distractions to facilitating medical care services and supports for care coordination, I... 7. When I work and communicate with interprofessional partners for care coordination of this case, I... 8. If I had the chance to redo the care coordination activities, I would do...instead of...because...

Monitoring behavior	**III. Reflect on your behaviors and reactions to the care coordination of this case.**
	9. My impression of my performance in evaluating capacity, energy, support, readiness, and skills to organize and manage the plan of care, is...
	10. I make sure I will update the needs assessment and individualized plan of care by...and if I need to make changes, I...
	11. I make sure I empower the patient/family for self-management of health care needs by...and if I need to make changes, I...
	12. Reaction to care coordination of this case...
	   a. My reaction to what I like about the care coordination of this case...
	   b. My reaction to what I do not like about the care coordination of this case...
	Optional prompt: Other comments I have about the care coordination of this case...

Adapted from Kuiper, Pesut, and Kautz (2009).

collaboration—creating, competing, and controlling—and involves managing shared knowledge; acknowledgment of values impacted; and the brokering, directing, coordinating, and monitoring of practice issues, interventions, and outcomes. The judgments made in this case are made by the team after the care coordination essential needs outcomes are evaluated. Each of the items in the judgment column corresponds to an essential need addressed in the CCCR systems model (Figure 13.3). Some key questions to ask, given the testing, are: What are the clinical judgments? Have the outcomes been achieved? Does the situation need to be reframed?

EXHIBIT 13.8 JUDGMENTS RELATED TO CARE COORDINATION VARIABLES

PLAN OF CARE

Encourage engagement in cardiac rehabilitation and treatment of hematoma

SAFETY

Prevent complications

NEEDS

Ongoing monitoring, education, and resources

CAPACITY

Support and empower

SKILLS

Support; adherence to regimen

RESOURCES

Diabetes educator, dietitian, cardiac rehabilitation nurse, support groups

SELF-MANAGEMENT

Maintain stability of medical conditions and prevent comorbid complications

Once the advanced practice nurse has experience coordinating care for acute care patients, the cases become part of a clinical reasoning learning history that become prototypes or schemas for other similar cases. These schemas and experience build on each other over time and result in the development of pattern recognition for future clinical reasoning applications. If the scenario results in a negative judgment, or progress is not being made to transition patients from present to desired states, the advanced practice nurse may have to reframe the situation, reconsider the keystone priority, reconsider the care coordination activities, and/or consult with members of the interprofessional team for the problem to be solved, and the outcome to be achieved. The key question to ask here is: How will this clinical learning experience impact future reasoning about similar cases?

CARE COORDINATION USING CCCR MODEL WORKSHEETS

The next step in the nursing diagnostic reasoning process is to augment the plan of care to include activities related to interprofessional care planning using the CCCR systems model framework (Exhibit 13.9) that builds on the OPT model of clinical

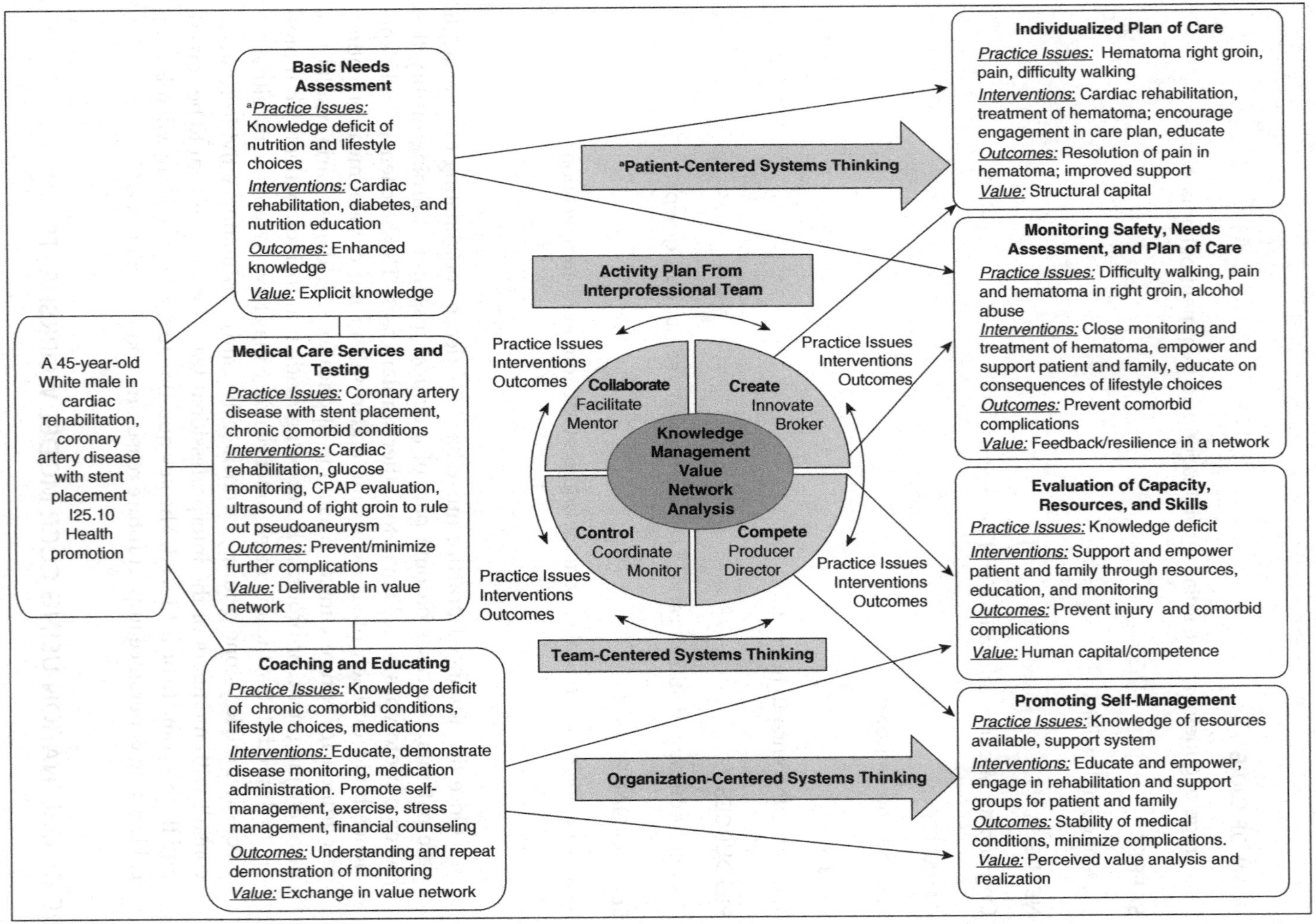
A 45-year-old White male in cardiac rehabilitation, coronary artery disease with stent placement I25.10 Health promotion
Basic Needs Assessment
ᵃPractice Issues: Knowledge deficit of nutrition and lifestyle choices
Interventions: Cardiac rehabilitation, diabetes, and nutrition education
Outcomes: Enhanced knowledge
Value: Explicit knowledge
Medical Care Services and Testing
Practice Issues: Coronary artery disease with stent placement, chronic comorbid conditions
Interventions: Cardiac rehabilitation, glucose monitoring, CPAP evaluation, ultrasound of right groin to rule out pseudoaneurysm
Outcomes: Prevent/minimize further complications
Value: Deliverable in value network
Coaching and Educating
Practice Issues: Knowledge deficit of chronic comorbid conditions, lifestyle choices, medications
Interventions: Educate, demonstrate disease monitoring, medication administration. Promote self-management, exercise, stress management, financial counseling
Outcomes: Understanding and repeat demonstration of monitoring
Value: Exchange in value network
ᵃPatient-Centered Systems Thinking
Activity Plan From Interprofessional Team
Practice Issues
Interventions
Outcomes
Collaborate
Facilitate
Mentor
Create
Innovate
Broker
Knowledge Management Value Network Analysis
Control
Coordinate
Monitor
Compete
Producer
Director
Team-Centered Systems Thinking
Organization-Centered Systems Thinking
Individualized Plan of Care
Practice Issues: Hematoma right groin, pain, difficulty walking
Interventions: Cardiac rehabilitation, treatment of hematoma; encourage engagement in care plan, educate
Outcomes: Resolution of pain in hematoma; improved support
Value: Structural capital
Monitoring Safety, Needs Assessment, and Plan of Care
Practice Issues: Difficulty walking, pain and hematoma in right groin, alcohol abuse
Interventions: Close monitoring and treatment of hematoma, empower and support patient and family, educate on consequences of lifestyle choices
Outcomes: Prevent comorbid complications
Value: Feedback/resilience in a network
Evaluation of Capacity, Resources, and Skills
Practice Issues: Knowledge deficit
Interventions: Support and empower patient and family through resources, education, and monitoring
Outcomes: Prevent injury and comorbid complications
Value: Human capital/competence
Promoting Self-Management
Practice Issues: Knowledge of resources available, support system
Interventions: Educate and empower, engage in rehabilitation and support groups for patient and family
Outcomes: Stability of medical conditions, minimize complications.
Value: Perceived value analysis and realization

FIGURE 13.3 Care Coordination Clinical Reasoning systems model worksheet.

[a] Practice issues can come from any discipline: nursing, medicine, pharmacy, social work, and so on.

CPAP, continuous positive airway pressure.

EXHIBIT 13.9 CARE COORDINATION CLINICAL REASONING DEFINITION

The authors define *care coordination clinical reasoning* as the application of critical, creative, systems, and complexity thinking to determine the practice issues, interdependencies, and interconnections of role relationships for collaborative work in service of caring for people to address problems, interventions, and outcomes through time and across health care contexts and services.

reasoning. The systems dynamics and interactions between and among the patient issues determine the care needed and the services provided. The complexities in this case are the issues related to Derek's lack of social support, substance abuse, noncompliance with medications, and comorbidities in his health status. The CCCR systems model web (Figure 13.4) visually represents the complexities in this case along with the essential care coordination practice issues that need attention to organize thinking that focuses on the patient's priority needs.

The CCCR systems model web (Exhibit 13.10) provides a blueprint for consideration of the care coordination practice issues so clinicians can determine interventions, outcomes, and the value exchange that supports safe, high-quality care. This process involves patient-centered systems thinking, team-centered systems thinking, and organization-centered systems thinking to thoroughly and efficiently manage all aspects of patient cases. The steps to create the web for this case start in the center with the patient description and medical diagnoses (Derek Roberts, a 45-year-old White male in a cardiac rehabilitation program) priority nursing domain (health promotion), and ICD-10 code (coronary artery disease I25.10) that show the overlap of patient issues that must be addressed by the advanced practice nurse and the care coordination interprofessional team.

Next, each large circle in this web represents the essential care coordination practice issues with evidence and defining characteristics for this patient story: needs assessment (nutritional needs, education needs of new diagnosis, medications, lifestyle choice consequences, and chronic comorbidities); individualized plan of care (encourage engagement in cardiac rehabilitation, support group, and rehabilitation education); medical care services and testing (cardiac rehabilitation monitoring, glucose monitoring of diabetes mellitus, and CPAP for sleep apnea); evaluation of capacity, resources, and skills (knowledge deficit, fatigued, unmotivated, and feels wife is "nagging" him); monitoring and safety (hematoma, pain in right groin, and difficulty walking); team collaboration (collaboration and communication among primary care provider, cardiologist, cardiac rehabilitation nurse, diabetes educator, and dietitian); coaching and educating (education regarding diagnosis, medications, lifestyle choices, alcohol use, and ongoing treatment); and self-management (knowledge of resources available, diabetes education and management).

The provider then reflects on the total picture on the worksheet and begins to draw lines of relationship, connection, or association among the essential needs. As directional lines are drawn to create the web, functional relationships between and among the needs are recognized. Clinical reasoning and thinking processes are used to explain and justify the reasons for connecting these care coordination needs as

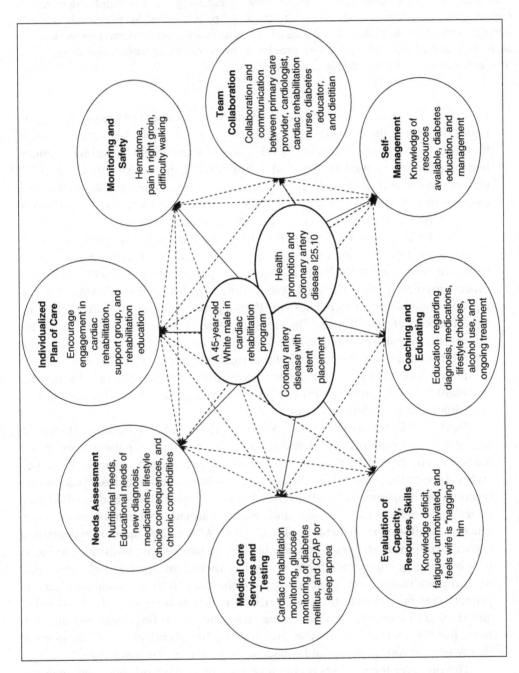

FIGURE 13.4 Care Coordination Clinical Reasoning systems model web.

CPAP, continuous positive airway pressure.

EXHIBIT 13.10 CCCR SYSTEMS MODEL WEB DEFINITION

The Care Coordination Clinical Reasoning systems model web enables one to visually represent the complexities and essential care coordination practice issues that need attention so as to organize thinking that focuses on the patient's and/or family's priority needs within the context of services provided within and between health care delivery systems.

central supporting elements in the patient's story, based on an analysis and synthesis of possible priorities as represented in the web. The priority care coordination needs that align with the patient story that would most efficiently and effectively represent the key issues of the patient are addressed. A key question to ask here is: Does the CCCR systems model web provide a comprehensive consideration of the most pertinent evidence for care coordination practice issues?

The CCCR systems model worksheet (see Figure 13.3) is the next worksheet in the framework designed to provide a graphic representation or visual map of the structure of the CCCR systems model and helps guide team-centered and organization-centered systems thinking. Some key questions to ask here are: What clinical decisions and interventions will help to achieve the outcomes identified on the OPT model of clinical reasoning (see Figure 13.2)? What specific interventions will the clinicians and members of the team implement? Why are providers considering these activities?

Writing each element on the worksheet shows how parts of the model relate to each other. In Figure 13.3, on the far left-hand side, there is space to write the description of the patient's health care situation that was at the center of the CCCR systems model web. Three essential needs are placed in the first boxes to the right of the description and include basic needs assessment, medical care services and testing, and coaching and education. Each of the care coordination needs identified in this model includes practice issues, interventions, outcomes, and value specification.

From patient-centered systems-thinking processes used to create the OPT clinical reasoning model worksheets for this patient story, the identified basic needs practice issues include knowledge deficit of nutrition and lifestyle choices. Targeted interventions for the team would be to promote cardiac rehabilitation and diabetes and nutrition education. The documented desired outcomes would be enhanced knowledge. A key question to ask here is: Have the basic needs been identified given the frame of the situation? Consider the value-impact analysis in this case using the questions from Table 13.4.

KNOWLEDGE MANAGEMENT AND VALUE ANALYSIS

The explicit value for role clarity, collaboration, and interaction of the team placed on the needs assessment is explicit knowledge. From Table 13.4, the value-networking reflection question for basic needs is: What knowledge is codified and conveyed to others through dialogue, demonstration, or media? Name three knowledge classification systems that could be used to represent the patient characteristics in this case:

1.
2.
3.

TABLE 13.4 Value Definitions and Reflection Questions

Deliverable	The specific values or objects that are conveyed from one role or participant to another role or participant. What are the deliverables that you offer and expect of others?
Exchange	This refers to two or more transactions between two or more roles or participants that evoke reciprocity. A process in which one role as agent receives resources from another role or agent and provides resources in return. What are the resource exchanges between roles or participants on your interprofessional health care team?
Explicit knowledge	The knowledge that is codified and conveyed to others through dialogue, demonstration, or media. What is the explicit knowledge shared among members of the team?
Feedback	This is the return of information about the impact of an activity. It can also mean the return of a portion of the output of a process as new input. What feedback is returned about activities or outputs in your care coordination activities? How does feedback influence team dynamics and goal attainment?
Human capital/ competence	The knowledge, skills, and competencies that reside in individuals who work in an organization or that are embedded in the organization's internal and external social networks. What human capital resources are needed in order for care coordination in your context to be successful?
Impact analysis	An assessment of how an input for a role is handled. What are the tangible/intangible costs, gains, or values from the input that generate a response or activity, or increase/decrease tangible assets?
Knowledge management	The degree to which the team facilitates and supports processes for creating, sustaining, sharing, and renewing organizational knowledge in order to generate social or economic gain or improve performance. Who is responsible and how is knowledge managed in the care coordination process?
Perceived value	The degree of value participants feel they receive from individual deliverables, which can come from roles, participants, or the network. What are the value-added dimensions of individual, collective, team, and organizational networks?
Resilience	The degree to which the network is able to reconfigure itself to respond to changing conditions and then return to its original form. What is the resilience capacity of the team and organization in which you work?
Structural capital	The infrastructure, routines, concepts, models, information systems, work systems, and business processes that support productivity and sustainability. To what degree do the structural capital and infrastructure support interprofessional teamwork and care coordination processes?
Systems thinking	An analysis and synthesis of the forces and interrelationships that shape the behavior of systems. To what degree do members of the team think about the system dynamics at the patient, group, team, or organizational levels?
Value realization	The degree to which tangible or intangible values turn the input into gains, benefits, capabilities, or assets that contribute to the success of an individual, group, organization, or network (Allee, 2008). To what degree do members of the team intentionally negotiate and manage competing values related to collaborating, creating, competing, and/or controlling?

Adapted from Allee, Schwabe, and Babb (2015).

From team-centered systems-thinking processes used for the basic needs assessment, the identified medical care services and testing practice issues include coronary artery disease with stent placement and chronic comorbid conditions. Targeted interventions for the team are cardiac rehabilitation, glucose monitoring, CPAP evaluation, and ultrasound of the right groin to rule out pseudoaneurysm. The documented desired outcomes are to prevent and minimize further complication. A key question to ask here is: Do the testing and interventions sufficiently manage the primary care needs? The explicit value for role clarity, collaboration, and interaction of the team placed on the medical care services and testing is to deliver evidence-based interventions based on the health care provider role. From Table 13.4, the value-networking reflection question for medical care services and testing basic needs is: What is the specific value or object that is conveyed from one role or participant to another role or participant? Name three deliverables that are essential for the care coordination success of this case:

1.
2.
3.

Organization-centered systems thinking is used by the team to enhance coaching and educating the patient. The identified coaching and educating practice issues include knowledge deficit of chronic comorbid conditions, lifestyle choices, and medications. Targeted interventions for the team are to educate; demonstrate disease monitoring; administer medication; and promote self-management, exercise, stress management, and financial counseling. The documented desired outcomes are to have the patient understand and repeat the demonstrations of monitoring health status. A key question to ask here is: Do the content and methods for coaching and teaching match the patients cognitive abilities and understanding? From Table 13.4, the value-networking reflection question for educating and coaching involves evaluating the transactions between two or more roles or participants in which one role as an agent receives resources from another role or agent and provides resources in return. The question would be: What is the exchange of resources and information between the providers and the patient regarding medication and available resources? Name three resources that could be exchanged between the providers and patient in this case:

1.
2.
3.

The diagram in the center of the worksheet is the activity plan from the interprofessional team (Exhibit 13.11). The team engages in collaborating, creating, competing, and controlling dynamics through communication (Quinn, Bright, Faerman, Thompson, & McGranth, 2014; Quinn, Heynoski, Thomas, & Spreitzer, 2014; Quinn & Quinn, 2015; Quinn & Rohrbough, 1983) to manage essential areas of organizational culture to realize the intangible value exchanges used to develop and manage an activity plan that considers interventions from the individualized plan of care, monitoring processes, evaluation of patient and family capacity with regard to resources and skills, and promotion of self-management. For example, in terms

EXHIBIT 13.11

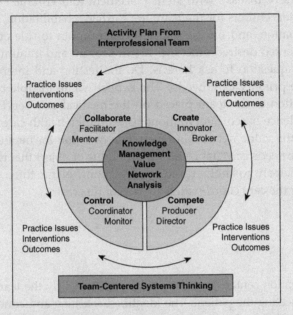

Key questions to consider for the four dimensions of the competing-values framework in the CCCR model are as follows:

- What are the desired outcomes in this case?
- What are the values I expect of myself and others?
- How are the feelings of the patient, family, and team considered in this case?
- What strategies could the team use to coordinate care?

of collaboration, people must understand themselves and communicate honestly and effectively. Individuals mentor and develop others collaboratively and know how to participate and lead teams. Often, this knowledge requires encouraging and managing constructive conflict. Competition enhances productivity and profitability. In this domain, vision and goal setting are a path to motivating self and others so that systems can be developed and organized to get results. Creating and promoting the adoption of new ideas or clinical innovations require attention to judicious use of power and ethics as well as championing new ideas and innovations through negotiating commitments and agreements for implementing and sustaining change. Control contributes to the development of stability and continuity as people work and manage across functions, organize information exchange, measure and monitor performance and quality, and enable compliance.

Key ingredients to team-centered systems thinking are that the members must be purpose centered, internally directed, other focused, and externally open to negotiation and communication surrounding competing values (Quinn, 2015; Quinn & Quinn, 2015). The activity plan from the interprofessional team in the CCCR model is guided by these principles and will promote the development of positive organizations and relationships. Each team member should be externally open to challenges, feedback and freedom from labels, higher performance, and the cultivation and development of communities of practice. When this outcome is challenged and false fixed, some team members are valued more than others in the context of competitive versus collaborative goals. Being other influenced cultivates empathy, rapport, energy, and calmness. Together, the team members feel safe and secure to take risks and act with trust, integrity, and resilience. Creating such a culture supports a spirit of inquiry, learning, and experimentation resulting in higher performance. Such behavior requires the activation of a reflective self in contrast to automatic self-justification and reactive modes of being and communicating. In order to be a positive influence and bring a state of leadership to the team, each member of the team needs to be vigilant about being purpose centered, choosing goals that create focus, energy, and meaning for the team. A focused purpose-centered team is likely to attract and create resources related to the reasoning required to communicate across settings to achieve CCCR goals.

The activity plan from the interprofessional team iteratively visits the practice issues that include communication among providers specific to this case, targeted interventions that are updated at team meetings across the contexts in which the providers are interacting, and documents the desired outcomes to maintain team support and keep the team equally informed about patient status. Some key questions to ask here are: Are the communication processes in place? Do they promote information exchange between and among the interprofessional health team members? The explicit value for role clarity, collaboration, and interaction of the team placed on the activity plan from the interprofessional team is determined by knowledge management and value impact analysis. From Table 13.4, the value-networking reflection questions for the activity plan from the interprofessional team are: What are the tangible/intangible costs, gains, or values from the input that generate a response or activity, or increase/decrease tangible assets? How does the team facilitate and support processes for collaborating, controlling, creating, and competiting to sustain, share, and renew organizational knowledge in order to generate social or economic gain or improve performance? Name a cost, gain, and value that would be generated from the activity plan of the team for this case:

1.
2.
3.

To the far right of the CCCR system model worksheet are four essential care coordination needs that evolve from the activity plan from the interprofessional team stemming from patient-centered systems thinking, team-centered systems thinking, and organization-centered systems thinking. These needs include the individualized plan of care; monitoring safety, needs assessment, and plan of care; evaluation of capacity, resources, and skills; and promoting self-management. Each of these care coordination essentials is defined as well by practice issues, interventions, outcomes, and values.

The patient-centered systems-thinking and team-centered systems-thinking activities are used for the individualized plan of care. The identified practice issues revolve around the hematoma of the right groin, pain, and difficulty walking. Targeted interventions for the provider and team are cardiac rehabilitation, treatment of the hematoma, encouraging engagement in the plan of care, and educating the patient. The documented desired outcomes are to resolve the pain from the hematoma and improved support services. Some key questions to ask here are: Does the individualized plan of care include team collaboration? Is there any input that was not yet considered? Are there providers who were overlooked? The explicit value for role clarity, collaboration, and interaction of the provider and team placed on the individualized plan of care is on structural capital. From Table 13.4, the value-networking reflection question for the individualized plan of care is: What are the infrastructure, routines, concepts, models, information systems, work systems, and business processes that support productivity and have sustainability? Name three routines, systems, or processes that support and sustain the productivity of the care coordination in this case:

1.
2.
3.

From the patient-centered systems-thinking and team-centered systems-thinking processes used for monitoring safety, needs assessment, and plan of care, identified practice issues include difficulty walking, pain and hematoma in the right groin, and alcohol abuse. Targeted interventions for the team are to closely monitor and treat the hematoma, empower and support the patient and family, and educate them on the consequences of lifestyle choices. The documented desired outcomes are to prevent comorbid complications. A key question to ask here is: Does the plan of care promote safety and meet the patient needs? The explicit value for role clarity, collaboration, and interaction of the team placed on monitoring safety, needs assessment, and plan of care is to obtain feedback and assess resilience in the network. From Table 13.4, the value-networking reflection questions for medical care services and testing basic needs are: What feedback is returned about activities or outputs? Was the network able to reconfigure itself to respond to changing conditions and then return to its original form? Name three areas of need and/or safety that were reassessed to determine whether the plan of care needed to be adjusted:

1.
2.
3.

Organization-centered systems-thinking processes, such as coaching and education, are used by the team to evaluate capacity, resources, and skills. The identified practice issues include knowledge deficit. Targeted interventions for the team are to support and empower the patient and family through resources, education, and monitoring. The documented desired outcomes are to prevent comorbid complications. A key question to ask here is: Do the interventions in the plan of care require skilled help and/or can the patient manage care needs independently? The explicit value for role clarity, collaboration, and interaction of the team placed on evaluating capacity, resources, and skills is identifying human capital and competence. From Table 13.4, the value-networking reflection question for educating and coaching involves evaluating the transactions between two or more roles or participants in which one role as an agent receives resources from another role or agent and provides resources in return. The question would be: What is the exchange of resources and information between the providers and the patient regarding medication and available resources? Name three exchanges of resources, skills, or information with the patient that are essential to the care coordination success of this case:

1.
2.
3.

Organization-centered systems thinking processes, such as coaching and education, are used by the team to promote self-management. The identified practice issues include knowledge of resources available to the patient and support systems. Targeted interventions for the team are to educate and empower the patient, engage the patient in rehabilitation, and make them aware of support groups. The documented desired outcomes are to have stability of medical conditions and minimize complications of disease conditions. A key question to ask here is: Is the patient able to identify the resources he needs and to navigate the health care system? The explicit value for role clarity, collaboration, and interaction of the team placed on promoting self-management is perceived value realization. From Table 13.4, the value-networking reflection question for promoting self-management is: What is the level of value that roles or participants feel they receive from individual deliverables, which can come from roles, participants, or the network? Name three examples of learned self-management that resulted from the care coordination of this case:

1.
2.
3.

With the use of the CCCR systems model, the advanced practice nurse and other providers address practice issues by using and developing evidence-based interventions, implementing measures of adherence, and evaluating processes and outcomes. This requires clinical reasoning at different levels of perspective—the individual patient needs, interprofessional team contributions, and attention to the systems in which people work and provide care. These practice issues, interventions, and outcomes for patient care coordination stem from the National Quality Forum (NQF, 2010a, 2010b) and the Agency for Healthcare Research and Quality (AHRQ, 2014).

As the center of attention for health care needs is managed by webs of relationships between and among providers, each interaction supports a specific value exchange as participant's partner for successful outcomes (Allee, 2003). The dynamic relationships that occurred, for this cardiac care patient, among the advanced practice nurse, cardiac rehabilitation nurse, physician, diabetes educator, dietitian, and support groups were collaborative, trusting, dynamic, and interdependent. Application of the competing-value competencies will relate to collaboration, creating, competing, and controlling, and help make explicit knowledge shared and managed to support innovation, coordination, and directing. Through the use of the electronic health record, connectivity impacted the value networking with greater access to knowledge and information. This process provided quick and effective feedback among team members for the complex needs this patient had related to complications from coronary artery disease and diabetes.

CLINICAL JUDGMENTS AND CCCR

The final phase of the clinical reasoning process is to determine whether outcomes were met and whether care coordination activities were successful. The CCCR model of clinical reasoning is revisited for the final phase of care coordination when judgments are made about achieving outcomes from the interprofessional team activity plan (see Exhibit 13.8). The worksheet (see Figure 13.2) is revisited to make judgments about the care coordination essentials (needs; individualized plan of care; safety; capacity, resources, and skills; and self-management). Shifting to the next level of perspective, using team-centered systems-thinking and organization-centered systems-thinking activities, collaboration and coordination of the plan of care reveal the ongoing planning and evaluation to provide appropriate patient support during this patient's recovery and rehabilitation from coronary artery disease. The goal is to provide a supportive environment with the appropriate resources for this married, 45-year-old White male. His coronary artery disease should be treated, and discharge planning from the rehabilitation unit should include resource personnel to help him manage his comorbid chronic illnesses. The patient will need education about abstaining from alcohol, taking antiplatelet medications, diabetes medications, dietary choices, and the role of rehabilitation. These resources lead to the best possible management and safety for this patient with coronary artery disease and diabetes.

Some remaining questions may arise as the evaluation of outcomes occurs such as: Can the organization provide continuing resources and reach care coordination outcomes for this patient? Were communication and the feedback loop effective between the health care providers and the patient? Did the complexity of the system hinder or enhance the achievement of outcomes? How do the competencies of the competing-values framework support the interprofessional dialogue and reasoning about the care coordination of this particular case? How do members of the team share and manage knowledge in service of care coordination? The advanced practice nurse as care coordinator views all the systems and is the key informant to communicate with the team regarding the efficiency and effectiveness of the processes for care outcomes. Judgments are made about whether the outcomes from case management have been achieved, and the information is recycled back to revise or enhance the plan of care.

The thinking processes used by the advanced practice nurse and other health care providers while implementing the CCCR systems model is promoted through monitoring of thinking, the environment, and behaviors for goal attainment (Zimmerman & Schunk, 2001). The courses of action chosen to manage issues and ensure that this patient remained safe revolve around behaviors and actions taken, thinking processes used, and environmental structuring. Critical reflective questions that can be used to prompt clinical reasoning to make judgments about the achievement of patient outcomes are shown in Table 13.5. Critical-, creative-, and systems-thinking processes are used for total care coordination, flow from patient-centered

TABLE 13.5 Team-Centered and Organization-Centered Systems-Thinking Reflection Questions

SELF-REGULATION ACTIVITIES	REFLECTION QUESTIONS

Monitoring thinking	**I. Reflect on the thinking processes the team used to navigate organizational systems for care coordination of this case.**
	1. The baseline needs identified by the team in this case are.... Adjustments in the plan of care for future successes include.... Difficulties were resolved by...
	2. Team reactions during the care coordination of this case in regard to organizational systems could be described as...and they were handled by...
	3. When the team was dealing with important facts to develop the plan to care, coach, and educate the patient/family about organizational systems it...
	4. Looking back on meaningful activities, the resources the team could have spent:
	  a. More time on...
	  b. Less time on...

Monitoring the environment	**II. Reflect on the environmental circumstances you encountered in the care coordination of this case.** 5. When the team prepares to carry out coaching and education activities for care coordination, it... 6. When the team considers particular distractions in the organizations that impede medical care services and supports for care coordination, it... 7. When the team works and communicates with organizational partners for care coordination of this case, it... 8. If the team had the chance to redo the care coordination activities, it would do...instead of...because...

Monitoring behavior	**III. Reflect on your behaviors and reactions to the care coordination of this case.**
	9. Impressions of the team performance in evaluating capacity, energy, support, readiness, and skills to organize and manage the plan of care within organizational systems are...
	10. The team assures that it will update the needs assessment and individualized plan of care by...and if it needs to make changes, it...
	11. The team makes sure it empowers the patient/family to navigate through organizational systems for management of health care needs by...and if it needs to make changes, it...
	12. The team reaction to care coordination of this case...
	  a. Reaction to what it likes about the navigation of organizational systems to facilitate the care coordination of this case...
	  b. Reaction to what it did not like about the navigation of organizational systems to facilitate the care coordination of this case...

	Optional prompt: Other comments about the care coordination of this case...

Adapted from Kuiper, Pesut, and Kautz (2009).

systems (Table 13.3), team-centered systems thinking (Table 13.5), and organization-centered systems thinking (Table 13.5) for case management.

SUMMARY

The clinical reasoning challenge for acute care begins with a description and understanding of the patient's story. The thinking strategies used in this case provided a safe and health-promoting environment for a middle-aged male patient with declining cardiac health. As the providers practice self-monitoring, self-evaluation, and self-correction, successful strategies are employed, and flaws in thinking are corrected as they collaborate and align interventions for patient success. The OPT clinical reasoning model provides the foundation and structure for clinical reasoning and systems thinking within an individual patient situation. The OPT structure and process can be used at several levels for care planning by the provider, by the team, and by the organization to discern alignment and coordination of care activities. The CCCR systems model provides the structure for clinical reasoning for the care coordination essential needs and their related practice issues, interventions, outcomes, and values.

KEY CONCEPTS

1. Clinical reasoning for care coordination with a patient in cardiac rehabilitation and chronic health problems can be promoted with a framework that includes structure, content, and process.
2. A supporting framework for CCCR extends case management using patient-centered systems thinking and the OPT clinical reasoning model across levels of perspective that also include team-centered systems thinking and organization-centered systems thinking to align care coordination activities.
3. The process of CCCR involves critical reflection for the individual provider and the team.
4. Attention to the dynamics of competing values and value-network analysis helps to define and describe the unique contributions that individual providers make to CCCR efforts supported through knowledge management and value-impact analysis.
5. A supporting framework for CCCR is completed by attending to the organization-centered systems thinking to make judgments about care coordination essentials.

STUDY QUESTIONS AND ACTIVITIES

1. Describe in your own words the benefits and processes of using the CCCR systems model with a rehabilitation patient.
2. Using the CCCR systems model, identify the care coordination essential needs of cases in cardiac rehabilitation.
3. To what degree can you explicitly identify and describe the value exchanges associated with care coordination in rehabilitation situations?

4. How can an interprofessional team use the competencies of the competing values of collaboration, creating, competing, and controlling to ensure efficiency and effectiveness of care coordination? How does your team negotiate roles of mentor, broker, director, and coordinator?

5. Identify all the possible standardized health care languages and communication strategies that could be considered in an acute care case. Does language impact on communication and the patient outcomes? How does a discipline-specific framework influence the feedback, decisions, and outcomes with rehabilitation?

6. Identify the relationship between critical reflection and thinking strategies as they are applied to the four levels of system-thinking perspectives that are required—patient, individual provider, team, and organization. What unique reflections are required to focus on team and organizational function with rehabilitation patients?

REFERENCES

Agency for Healthcare Research and Quality (AHRQ). (2014). *What is care coordination? Care coordination measures atlas update.* Rockville, MD: Author. Retrieved from http://www.ahrq.gov/professionals/prevention-chronic-care/improve/coordination/index.html

Allee, V. (2003). *The future of knowledge: Increasing prosperity through value networks.* Burlington, MA: Butterworth-Heinemann.

Allee, V. (2008). Value network analysis and value conversion of tangible and intangible assets. *Journal of Intellectual Capital, 9*(1), 5–24.

Allee, V., Schwabe, O., & Babb, M. K. (Eds.). (2015). *Value networks and the true nature of collaboration.* Tampa, FL: Megher–Kifer Press ValueNet Works and Verna Allee Associates.

Haas, S. A., Swan, B. A., & Haynes, T. S. (2014). *Care coordination and transition management core curriculum.* Pitman, NJ: American Academy of Ambulatory Care Nursing.

Kuiper, R., Pesut, D., & Kautz, D. (2009). Promoting the self-regulation of clinical reasoning skills in nursing students. *Open Nursing Journal, 3,* 76–85. Retrieved from http://www.ncbi.nlm.nih.gov/pmc/articles/PMC2771264

National Quality Forum (NQF). (2010a). *Preferred practices and performance measures for measuring and reporting care coordination: A consensus report.* Washington, DC: Author.

National Quality Forum (NQF). (2010b). *Quality connections: Care coordination.* Washington, DC: Author.

Pesut, D. J. (2008). Thoughts on thinking with complexity in mind. In C. Lindberg, S. Nash, & C. Lindberg (Eds.), *On the edge: Nursing in the age of complexity* (pp. 211–238). Bordentown, NJ: Plexus Press.

Quinn, R. (2015). *The positive organization: Breaking free from conventional cultures, constraints, and beliefs.* Oakland, CA: Berrett-Koehler.

Quinn, R., & Quinn, R. E. (2015). *Lift: Becoming a positive force in any situation.* San Francisco, CA: Berrett-Koehler.

Quinn, R. E., Bright, D., Faerman, S. R., Thompson, M. P., & McGrath, M. R. (2014). *Becoming a master manager: A competing values approach.* Hoboken, NJ: John Wiley & Sons.

Quinn, R. E., Heynoski, K., Thomas, M., & Spreitzer, G. M. (2014). *The best teacher in you: How to accelerate learning and change lives.* San Francisco, CA: Berrett-Koehler.

Quinn, R. E., & Rohrbough, J. (1983). A spatial model of effectiveness criteria: Towards a competing values approach to organizational analysis. *Management Science, 29,* 363–377.

World Health Organization (WHO). (2015). *Manual of the International Classification of Diseases and related health problems* (10th rev. ed.). Geneva, Switzerland: Author. Retrieved from http://www.icd10data.com

Zimmerman, B., & Schunk, D. S. (2001). *Self-regulated learning and academic thought*. Mahwah, NJ: Lawrence Erlbaum.

CHAPTER 14

CARE COORDINATION FOR LONG-TERM CARE OF THE ADULT PATIENT

In this chapter, we use the Care Coordination Clinical Reasoning (CCCR) systems model, as described in Part I, and explain how the model can be used to reason about a case, given the context of long-term care. The advanced practice nurse is working with a family that is in need of support services to promote quality outcomes at the end of life. The provider–clinic is the point of access for patients–families. The advanced practice nurse provides care coordination through the application and use of critical-, creative-, systems-, and complexity-thinking processes to manage patient problems with an interprofessional team to design appropriate interventions and establish patient-centered outcomes. Depending on the nature of need involved in the case, referrals to other specialty or primary care providers, community services, and living environments are determined and considered in managing care coordination and transitions (Haas, Swan, & Haynes, 2014).

The CCCR systems model framework begins with the patient story, which is derived from gathering data and evidence from an interview, history, physical examination, and the health record. The advanced practice nurse then develops an individual plan of care using the Outcome-Present State-Test (OPT) model worksheets. In order to do this, one activates the patient-centered systems-thinking skills for complex patient stories and habitually uses key questions to reflect on the specific sections of the model (Pesut, 2008), as well as the dimensions of the care coordination processes.

LEARNING OUTCOMES

After completing this chapter, the reader should be able to:

1. Explain the components of a care coordination framework that are needed to manage the problems, interventions, and outcomes of people at the end of life navigating long-term care issues
2. Describe the different thinking processes that support clinical reasoning skills and strategies for determining priorities for end-of-life and long-term care coordination

3. Define the cognitive and metacognitive self-regulatory processes that support individual provider critical reflection related to levels and perspectives associated with clinical reasoning for end of life and long-term care coordination

4. Describe how the communication between interprofessional health care team members is essential for care coordination to address patient and family needs during end of life and long-term care issues

5. Describe the critical meta-reflective processes that support team reflection related to levels and perspectives associated with the care coordination challenges and clinical reasoning required to navigate patient care plans with end of life and long-term care issues

THE PATIENT STORY

We begin with the history and story of an 81-year-old African American female, Fanny White, who is a resident in a long-term care skilled nursing facility. She has been on the memory care unit for the past year and her care is managed by a geriatric nurse practitioner. One day a certified nursing assistant reported that he was having difficulty getting her out of bed to go to the dining room for lunch because of increased fatigue and lethargy. The baseline at this facility is to use one assist for transfers. On this day, Ms. White required two assists to transfer from the bed to the wheelchair. The staff reports a progressive general functional decline after Ms. White was admitted to the hospital for pneumonia 4 months ago. She has been experiencing decreased appetite and weight loss. Ms. White's history includes 25-pack-years of smoking; however, she quit 2 months ago. Other comorbidities are Alzheimer's-type dementia, hypertension, rheumatoid arthritis, impaired fasting glucose, chronic obstructive pulmonary disease, and depression.

The physical examination reveals an elderly African American female slumped over in a wheelchair. She has oxygen therapy at 2 L/min via nasal cannula. She responds to her name by attempting to lift her head and open her eyes. Her speech is garbled and incoherent compared to her usual baseline status. Demographic characteristics include height of 62 inches, blood pressure of 70/40 mmHg, heart rate of 70 beats/minute, weak and thready radial pulse, and oxygen saturation of 85%. Her body mass index for the past 5 months is described in Table 14.1.

Laboratory values are as follows—white blood count: $4.60/mm^3$, hemoglobin: 12.5 g/dL, hematocrit: 38.4%, blood urea nitrogen: 12 mg/dL, creatinine: 0.9 g/dL, estimated glomerular filtration rate: 73 mL/min, glucose: 93 g/dL, potassium: 4.8 mEq/L, calcium: 8.3 mEq/L, chloride: 97 mEq/L, sodium: 130 mEq/L, carbon dioxide: 23 mEq/L, prealbumin: 10 mg/dL, and albumin: 2.6 g/dL. The patient's daily oral medications include Norvasc, naproxen sodium, Prilosec, Zoloft, Zofran, Marinol, and Mighty protein shakes.

PATIENT-CENTERED PLAN OF CARE USING OPT WORKSHEETS

Once the story is obtained from all possible sources, care planning proceeds using the OPT clinical reasoning web worksheet (Figure 14.1), which helps determine relationships among issues and highlights potential keystone issues. The OPT clinical

TABLE 14.1 Body Mass Index

TIME	WEIGHT (lb.)	BODY MASS INDEX
5 months ago	124	22.7
4 months ago (after hospitalization)	107	
2 months ago	106	19.4
1 month ago	90	16.5
Today	85	15.5

reasoning web is a graphic representation of the functional relationships between and among diagnostic hypotheses derived from the analysis and synthesis regarding how each element of the story and issues relate to one another. This activates critical and creative thinking. The visual diagram that results illustrates dynamics among issues and a convergence helps to pinpoint central issues that require nursing care. As one thinks about this case, and begins to spin and weave a clinical reasoning web, relationships are identified among nursing domains and diagnoses as they are combined with medical conditions. The long-term care conditions in this case are history of Alzheimer's dementia, chronic obstructive pulmonary disease, and comorbidities. Once the advanced practice nurse considers these diagnoses, the nursing care domains associated with them are identified. The complementary nursing diagnoses most impacted in this case are adult failure to thrive and imbalanced nutrition: less than body requirements.

To spin and weave the web providers use thinking processes to analyze and synthesize relationships among diagnostic hypotheses associated with a patient's health status. The visual representation and mapping of these relationships support the development of systems thinking and making connections between and among the medical and nursing diagnoses under consideration, given the patient story.

The steps to the creation of the OPT clinical reasoning web using the worksheet are as follows:

1. Place a general description of the patient in the respective middle circle—81-year-old African American female (Fanny White) patient.
2. Place the major medical diagnoses in the respective middle circle—history of Alzheimer's-type dementia, chronic obstructive pulmonary disease, and comorbidities.
3. Place the major nursing diagnoses in the respective middle circle—adult failure to thrive and imbalanced nutrition: less than body requirements.
4. Choose the nursing domains for which each medical and nursing diagnosis is appropriate—perception and cognition, coping and stress tolerance, nutrition, safety and protection, elimination and exchange, role relationship, comfort, activity and rest, and health promotion.
5. Generate all the International Classification of Diseases-10 (ICD-10) codes that are appropriate for the particular patient and family story that coincide with the nursing domains—Alzheimer's dementia (F02.80), depression (F03.90),

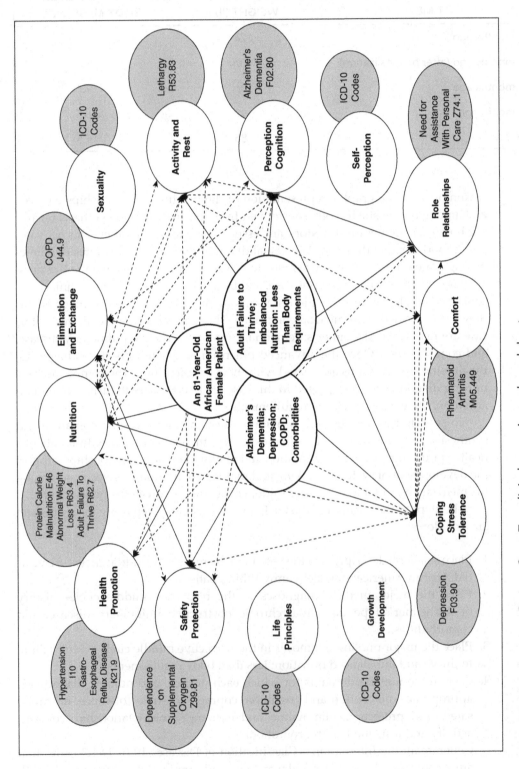

FIGURE 14.1 Outcome-Present State-Test clinical reasoning web worksheet.

COPD, chronic obstructive pulmonary disease; ICD-10, International Classification of Diseases, 10th edition.

TABLE 14.2 Relationships Among Nursing Domains, Medical Diagnoses, and Web Connections

NURSING DOMAINS	MEDICAL DIAGNOSES (ICD-10 CODES)	WEB CONNECTIONS
Perception/cognition	Alzheimer's dementia F02.80	10
Coping/stress tolerance	Depression F03.90	10
Nutrition	Abnormal weight loss R63.4 Protein calorie malnutrition E46 Adult failure to thrive R62.7	9
Activity/rest	Lethargy R53.83	8
Elimination and exchange	Chronic obstructive pulmonary disease J44.9	7
Safety/protection	Dependence on supplemental oxygen Z99.81	6
Role relationship	Need for personal assistance Z74.1	5
Comfort	Rheumatoid arthritis M05.449	4
Health promotion	Hypertension I10 Gastroesophageal reflux disease K21.9	3

Source: World Health Organization (2015).

abnormal weight loss (R63.4), protein calorie malnutrition (E46), adult failure to thrive (R62.7), dependence on supplemental oxygen (Z99.81), chronic obstructive pulmonary disease (J44.9), rheumatoid arthritis (M05.449), need for personal assistance (Z74.1), rheumatoid arthritis (M05.449), lethargy (R53.83), hypertension (I10), and gastroesophageal reflux disease (K21.9).

6. Once the nursing domains, diagnoses, and ICD-10 codes are identified, reflect on the total web worksheet and concurrently consider and explain how each of the issues is or is not related to the other issues. Draw lines of relationship to spin and weave the web connections or associations among the ICD-10 codes/diagnoses. As the you draw the lines, think out loud, justify the reasons for the connections, and explain specifically how the diagnoses may or may not be connected or related.

7. After you have spent some time connecting the relationships, determine which domain/domains have the highest priority for care coordination and most efficiently and effectively represent the keystone nursing care needs of the patient by counting the arrows that connect the medical problems (ICD-10 codes). In this case, counting 10 lines (Table 14.2), pointing to or from the nursing domains of perception/cognition, coping/stress tolerance, and role relationships represents the priority present-state keystone issues resulting from Alzheimer's disease and depression.

8. Look once again at the sets of relationships and determine the theme or keystone that summarizes the patient-in-context or the patient story—the problems related to perception and cognition and coping and stress tolerance are the keystone issues for this case.

The OPT clinical reasoning web worksheet in Figure 14.1 shows a template with the patient health care situation, medical diagnoses, and nursing diagnoses in the center. Around the outer edges of the web are nursing domains with ICD-10 codes derived from history and physical assessment associated with the patient story. The directional arrows that create the web effect represent connections, explanations, and functional relationships between and among the diagnostic possibilities. As one can see, the domains and ICD-10 codes with more connections converging on one of the circles display the priority problem or keystones, in this case perception and cognition and coping and stress tolerance. A keystone issue is one or more central supporting elements of the patient's story that help focus and determine a root cause or center of gravity of the system dynamics and helps guide reasoning and care coordination based on an analysis (breaking things down into discrete parts) and synthesis (putting the parts together in a greater whole) of diagnostic possibilities as represented in the web. Some key questions to ask here are: How does the clinical reasoning web reveal relationships between and among the identified diagnoses? To what degree do these relationships make practical clinical sense according to the evidence and patient story? Table 14.2 shows a summary of the connections highlighting the priority with the most connections.

After considering the full picture using the clinical reasoning web worksheet, the next step is to use the OPT clinical reasoning model worksheet to facilitate and structure the patient-centered systems thinking about the care coordination of the identified problems highlighted in Table 14.2. As the advanced practice nurse thinks about the patient, he or she will concurrently consider the frame, outcome state, and present state. Each aspect of the OPT clinical reasoning model contributes to the other. The OPT clinical reasoning model worksheet is a map of the structure designed to provide an illustrative representation and guide thinking processes about relationships between and among competing issues and problems. Some questions that guide the use of the OPT clinical reasoning model are shown in Table 14.3 (Pesut, 2008).

By writing each element on the worksheet, all the parts of the model become related to each other. As the health care provider moves from right to left, the model structures the plan of care. Critical thinking skills are used to consider the patient story and creative thinking is used to identify and reason about the keystone issues/themes/cues to determine the most significant evidence in the present state. Complexity thinking helps the provider to consider the outcomes desired and the gaps between the present and outcome states. Once interventions and tests are decided, the plan of care transitions over to a care coordination model and team-centered systems thinking that considers patient and family preferences within the frame of the situation.

The patient-in-context story (Exhibit 14.1) is on the far right-hand side, as depicted in Figure 14.2. The advanced practice nurse notes relevant facts of the story, which in this case include the patient demographics and characteristics; 81-year-old African American female residing in a long-term care facility on a memory unit. She has a diagnosis of Alzheimer's dementia, depression, malnutrition, and several comorbidities. Her failure to thrive has placed her in the caseload of a geriatric nurse practitioner who is to assist the family in making some end-of-life decisions about resuscitation as a result of Ms. White's functional decline. Significant

TABLE 14.3 Questions That Guide the Use of the OPT Model

Patient-in-context	What is the patient story?
Diagnostic cue/ web logic	What diagnoses have you generated?
	What outcomes do you have in mind, given the diagnoses?
	What evidence supports those diagnoses?
	How does a reasoning web reveal relationships among the identified problems (diagnoses)?
	What keystone issue(s) emerge?
Framing	How are you framing the situation?
Present state	How is the present state defined?
Outcome state	What are the desired outcomes?
	What are the gaps or complementary pairs (~) of outcomes and present states?
Test	What are the clinical indicators of the desired outcomes?
	On what scales will the desired outcomes be rated?
	How will you know when the desired outcomes are achieved?
	How are you defining your testing in this particular case?
Decision making (interventions)	What clinical decisions or interventions help to achieve the outcomes?
	What specific intervention activities will you implement?
	Why are you considering these activities?
Judgment	Given your testing, what is your clinical judgment?
	Based on your judgment, have you achieved the outcome or do you need to reframe the situation?
	How, specifically, will you take this experience and learning with you into the future as you reason about similar cases?

OPT, Outcome-Present State-Test.
Adapted from Pesut (2008).

EXHIBIT 14.1 PATIENT-IN-CONTEXT STORY

An 81-year-old African American female (Fanny White) with a diagnosis of Alzheimer's dementia and depression. She shows functional decline since a hospitalization for pneumonia 4 months ago. This end-of-life decline is exhibited by protein malnutrition, significant weight loss, and adult failure to thrive. Her son holds the health care power of attorney; he has decided to change the resuscitation status to do not resuscitate.

Blood pressure: 70/40 mmHg, O_2 sat: 85%, sodium: 130 mEq/L, prealbumin: 10 mg/dL, albumin: 2.6 g/dL

BP, blood pressure; O_2 sat: oxygen saturation.

laboratory data show hypotension and oxygen dependency caused by chronic obstructive pulmonary disease and poor nutritional status, which has affected electrolyte levels, protein balance, and body mass index. Assessment of her medication regimen requires some needed adjustments as a result of hypotension and lethargy

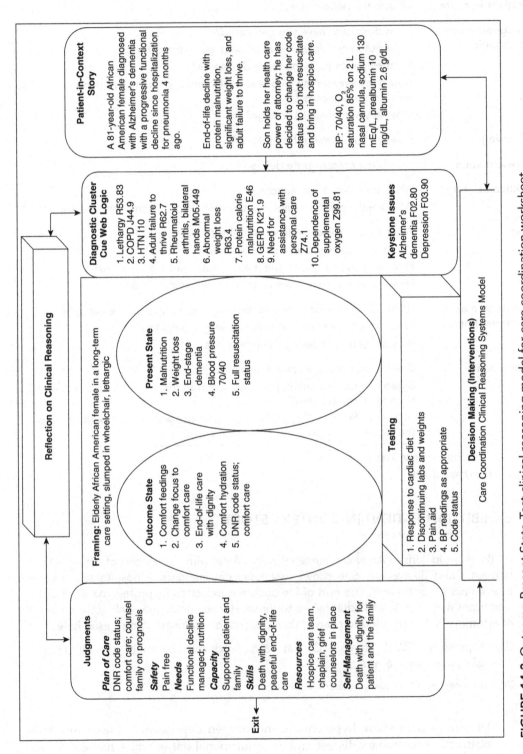

FIGURE 14.2 Outcome-Present State-Test clinical reasoning model for care coordination worksheet.

BP, blood pressure; COPD, chronic obstructive pulmonary disease; DNR, do not resuscitate; GERD, gastroesophageal reflux disease; HTN, hypertension.

EXHIBIT 14.2 DIAGNOSTIC CLUSTER CUE WEB LOGIC

1. Lethargy R53.83
2. COPD J44.9
3. Hypertension I10
4. Adult failure to thrive R62.7
5. Rheumatoid arthritis, hands M05.449
6. Abnormal weight loss R63.4
7. Protein calorie malnutrition E46
8. GERD K21.9
9. Need for personal care assistance Z74.1
10. Dependence on O_2 Z99.81

KEYSTONE ISSUE/THEME

1. Alzheimer's dementia F02.80
2. Depression F03.90

COPD, chronic obstructive pulmonary disease; GERD, gastroesophageal reflux disease.

EXHIBIT 14.3 FRAMING

An elderly African American female in a long-term care unit admitted with failure to thrive.

on physical examination. A key point at this juncture is to review and reflect on the patient story for accuracy and thoroughness to be able to proceed with care planning for care coordination.

Moving to the left, there is a place to list the diagnostic cluster cues on the web of medical diagnoses and ICD-10 codes (Exhibit 14.2). At the bottom of this box are placed the designated keystone issues or themes that fall under the most significant nursing domain—Alzheimer's dementia F02.80 and depression F03.90. Remember diagnostic cluster cue web logic is the use of inductive and deductive thinking skills. Some key questions to ask here are: What diagnoses were generated? Is there evidence to support those diagnoses? Is the keystone issue appropriate, given this patient story?

In the center and background of the worksheet are places to indicate the frame or theme that best represents the background issues regarding thinking about the patient story (Exhibit 14.3). The frame of this case is an elderly African American female in a long-term care unit admitted with failure to thrive. This helps to organize the present state, outcome state, illustrates the gaps, and provides insights about what tests need to be considered to fill the gap. Decision making and reflection surround the framing as the advanced practice nurse thinks of many things simultaneously. Reflective thinking is used to monitor thinking and behavior. A key question to ask here is: How do I frame the situation and does the frame agree with the patient–family view of the situation?

At the center of the sheet are spaces to place the present state (Exhibit 14.4) and outcome state (Exhibit 14.5) side by side. The present state in this case shows

EXHIBIT 14.4 PRESENT STATE

1. Malnutrition
2. Weight loss
3. End-stage dementia
4. Blood pressure: 70/40 mmHg
5. Full resuscitation status

EXHIBIT 14.5 OUTCOME STATE

1. Comfort feedings
2. Change focus to comfort care
3. End-of-life care with dignity
4. Comfort hydration
5. Do-not-resuscitate status—comfort care

EXHIBIT 14.6 TESTING

1. Response to discontinuing cardiac diet
2. Discontinuing laboratory tests and weights
3. Supply pain aid
4. Blood pressure readings as appropriate
5. Resuscitation status

five primary health care problems related to the keystone issues: malnutrition, weight loss, end-stage dementia, blood pressure 70/40 mmHg, and full resuscitation status. The outcome state shows five matching goals to be achieved through care coordination: comfort feedings, change focus to comfort care, end-of-life care with dignity, comfort hydration, and do-not-resuscitate status—comfort care. Putting the two states together creates a gap analysis that naturally shows where the patient is and what the goals are in terms of the patient's care. Some key questions to ask here are: Are the outcomes appropriate given the diagnoses? Are there gaps between the outcomes and present state? Are there clinical indicators of the desired outcome state?

The gap between where the patient is and where the advanced practice nurse wants the patient to be is one way to create a test (Exhibit 14.6). Clinical decisions are choices made about interventions that will help the patient transition from present state to a desired outcome state. As interventions are tested, the advanced practice nurse evaluates the degree to which outcomes are or are not being achieved. The tests chosen in this case include response to discontinuing a cardiac diet, discontinuing laboratory tests and weights, supply of pain aids, blood pressure readings as appropriate, and resuscitation status.

EXHIBIT 14.7 REFLECTION ON CLINICAL REASONING

What clinical decisions or interventions help to achieve the outcomes?

What specific intervention activities will you implement?

Why are you considering these activities?

Testing is concurrent and iterative as one gets closer and closer in successive increments toward goal achievement. Some key questions to ask here are: How the advanced practice nurse is defining *testing*? On what scales will the desired outcome be rated? How will the advanced practice nurse know when the desired targeted outcomes are achieved?

The reflection box at the top of Figure 14.2 (Exhibit 14.7) reminds the advanced practice nurse of the thinking strategies used for the patient situation. These strategies also help make explicit many of the relationships among ideas and issues associated with the patient problems. Examples of clinical reasoning reflection questions that could be used during patient-centered systems thinking are listed in Table 14.4.

Finally, the judgment space on the far left-hand side of the model (Exhibit 14.8) is the place to write in the results of the conclusions drawn from the CCCR model. Based on the degree of gap or comparison of where the patient is, and where the health care team wants the patient to be, there may or may not be an evidence gap. Once there is evidence that fills that gap, the nurse has to attribute meaning to the data. Making judgments about clinical issues is about the meaning the advanced practice nurse attributes to the evidence derived from the test or gap analysis of the present to the desired state. Complexity thinking, team-centered systems thinking, and organization-centered systems-thinking skills are used by the care coordination team at this point to evaluate and judge the successes or deficits from the plan of care. Interprofessional team activity requires negotiation of the competing values of collaborating, creating, competing, and controlling, and involves managing shared knowledge; acknowledgment of values impacted; and the brokering, directing, coordinating, and monitoring of practice issues, interventions, and outcomes. The judgments made in this case are made by the team after the care coordination essential needs outcomes are evaluated. Each of the items in the judgment column corresponds to an essential need addressed in the CCCR systems model (Figure 14.3). Some key questions to ask here are: Given the testing, what are the clinical judgments? Have the outcomes been achieved? Does the situation need to be reframed?

Once the advanced practice nurse has experience coordinating care for patients at the end of life, the cases become part of a clinical reasoning learning history, which become prototypes or schemas for other similar cases. These schemas and experience build on each other over time and result in the development of pattern recognition for future clinical reasoning applications. If the scenario results in a negative judgment, or progress is not being made to transition patients from present

TABLE 14.4 Patient-Centered Systems-Thinking Reflection Questions

SELF-REGULATION ACTIVITIES	REFLECTION QUESTIONS
Monitoring thinking	I. Reflect on the thinking processes you used with the care coordination of this case.
	1. The baseline needs I identify in this case are.... I think I can identify future adjustments in the plan of care by...if I have difficulty I...
	2. When I think about my feelings during the care coordination of this case, I describe them as...and I handle them by...
	3. When I try to remember or understand important facts to develop the plan of care, coach, and educate the patient/family I....
	4. As I look back on meaningful activities, the resources I could have spent:
	a. More time on....
	b. Less time on....
Monitoring the environment	II. Reflect on the environmental circumstances you encountered in the care coordination of this case.
	5. When I prepare to carry out coaching and education activities for care coordination, I...
	6. When I think about particular distractions to facilitating medical care services and supports for care coordination, I...
	7. When I work and communicate with interprofessional partners for care coordination of this case, I....
	8. If I had the chance to redo the care coordination activities, I would do.... instead of.... because ....
Monitoring behavior	III. Reflect on your behaviors and reactions to the care coordination of this case.
	9. My impression of my performance in evaluating capacity, energy, support, readiness, and skills to organize and manage the plan of care, I...
	10. I make sure I will update the needs assessment and individualized plan of care by.... and if I need to make changes, I....
	11. I make sure I empower the patient–family for self-management of health care needs by...and if I need to make changes, I...
	12. Reaction to care coordination of this case...
	a. My reaction to what I like about the care coordination of this case...
	b. My reaction to what I do not like about the care coordination of this case...
	Optional prompt: Other comments I have about the care coordination of this case...

Adapted from Kuiper, Pesut, and Kautz (2009).

to desired states, the advanced practice nurse may have to reframe the situation, reconsider the keystone priority, reconsider the care coordination activities for the problem to be solved and the outcome to be achieved. The key question to ask here is: How will the advanced practice nurse specifically take this clinical learning experience into the future to reason about similar cases?

EXHIBIT 14.8 JUDGMENTS RELATED TO CARE COORDINATION VARIABLES

PLAN OF CARE

Do-not-resuscitate status, comfort care, and counsel family on prognosis

SAFETY

Pain free

NEEDS

Functional decline and nutrition managed

CAPACITY

Support patient and family

SKILLS

Death with dignity, peaceful end-of-life care

RESOURCES

Hospice care team, chaplain, grief counselors

SELF-MANAGEMENT

Death with dignity for patient and the family

CARE COORDINATION USING CCCR MODEL WORKSHEETS

The next step in the nursing diagnostic reasoning process is to augment the plan of care to include activities related to interprofessional care planning using the CCCR systems model framework that builds on the OPT model of clinical reasoning (see Exhibit 14.9). The systems dynamics and interactions between and among the patient issues determine the care needed and the services provided. The complexities in this case are the overlapping issues related to the physical and mental comorbidities this patient is experiencing. The CCCR systems model web (Figure 14.4) visually represents the complexities in this case along with the essential care coordination practice issues that need attention so as to organize thinking that focuses on the patients and/or family's priority needs.

The CCCR systems model web (Exhibit 14.10) provides a blueprint for consideration of the care coordination practice issues so clinicians can determine interventions, outcomes, and the value exchange that supports safe, high-quality care. This process involves patient-centered systems thinking, team-centered systems thinking, and organization-centered systems thinking to thoroughly and efficiently

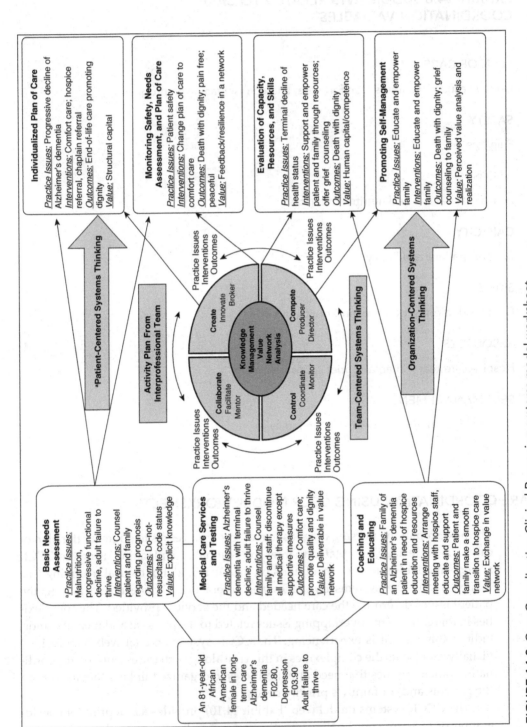

FIGURE 14.3 Care Coordination Clinical Reasoning systems model worksheet.

[a] Practice issues can come from any discipline: nursing, medicine, pharmacy, social work, and so on.

EXHIBIT 14.9 CARE COORDINATION CLINICAL REASONING DEFINITION

The authors define *care coordination clinical reasoning* as the application of critical, creative, systems, and complexity thinking to determine the practice issues, interdependencies, and interconnections of role relationships for collaborative work in service of caring for people to address problems, interventions, and outcomes through time and across health care contexts and services.

manage all aspects of patient and family cases. The steps to creating the web for this case start in the center, with the patient description and medical diagnoses (81-year-old African American [Fanny White] elderly female with a failure to thrive), priority nursing domain (perception/cognition, coping/stress tolerance), and ICD-10 codes (Alzheimer's dementia F02.80 and depression F03.90) that show the overlap of patient issues that must be addressed by the advanced practice nurse and the care coordination interprofessional team.

Next, each large circle in this web represents the essential care coordination practice issues with evidence and defining characteristics for this patient story: needs assessment (nutrition, progressive terminal decline); individualized plan of care (resuscitative code status, comfort care); medical care services and testing (resuscitative code status, hospice care referral); evaluation of capacity, resources, and skills (general progressive failure to thrive); monitoring and safety (supplemental oxygen dependent); team collaboration (collaboration and communication among providers, skilled facility staff, social worker, hospice care chaplain); coaching and educating (education to patient and family regarding prognosis); and self-management (knowledge of resources available to patient and family).

The provider then reflects on the total picture on the worksheet and begins to draw lines of relationship, connection, or association among the essential needs. As directional lines are drawn to create the web, functional relationships between and among the needs are recognized. Clinical reasoning and thinking processes are used to explain and justify the reasons for connecting these care coordination needs as central supporting elements in the patient's story based on an analysis and synthesis of possible priorities as represented in the web. The priority care coordination needs that align with the patient story that would most efficiently and effectively represent the key issues of the patient are addressed. A key question here is: Does this CCCR systems model web provide a comprehensive consideration of the most pertinent evidence for care coordination practice issues?

The CCCR systems model worksheet (see Figure 14.3) is the next worksheet in the framework designed to provide a graphic representation or visual map of the structure of the CCCR systems model and help guide team-centered systems and organization-centered systems thinking. Some key questions to ask are: What clinical decisions and interventions will help to achieve the outcomes identified on the OPT model of clinical reasoning (see Figure 14.2)? What specific interventions will the advanced practice nurse and/or the team implement? Why consider these activities?

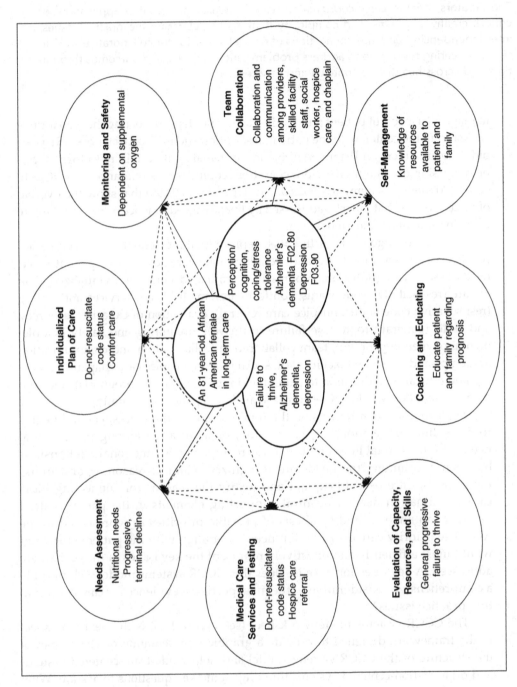

FIGURE 14.4 Care Coordination Clinical Reasoning systems model web.

EXHIBIT 14.10 CCCR SYSTEMS MODEL WEB DEFINITION

The Care Coordination Clinical Reasoning systems model web enables one to visually represent the complexities and essential care coordination practice issues that need attention so as to organize thinking that focuses on the patient's and/or family's priority needs within the context of services provided within and between health care delivery systems.

Writing each element on the worksheet shows how parts of the model relate to each other. In Figure 14.3, on the far left-hand side, there is space to write the description of the patient's health care situation that was at the center of the CCCR systems model web. Three essential needs are placed in the first boxes to the right of the description and include basic needs assessment, medical care services and testing, and coaching and education. Each of the care coordination needs identified in this model include practice issues, interventions, outcomes, and value specification.

From patient-centered systems-thinking processes used to create the OPT clinical reasoning model worksheets for this patient story the identified basic needs practice issues include malnutrition, progressive functional decline, and adult failure to thrive. Targeted interventions for the team would be to counsel the patient and family regarding the prognosis. The documented desired outcomes would be to change end-of-life care to include a do-not-resuscitate code status. A key question to ask is: Have the basic needs been identified, given the frame of the situation? Consider the value-impact analysis in this case using the questions from Table 14.5.

KNOWLEDGE MANAGEMENT AND VALUE ANALYSIS

The explicit value for role clarity, collaboration, and interaction of the team placed on the needs assessment is explicit knowledge. From Table 14.5, the value-networking reflection question for basic needs is: What knowledge is codified and conveyed to others through dialogue, demonstration, or media? Name three knowledge classification systems that could be used to represent the patient characteristics in this case:

1.
2.
3.

From team-centered systems-thinking processes used for the basic needs assessment, the identified medical care services and testing practice issues include Alzheimer's dementia with terminal decline and adult failure to thrive. Targeted interventions for the team are counseling the family and staff and discontinue all medical therapy except supportive measures. The documented desired outcomes are to provide comfort care and promote quality of life with dignity. A key question to ask is: Do the testing and interventions sufficiently manage the primary care needs? The explicit value for role clarity, collaboration, and interaction of the

TABLE 14.5 Value Definitions and Reflection Questions

Deliverable	The specific values or objects that are conveyed from one role or participant to another role or participant. What are the deliverables that you offer and expect of others?
Exchange	Refers to two or more transactions between two or more roles or participants that evoke reciprocity. A process in which one role as agent receives resources from another role or agent and provides resources in return. What are the resource exchanges between roles or participants on your interprofessional health care team?
Explicit knowledge	The knowledge that is codified and conveyed to others through dialogue, demonstration, or media. What is the explicit knowledge shared among members of the team?
Feedback	Refers to the return of information about the impact of an activity. It can also mean the return of a portion of the output of a process as new input. What feedback is returned about activities or outputs in your care coordination activities? How does feedback influence team dynamics and goal attainment?
Human capital/ competence	The knowledge, skills, and competencies that reside in individuals who work in an organization or that are embedded in the organization's internal and external social networks. What human capital resources are needed in order for care coordination in your context to be successful?
Impact analysis	An assessment of how an input for a role is handled. What are the tangible–intangible costs, gains, or values from the input that generate a response or activity, or increase/decrease tangible assets?
Knowledge management	The degree to which the team facilitates and supports processes for creating, sustaining, sharing, and renewing organizational knowledge in order to generate social or economic gain or improve performance. Who is responsible and how is knowledge managed in the care coordination process?
Perceived value	The degree of value participants feel they receive from individual deliverables that can come from roles, participants, or the network. What are the value-added dimensions of individual, collective, team, and organizational networks?
Resilience	The degree to which the network is able to reconfigure to respond to changing conditions and then return to original form. What is the resilience capacity of the team and organization in which you work?
Structural capital	The infrastructure, routines, concepts, models, information systems, work systems, and business processes that support productivity and sustainability. To what degree does the structural capital and infrastructure support interprofessional teamwork and care coordination processes?
Systems thinking	Refers to an analysis and synthesis of the forces and interrelationships that shape the behavior of systems. To what degree do members of the team think about the system dynamics at the patient, group, team, or organizational levels?
Value realization	The degree to which tangible or intangible values turn the input into gains, benefits, capabilities, or assets that contribute to the success of an individual, group, organization, or network (Allee, 2008). To what degree do members of the team intentionally negotiate and manage competing values related to collaborating, creating, competing, and controlling?

Adapted from Allee, Schwabe, and Babb (2015).

team placed on the medical care services and testing is to deliver evidence-based interventions based on the health care provider role. From Table 14.5, the value-networking reflection question for medical care services and testing basic needs is: What is the specific value or object that is conveyed from one role or participant to another role or participant? Name three deliverables that are essential for the care coordination success of this case:

1.
2.
3.

Organization-centered systems thinking is used by the team to enhance coaching and education of the patient and family. The identified coaching and educating practice issues include informing the family of an Alzheimer's dementia patient of the need for hospice education and resources. Targeted interventions for the team are to arrange a meeting with hospice staff and educate patient and family. The documented desired outcomes are to assist the patient and family to make a smooth transition to hospice care. A key question to ask is: Do the content and methods for coaching and teaching match the patient and family cognitive abilities and understanding? From Table 14.5, the value-networking reflection question for educating and coaching involves evaluating the transactions between two or more roles or participants in which one role as an agent receives resources from another role or agent and provides resources in return. The question would be: What is the exchange of resources and information between the providers and the patient and family regarding medication and available resources? Name three resources that could be exchanged between the providers and family and patient in this case:

1.
2.
3.

The diagram in the center of the worksheet is the activity plan from the interprofessional team (Exhibit 14.11). The team engages in collaborating, creating, competing, and controlling dynamics through communication (Quinn, Bright, Faerman, Thompson, & McGrath, 2014; Quinn, Heynoski, Thomas, & Spreitzer, 2014; Quinn & Quinn, 2015; Quinn & Rohrbough, 1983) to manage essential areas of organizational culture to realize the intangible value exchanges used to develop and manage an activity plan that considers interventions from the individualized plan of care, monitoring processes, evaluation of patient and family capacity with regard to resources and skills, and promotion of self-management. For example, in terms of collaboration, people must understand themselves and communicate honestly and effectively. Individuals mentor and develop others collaboratively and know how to participate and lead teams. Often this knowledge requires encouraging and managing constructive conflict. Competition enhances productivity and profitability. In this domain, vision and goal setting are a path to motivating self and others so that systems can be developed and organized to get

EXHIBIT 14.11

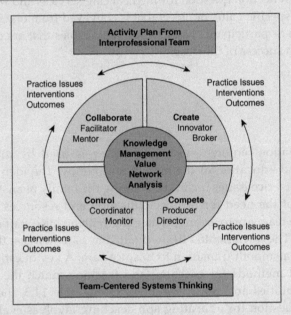

Key questions to consider for the four dimension of the competing-values framework in the CCCR model.

- What are the desired outcomes in this case?
- What are the values I expect of myself and others?
- How are the feelings of the patient, family, and team considered in this case?
- What strategies could the team use to coordinate care?

results. Creating and promoting the adoption of new ideas or clinical innovations requires attention to judicious use of power and ethics as well as championing new ideas and innovations through negotiating commitments and agreements for implementing and sustaining change. Control contributes to the development of stability and continuity as people work and manage across functions, organize information exchange, measure and monitor performance and quality, and enable compliance.

Key ingredients to team-centered systems thinking are that the members must be purpose centered, internally directed, other focused, and externally open to negotiation and communication surrounding competing values (Quinn, 2015; Quinn & Quinn, 2015). The activity plan from the interprofessional team in the CCCR model is guided by these principles and will promote the development of positive organizations and relationships. Each team member should be externally open to challenges, feedback, and freedom from labels, higher performance, and the cultivation and development of communities of practice. When this outcome is challenged and false fixed, some team members are valued more than others in the context of competitive versus collaborative goals. Being other influenced cultivates empathy, rapport, energy, and calmness. Together, the team members feel safe and secure enough to take risks and act with trust, integrity, and resilience. Creating such a culture supports a spirit of inquiry, learning, and experimentation that results in higher performance. Such behavior requires the activation of a reflective self in contrast to automatic self-justification and reactive modes of being and communicating. In order to be a positive influence and bring a state of leadership to the team, each member of the team needs to be vigilant about being purpose centered, choosing goals that create focus, energy, and meaning for the team. A focused, purpose-centered team is likely to attract and create resources related to the reasoning required to communicate across settings to achieve CCCR goals.

The activity plan from the interprofessional team iteratively visits the practice issues that include communication between providers specific to this case, targeted interventions that are updated at team meetings across the contexts in which the providers are interacting, and documents the desired outcomes to maintain team support and keep the team equally informed about patient status. Some key questions to ask are: Are the communication processes in place? Do they promote information exchange between and among the interprofessional health team members? The explicit value for role clarity, collaboration, and interaction of the team placed on the activity plan from the interprofessional team is determined by knowledge management and value impact analysis. From Table 14.5, the value-networking reflection questions for the activity plan from the interprofessional team are: What are the tangible–intangible costs, gains, or values from the input that generate a response or activity, or that increase/decrease tangible assets? How does the team facilitate and support processes for collaborating, controlling, creating, and competing to sustain, share, and renew organizational knowledge in order to generate social or economic gain or improve performance? Name a cost, gain, and value that would be generated from the activity plan of the team for this case:

1.
2.
3.

To the far right of the CCCR system model worksheet are four essential care coordination needs that evolve from the activity plan from the interprofessional team stemming from patient-centered systems thinking, team-centered systems thinking, and organization-centered systems thinking. These needs include the individualized plan of care; monitoring safety, needs assessment, and plan of care; evaluating capacity, resources, and skills; and promoting self-management. Each of these care coordination essentials is defined as well by practice issues, interventions, outcomes, and values.

The patient-centered systems-thinking and team-centered systems-thinking activities are used for the individualized plan of care. The identified practice issues revolve around the progressive decline of an Alzheimer's dementia patient. Targeted interventions for the provider and team are to provide comfort care, hospice referral, and chaplain referral. The documented desired outcomes are to provide end-of-life care promoting dignity. Some key questions to ask are: Does the individualized plan of care include team collaboration? Is there any input that was not yet considered? Are there providers who were overlooked? The explicit value for role clarity, collaboration, and interaction of the provider and team placed on the individualized plan of care is on structural capital. From Table 14.5, the value-networking reflection question for the individualized plan of care is: What are the infrastructure, routines, concepts, models, information systems, work systems, and business processes that support productivity and have sustainability? Name three routines, systems, or processes that support and sustain the productivity of the care coordination in this case:

1.
2.
3.

From the patient-centered systems-thinking and team-centered systems-thinking processes used for monitoring safety, needs assessment, and plan of care, identified practice issues include patient safety. Targeted interventions for the team are to change the plan of care to comfort care. The documented desired outcomes are for a death with dignity, to be pain free, and peaceful. A key question to ask is: Does the plan of care promote safety and meet the patient and family needs? The explicit value for role clarity, collaboration, and interaction of the team placed on monitoring safety, needs assessment, and plan of care is to obtain feedback and assess resilience in the network. From Table 14.5, the value-networking reflection questions for medical care services and testing basic needs are: What feedback is returned about activities or outputs? Was the network able to reconfigure itself to respond to changing conditions and then return to its original form? Name three areas of need and/or safety that were reassessed to determine whether the plan of care needed to be adjusted:

1.
2.
3.

Organization-centered systems-thinking processes, such as coaching and education, are used by the team to evaluate capacity, resources, and skills. The identified practice issues include the identification of terminal decline of health status. Targeted interventions for the team are to support and empower the patient and family through resources and to offer grief counseling. The documented desired outcomes are a death with dignity. Some key questions to ask are: Do the interventions in the plan of care require skilled help? Can the patient and family manage care needs independently? The explicit value for role clarity, collaboration, and interaction of the team placed on evaluating capacity, resources, and skills is identifying human capital and competence. From Table 14.5, the value-networking reflection question for educating and coaching involves evaluating the transactions between two or more roles or participants in which one role as an agent receives resources from another role or agent and provides resources in return. The question would be: What is the exchange of resources and information between the providers and the patient and family regarding medication and available resources? Name three exchanges of resources, skills, or information with the patient and family that are essential to the care coordination success of this case:

1.
2.
3.

Organization-centered systems-thinking processes, such as coaching and education, are used by the team to promote self-management. The identified practice issues include knowledge of resources available to the family. Targeted interventions for the team are to educate and empower the family. The documented desired outcomes are death with dignity for the patient and grief counseling for the family. A key question to ask is: Are the patient and family able to identify the resources they need and to navigate the health care system? The explicit value for role clarity, collaboration, and interaction of the team placed on promoting self-management is perceived value realization. From Table 14.5, the value-networking reflection question for promoting self-management is: What is the level of value that roles or participants feel they receive from individual deliverables that can come from roles, participants, or the network? Name three examples of learned self-management that resulted from the care coordination of this case:

1.
2.
3.

With the use of the CCCR systems model, the advanced practice nurse and other providers address practice issues by using and developing evidence-based interventions, implementing measures of adherence, and evaluating processes and outcomes. This requires clinical reasoning at different levels of perspective—the individual patient needs, interprofessional team contributions, and attention to the systems in which people work and provide care. These practice issues, interventions, and outcomes for patient and family care coordination stem from the National Quality Forum (NQF, 2010a, 2010b) and the Agency for Healthcare Research and Quality (AHRQ, 2014).

As the center of attention for health care needs is managed by webs of relationships between and among providers, each interaction supports a specific value exchange as the participant's partner for successful outcomes (Allee, 2003). The dynamic relationships that occurred for this elderly patient in a skilled facility among the advanced practice nurse, nursing staff, physician, hospice staff, chaplain, and social worker were collaborative, trusting, dynamic, and interdependent. Application of the competing-value competencies will relate to collaboration, creating, competing, and controlling, and help make explicit knowledge shared and managed to support innovation, coordination, and directing. Through the use of the electronic health record, connectivity impacted the value networking with greater access to knowledge and information. This process provided quick and effective feedback between team members for the complex needs this patient had related to end-of-life issues.

CLINICAL JUDGMENTS AND CCCR

The final phase of the clinical reasoning process is to determine whether outcomes were met and whether care coordination activities were successful. The OPT model of clinical reasoning is revisited for the final phase of care coordination when judgments are made about achieving outcomes from the interprofessional team activity plan (see Exhibit 14.8). The worksheet (see Figure 14.2) is revisited to make judgments about the care coordination essentials (needs, individualized plan of care; safety; capacity, resources, skills, and self-management). Shifting to the next level of perspective, using team-centered systems and organization-centered systems-thinking activities, collaboration, and coordination of the plan of care, reveals ongoing planning and evaluation to provide appropriate patient and family support during this end-of-life situation. The goal is to provide a safe and peaceful environment to achieve death with dignity for the patient. The appropriate hospice facility should be identified. Family support is needed to educate about hospice care and grief counseling. Resources identified for this case would be the hospice staff, chaplain, and support groups. These resources lead to the best possible management of this end-of-life situation for this patient and self-management of a peaceful death for the family.

Some remaining questions may arise as the evaluation of outcomes occurs such as: Can the organizations provide continuing resources and reach care coordination outcomes for this patient? Were communication and feedback loops effective between the health care providers and patient and family? Did the complexity of the system hinder or enhance the achievement of outcomes? The advanced practice nurse as care coordinator views all the systems and is the key informant to communicate with the team regarding the efficiency and effectiveness of the processes for care outcomes. Judgments are made about whether the outcomes from case management have been achieved, and the information is recycled back to revise or enhance the plan of care.

The thinking processes used by the advanced practice nurse and other health care providers while implementing the CCCR systems model are promoted through monitoring of thinking, the environment, and behaviors for goal attainment (Zimmerman & Schunk, 2001). The courses of action chosen to manage issues and ensure that this patient remained safe revolve around behaviors and actions taken, thinking processes used, and environmental structuring. Critical reflective questions that can be used to prompt clinical reasoning to make judgments about the achievement of patient and family outcomes are listed in Table 14.6. Critical-, creative-, and systems-thinking processes are used for total care coordination, flow from patient-centered systems (Table 14.4), team-centered systems thinking (Table 14.6), and organization-centered systems thinking (Table 14.6) for case management.

TABLE 14.6 Team-Centered and Organization-Centered Systems-Thinking Reflection Questions

SELF-REGULATION ACTIVITIES	REFLECTION QUESTIONS

Monitoring thinking	I. **Reflect on the thinking processes the team used to navigate organizational systems for care coordination of this case.**
	
	1. The baseline needs identified by the team in this case are.... Adjustments in the plan of care for future successes include.... Difficulties were resolved by...
	
	2. Team reactions during the care coordination of this case in regard to organizational systems could be described as...and they were handled by...
	
	3. When the team was dealing with important facts to develop the plan of care, coach, and educate the patient–family about organizational systems, it....
	
	4. Looking back on meaningful activities, the resources the team could have spent:
	  a. More time on...
	  b. Less time on...

Monitoring the environment	II. **Reflect on the environmental circumstances you encountered in the care coordination of this case.** 5. When the team prepares to carry out coaching and education activities for care coordination, it... 6. When the team considers particular distractions in the organizations that impede medical care services and supports for care coordination, it... 7. When the team works and communicates with organizational partners for care coordination of this case, it... 8. If the team had the chance to redo the care coordination activities, it would do... instead of... because ...

Monitoring behavior	III. **Reflect on your behaviors and reactions to the care coordination of this case.**
	
	9. Impressions of the team performance in evaluating capacity, energy, support, readiness, and skills to organize and manage the plan of care within organizational systems are...
	
	10. The team assures that it will update the needs assessment and individualized plan of care by... and if it needs to make changes, it...
	
	11. The team makes sure that it empowers the patient–family to navigate through organizational systems for management of health care needs by...and if it needs to make changes, it...
	
	12. The team reaction to care coordination of this case...
	  a. Reaction to what it likes about the navigation of organizational systems to facilitate the care coordination of this case...
	  b. Reaction to what it did not like about the navigation of organizational systems to facilitate the care coordination of this case...

Optional prompt: Other comments about the care coordination of this case...

Adapted from Kuiper, Pesut, and Kautz (2009).

SUMMARY

The clinical reasoning challenge for long-term care begins with a description and understanding of the patient's story. The thinking strategies used in this case provided a safe and health-promoting environment for a patient who was declining in health and exhibiting a failure to thrive. As the providers practice self-monitoring, self-evaluation, and self-correction, successful strategies are employed, and flaws in thinking are corrected as they collaborate and align interventions for patient and family success. The OPT clinical reasoning model provides the structure for clinical reasoning and systems thinking within an individual patient and family situation. The OPT structure and process can be used at several levels for care planning by the provider, by the team, and by the organization to discern alignment and coordination of care activities. The CCCR systems model provides the structure for clinical reasoning for the care coordination essential needs and their related practice issues, interventions, outcomes, and values.

KEY CONCEPTS

1. Clinical reasoning for care coordination with long-term care and end-of-life issues can be promoted with a framework that includes structure, content, and process.
2. A supporting framework for CCCR extends case management using patient-centered systems thinking and the OPT clinical reasoning model across levels of perspective that also includes team-centered systems thinking and organization-centered systems thinking to align care coordination activities.
3. The process of CCCR involves critical reflection for the individual provider and team.
4. Value-network analysis helps to define and describe the unique contributions that individual providers make to CCCR efforts supported through knowledge management and value-impact analysis.
5. A supporting framework for CCCR is completed by attending to the organization-centered systems thinking to make judgments about care coordination essentials.

STUDY QUESTIONS AND ACTIVITIES

1. Describe in your own words the benefits and processes of using the CCCR systems model with long-term care cases.
2. Using the CCCR systems model, identify the care coordination essential needs of cases in long-term care.
3. To what degree can you explicitly identify and describe the value exchanges associated with care coordination in long-term care situations.
4. How can an interprofessional team use the competencies of the competing values of collaboration, creating, competing, and controlling to ensure efficiency

and effectiveness of care coordination? How does your team negotiate roles of mentor, broker, director, and coordinator?

5. Identify all the possible standardized health care languages and communication strategies that could be considered in a long-term care and end-of-life case. Does language impact on communication and the patient outcomes? How does a discipline-specific framework influence the feedback, decisions, and outcomes with end-of-life care?

6. Identify the relationship between critical reflection and thinking strategies as they are applied to the three levels of system-thinking perspectives that are required—individual provider, team, and organization. What unique reflections are required to focus on team and organizational function with long-term care?

REFERENCES

Agency for Healthcare Research and Quality (AHRQ). (2014). *What is care coordination? Care coordination measures atlas update.* Rockville, MD: Author. Retrieved from http://www.ahrq.gov/professionals/prevention-chronic-care/improve/coordination/index.html

Allee, V. (2003). *The future of knowledge: Increasing prosperity through value networks.* Burlington, MA: Butterworth-Heinemann.

Allee, V. (2008). Value network analysis and value conversion of tangible and intangible assets. *Journal of Intellectual Capital, 9*(1), 5–24.

Allee, V., Schwabe, O., & Babb, M. K. (Eds.). (2015). *Value networks and the true nature of collaboration.* Tampa, FL: Megher–Kifer Press ValueNet Works and Verna Allee Associates.

Haas, S. A., Swan, B. A., & Haynes, T. S. (2014). *Care coordination and transition management core curriculum.* Pitman, NJ: American Academy of Ambulatory Care Nursing.

Kuiper, R., Pesut, D., & Kautz, D. (2009). Promoting the self-regulation of clinical reasoning skills in nursing students. *Open Nursing Journal, 3,* 76–85. Retrieved from http://www.ncbi.nlm.nih.gov/pmc/articles/PMC2771264

National Quality Forum. (2010a). *Preferred practices and performance measures for measuring and reporting care coordination: A consensus report.* Washington, DC: Author.

National Quality Forum. (2010b). *Quality connections: Care coordination.* Washington, DC: Author.

Pesut, D. J. (2008). Thoughts on thinking with complexity in mind. In C. Lindberg, S. Nash, & C. Lindberg (Eds.), *On the edge: Nursing in the age of complexity* (pp. 211–238). Bordentown, NJ: Plexus Press.

Quinn, R. (2015). *The positive organization: Breaking free from conventional cultures, constraints, and beliefs.* Oakland, CA. Berrett-Koehler.

Quinn, R., & Quinn, R. E. (2015). *Lift: Becoming a positive force in any situation.* San Francisco, CA: Berrett-Koehler.

Quinn, R. E., Bright, D., Faerman, S. R., Thompson, M. P., & McGrath, M. R. (2014). *Becoming a master manager: A competing values approach.* Hoboken, NJ: John Wiley & Sons.

Quinn, R. E., Heynoski, K., Thomas, M., & Spreitzer, G. M. (2014). *The best teacher in you: How to accelerate learning and change lives.* San Francisco, CA: Berrett-Koehler.

Quinn, R. E., & Rohrbough, J. (1983). A spatial model of effectiveness criteria: Towards a competing values approach to organizational analysis. *Management Science, 29,* 363–377.

World Health Organization (WHO). (2015). *Manual of the International Classification of Diseases and related health problems* (10th rev. ed.). Geneva, Switzerland: Author. Retrieved from http://www.icd10data.com

Zimmerman, B., & Schunk, D. S. (2001). *Self-regulated learning and academic thought*. Mahwah, NJ: Lawrence Erlbaum.

PART III

CARE COORDINATION CLINICAL REASONING INTO THE FUTURE

CHAPTER 15

FUTURE TRENDS AND CHALLENGES

FUTURE TRENDS

In this chapter, we identify, describe, and discuss future trends and challenges associated with the Care Coordination Clinical Reasoning (CCCR) model proposed in this book. Transformation and redesign of a 21st-century health care system requires understanding the driving forces that make a difference between change and transformation. Change efforts focused on the past may or may not help create inspired futures. Transformation is about creating a desired future and requires futures literacy. Futures literacy invites people to create and share stories about the future to inform current practice and realities. Advanced practice clinicians ought to have some grasp of anticipated future trends and consequences related to the work that they do. The National Center for Healthcare Leadership convened futurists to discern trends related to the state of health in the 21st century. Here are some of the trends futurists believe are likely:

- The United States will become part of a global system focusing on wellness and preventive care worldwide.
- Patients will receive care from "virtual" centers of excellence around the world.
- Deeper understanding of the human genome will create exciting new forms of drugs that will prevent disease from developing. Treatment will evolve from disease management to prevention or minimization.
- As people become senior citizens the issue of rising costs, resource allocation, and priorities will be exacerbated.
- Fueled by access to information through the Internet, people will take more responsibility for their personal health decisions and demand that the system treat them as customers rather than users.
- Most Americans will receive care from specialized centers for chronic diseases (cancers, women's health, heart, etc.)
- Standard diagnostic health will largely be electronic, with people conducting their own "doctor visits" from home through miniature data-collection and monitoring devices.

Practicing nurses will have to be flexible and open to changes that may come to the forefront of health care quickly and lead the way in care coordination. Their leadership skills will have to be honed and current in order to be flexible in guiding patients and other providers through these changes. The National Center for Healthcare Leadership (2015) has developed a Leadership Competency model that focuses on three essential domains and defines 26 competencies within those domains that demonstrate the essential skills and competencies for future leadership. The domains and competencies are:

- **Transformation** that supports visionary thinking, and that energizes, and stimulates change processes that engage people and communities in the design and development of new models of health care and wellness. Competencies that support this domain are a strategic orientation, innovative thinking, information seeking, analytic thinking, a community orientation, financial knowledge management, and an achievement orientation.
- **People skills** that engage and energize employees in service of valuing people's capabilities and appreciating the impact and influence that people have on each other and on stakeholders with whom they engage. Competencies that support this domain are relationship building, interpersonal understanding, professionalism, self-confidence, self-development, talent development, team leadership, and human resources management.
- **Execution** of the skill and abilities to translate vision and strategy into organizational performance. Competencies that support this domain are organizational awareness, change leadership, impact and influence, accountability, collaboration, communication skills, initiative, information technology management, performance measurement, process management/organizational design, and project management.

In addition to the national Leadership Competency models that exist, the American Nurses Association (ANA) has established a leadership institute and developed a leadership competency model that supports quality, safety, and evidence-based practice. The ANA Leadership Competency model builds on the following standards of nursing performance competency expectations associated with collaboration, communication, education, environmental health, ethics, evidence-based practice and research, leadership, practice evaluation, quality nursing practice, and resource utilization (ANA, 2013). The ANA Leadership Institute Competency Framework is organized around the belief that nurse leaders must actively lead themselves, lead others, and lead the organizations in which they work. Leading self requires adaptability, flexibility, being open to influence, projecting an executive image, motivating self, building relationships with integrity, maximizing learning, and self-awareness. Leading others requires effective communication skills, building collaborative relationships, communicating effectively to leverage differences, managing competing values, and developing and empowering others. Leading the organization requires systems thinking, business acumen, and the ability to turn vision into action through project management skills, sense making, and decisiveness as leaders navigate change. Each of the competency clusters are defined, described, and linked with specific behavioral objectives that help one craft a professional leadership development plan.

The purposes of education programs will change as curricula are designed to prepare future health care providers for these domains and for mastery of the related competencies. New pedagogies and models of instruction in clinical reasoning will be required to prepare the workforce.

Couple these future trends with the work of the Institute for the Future for the Phoenix Research Institute which identified six drivers and 10 skills necessary for a 2020 workforce. The drivers are increasing global life spans, the rise of smart machines and automation, an increase in sensors and big-data collection, new media tools and literacy expectations, and social technologies that connect communities of practice, learning, and research.

These drivers require advance skills in order to be successful in the evolving and developing workforce. Essential 2020 workforce skills include:

- Sense making: ability to determine the deeper meaning or significance of what is being expressed.
- Social intelligence: ability to connect to others in a deep and direct way, to sense and stimulate reactions and desired interactions.
- Novel and adaptive thinking: proficiency at thinking and coming up with solutions and responses beyond that which is rote or rule based.
- Cross-cultural competency: ability to operate in different cultural settings.
- Computational thinking: ability to translate vast amounts of data into abstract concepts and to understand data based reasoning.
- New media literacy: ability to critically assess and develop content that uses new media forms, and to leverage these media for persuasive communication.
- Transdisciplinarity: literacy in and ability to understand concepts across multiple disciplines.
- Design mind-set: ability to represent and develop tasks and work processes for desired outcomes.
- Cognitive load management: ability to discriminate and filter information for importance, and to understand how to maximize cognitive functioning using a variety of tools and techniques.
- Virtual collaboration: ability to work productively, drive engagement, and demonstrate presence as a member of a virtual team.

The authors believe that the CCCR model proposed in this text supports the development and mastery of the projected future workforce skills. In specific, the model supports sense making through the application and reinforcement of critical-, creative-, systems-, and complexity-thinking skills. The model values inclusion and social intelligence concerning patient preferences and team and interprofessional dynamics. The model supports adaptive and novel thinking based on analysis and synthesis of competing values and relationships between and among competing nursing care needs and concurrent International Classification of Diseases (ICD)-10 diagnostic categories. The model underscores the importance of cultural considerations in care planning. Data related to diagnostic tests and medical services and testing influence and inform computational thinking. The challenges of electronic health record use and new forms of communication with patients and team members as well as providers across service delivery lines, necessitates the development of new media literacy skills. The different levels of perspectives highlighted in the model encourage transdisciplinarity as clinicians consider patient-centered, team-centered, and health care system–centered issues and challenges. The activity plans associated with practice issues, interventions, and outcomes as well as the negotiation of competing values and roles and team relationships support interprofessional collaboration and teamwork. The creative thinking required in the model supports a design-thinking mind-set. Attention to the issues of framing, filter, and focus relate to cognitive load and knowledge management. Finally, the evolving nature and use of electronic health records and the rise of consumerism in regard to self-management and expectations of shared health care information (Topol, 2015) will drive developments in virtual collaboration and communication.

Digital health futurists Rohit Bhargava and Fard Johnmar (2013/2014) have identified three themes and 15 trends that will influence health care and care coordination clinical reasoning into the future. The first theme is health hyperficiency, which is emerging as a result of innovations in computing. The first trend within this theme relate to empathetic interfaces as health technologies become more intuitive and human-like. A second trend in this category is unhealthy surveillance, which relates to the fact that more health data is being collected about individuals, families, and communities—such massive data collections raise issues about privacy and security. A third trend in this category is predictive psychohistory—because big data and powerful computers are being used to generate and make small- and large-scale predictions.

A second theme likely to influence and affect the nature of care coordination into the future is the personalized health movement. Within this theme there are eight trends emerging and developing: the over-quantified self related to frustration and confusion associated with wearable health devices, augmented nutrition that enables people to make better food choices, the device divide that may prevent some people from gaining access to the latest health innovations, microhealth rewards, and multicultural misalignment that may prevent some cultures from effectively using health technologies. Three more trends in this category include medical genealogy, where genetic information can be used to predict disease and drive medication decisions, neuro-influence mapping in which advances in brain mapping may help treatment especially in mental illness, and the notion of health real estate where zip codes matter in terms of health and wellness living choices.

Finally, the third theme and constellation of trends relate to digital peer-to-peer health care. Three of the most significant trends in this category are care-hacking, in which caregivers and patients use digital tools to "hack" the health system in service of access and better care; accelerated trial sourcing, in which patients use social tools to find one another, prepare for clinical trials, and recruit pharma firms to conduct research; and virtual counseling via the Internet, which is also an emerging trend within the digital peer-to-peer health care theme. In fact, virtual counseling may support care coordination as social and other digital technologies will help patients and caregivers mentor each other and navigate and evaluate care delivery and expectations.

As clinicians look to the future, Lamb, Zimring, Chuzi, and Dutcher (2010) suggest that there is another set of interprofessional competencies clinicians ought to master related to health care design. Specifically, clinicians ought to be sensitized to the science of health care design, issues and challenges associated with health care systems and environments, the essential aspects of patient- and family-centered care, teamwork, and the culture of health professionals as well as design professions. The knowledge, skills, and attitudes associated with these competencies and skill sets provide the foundation for the domains of integration of competencies into the interprofessional team and innovation in approaches to care coordination of the future.

CHALLENGES FOR NURSING EDUCATION

Education Issues for Care Coordination

The care coordination trends and models require that educational measures be in place to prepare the advanced practice nurse for leadership roles in care coordination with an interprofessional team and the recipients of care: the patient and the family. The educational mandates stated by the ANA (2015) in *The ANA Scope and Standards of Practice* include nurses' preparation for essential roles in care coordination in future health care contexts. Educational strategies are needed to teach the foundational competencies of care coordination (Lamb, 2013), Quality and Safety Education for Nurses (QSEN; Cronenwett et al., 2007), and interprofessional clinical collaboration (American Association of Colleges of Nursing [AACN], 2015) during didactic and clinical experiences to facilitate team-based patient-centered care.

The Advanced Practice Registered Nurse (APRN) Consensus model was designed to provide a framework to prepare clinicians to meet the demands of patient populations and has been endorsed by 41 professional organizations. To facilitate APRN practice roles, education, licensure, certification, and practice must go hand in hand to ensure patient safety and high levels of expert decision making (Bolick et al., 2013). In addition, the statements put forth for competency-based education from the Institute of Medicine (IOM; 2010) report clearly specify competencies that should be included in curricula to prepare RNs for expert decision making, quality-enhancement skills, systems thinking, and team leadership at all levels of preparation. The IOM competencies include knowledge, skills, and abilities related to interprofessional teamwork, patient-centered care, using information technologies, ethical standards, and leadership for health promotion and disease management. Nurse educators are obligated to develop master teaching skills by keeping pace with knowledge development, evidence-based teaching strategies, and new technologies.

At the graduate level, nurses need to develop an even deeper understanding of care coordination, quality improvement, systems thinking, and policy (National Organization of Nurse Practitioner Faculty [NONPF], 2014). Individuals who have the appropriate graduate education sit for a certification examination to assess national competencies in their specialty area of practice for regulatory purposes. The advanced practice graduate is prepared to assume responsibility and accountability for health promotion and/or maintenance as well as the assessment, diagnosis, and management of complex patient problems.

Some authors also suggest that nursing analytics be taught to help the practitioner solve complex health problems (Ritt, 2014). Analytics is defined as the extensive use of data to describe, predict, prescribe, and compare data that drives decision making with the goal of improving results. The significance of embedding analytics into clinical practice improves workflow, enhances decision making, increases productivity, reduces costs, and promotes desired patient outcomes. With all these changes in the advanced practice nurse's role, there has been some recent seminal work to promote educational programs in care coordination and transition management in clinical settings so that professional nursing can assume leadership roles.

The CCCR model was developed based on the success of the Outcome-Present State-Test (OPT) model of clinical reasoning, which has been evaluated as a useful educational strategy to promote clinical reasoning with undergraduate students for over 10 years. Discoveries with student samples in a variety of clinical circumstances revealed that using the model worksheets as a scaffold for reasoning in clinical contexts resulted in improved self-efficacy in the use of clinical reasoning skills over time (Kuiper, Pesut, & Kautz, 2009).

The OPT worksheets also promoted the use of a standardized nursing language and was associated with higher ratings on safety interventions on the OPT worksheets (Kautz, Kuiper, Pesut, & Williams, 2006). Evaluation of self-regulated learning (SRL) reflections with the OPT model use revealed consistent use of thinking strategies, attention to environmental situations, and self-monitoring (Kuiper, 2002). A recent Delphi study subjected the pedagogical model with components of the OPT model and SRL reflections to a group of educational experts. The OPT model was found to promote the cognitive domain, and the SRL reflections promoted the metacognitive domain (Rahim & Goolamally, 2014). Used as a whole it is suggested that these models would indeed enhance clinical reasoning and clinical judgment skills (Bartlett et al., 2008; Kautz, Kuiper, Pesut, Knight-Brown, & Daneker, 2005; Rahim & Goolamally, 2014).

Care Coordination Curricula

The adoption and diffusion of the OPT model worksheets and the use of SRL reflection strategies in preparing advanced practice graduate students for care coordination is well timed because of the recent development of some care coordination curricula. The CCCR model described and developed in this text helps to operationalize the American Academy of Ambulatory Care Nursing care coordination and transition management core curriculum (Haas, 2014). The Care Coordination and Transition Management (CCTM) model offers a curriculum framework for care coordination and integrates the QSEN format (Cronenwett et al., 2007). The model curriculum and logic model focus and extend learning about the knowledge, skills, and abilities clinicians need to activate and operationalize the care coordination management and transition process. Evidence-based dimensions and activities are developed into a curriculum and include the concepts, principles, and strategies related to self-management; education and engagement of patient and family; cross-setting of communication and transition; coaching and counseling of patients and families; use of the nursing process (assessment, plan, intervention, evaluation); teamwork and collaboration; patient-centered planning; population health management; and advocacy (Haas, Swan, & Haynes, 2013). In addition, chapters and resources are also provided that explore population health management, care coordination and transition management between acute and ambulatory care, and informatics in nursing practice and telehealth nursing practice. These care coordination dimensions are similar to the care coordination model concepts presented by Schraeder and Shelton (2013) and the coordination practice issues put forth in the CCCR model described in this book. The core curriculum presented by Haas, Swan, and Haynes (2013) was designed for the RN working in any care coordination and transitions management setting.

The interprofessional literature also suggests an educational and research agenda surrounding health care curricula for interprofessional education. The goal is to educate and equip graduate students with interprofessional capabilities, the ability to recognize professional boundaries, comfort with reflecting on interprofessional relationships during work on a health care delivery team, and awareness of stereotypes that exist within the self and others (Thistlewaite, 2012).

One of the most important challenges in the area of interprofessional education for care coordination is to negotiate and manage the dynamic tensions between and among different disciplines (Jacobsen & Lindqvist, 2009). The CCCR model supports education for advanced practice nurses and the interprofessional team by serving as a platform and blueprint for the goal of reinforcing the frame and focus on patient and families while enhancing teamwork (Morphet et al., 2014), systems thinking (Cabrera & Cabrera, 2015), and value networking (Allee, Schwabe, & Babb, 2015). The CCCR model is a collaborative model we propose to help meet the challenges nurse educators will face in order to promote CCCR. The authors believe that the CCCR model and the worksheets related to the different levels and perspective of patient-centered, team-centered, and organization-centered systems thinking support interaction and dialogue among interprofessional team members. In one study, stereotyping was decreased in the group of health care students who experienced interprofessional education (IPE; Ekmekci, 2013). Hence, there are reasons to develop interprofessional curricula and tools for future health care students because when students learn together in interprofessional clinical learning experiences, they develop confidence, competence, communication, and understanding of role clarity for teamwork, which improves patient care (Morphet et al., 2014).

Teaching–Learning Strategies

Some of the pedagogical strategies used to assist faculty in promoting clinical reasoning for care coordination include creating situations in which students work and interact together in interprofessional teams in simulation or authentic clinical settings.

Research surrounding the OPT model and SRL reflection pedagogies reveals that the scaffolding provided by worksheets is necessary in order to promote habitual thinking skills and activities. Using the tools and strategies described in this text, nurse educators can assist students in developing the clinical reasoning skills unique to the care coordination role. Faculty development with the CCCR model worksheets provided in this text is likely to support situated cognition in students so that they form habitual ways of thinking, reasoning, communicating, and recognizing the value-network impact of teamwork and analytics for complex problem solving.

For example, evaluating the use of the worksheets over time is likely to reveal the progression and growth of clinical thinking and reasoning as it relates to care coordination and transition management. The OPT model clinical reasoning web can be evaluated to determine the mastery of identifying nursing problems by domains and diagnoses and matching them to medical problems identified though ICD-10 codes. Choosing the priority patient and family needs can then be arranged into the OPT clinical reasoning model for care coordination. Practicing with this worksheet helps the student develop schema and prototypes that can be recalled for subsequent cases in clinical settings. The recall process can be evaluated with think-aloud techniques and case study exercises. Reflection on these clinical reasoning activities can be prompted and evaluated through a variety of qualitative methods for themes and types of thinking skills used. Then, as the student transitions to the CCCR systems model web, particular attention is given to the coordination of practice issues. The work of the interprofessional team under each of these issues can be promoted and evaluated to check for accuracy and specificity as they relate to each patient and family case. The culmination of all the preparatory work from the other worksheets is pulled together in the CCCR systems model to prioritize patient and family needs and collaborate, create, control, and compete surrounding the practice issues, interventions, and outcomes for each coordination practice issue. Helping the student understand the values embedded in each issue, communicating across settings, and switching among patient-centered, team-centered, and organization-centered systems thinking is a challenge to learn, and for faculty to teach. Observing, evaluating, and measuring the achievement of these skills over time determines the usefulness of the pedagogies used and the curriculum needed to support role development for care coordination and transition management. As students work through these exercises, faculty will be able to track their thinking, observe their progression, and evaluate growth as skills are developed for the role of a care coordinator.

Some teaching strategies for patient-centered, team-centered, and organization-centered systems thinking include clinical practice assignments that survey interprofessional staff knowledge and practice, discussion boards, unfolding case studies, peer learning, and simulations that are face to face or online (Phillips, Stalter, Dolansky, & Lopez, 2015). The safety of having clinical-simulation experiences with standardized patient scenarios would help incorporate analytic data into decision making (Ritt, 2014). Web-based learning experiences also have merit in dealing with the work-schedule conflicts of advanced practice students and enable content to be repeated at will. Educational research can include the use of quantitative measures, such as psychometric testing and repeated measures, and qualitative measures, such as think-aloud protocols and narrative reflection analyses. The ANA (2015) has also suggested clinical-improvement projects to evaluate student understanding of care coordination efforts and outcomes.

CHALLENGES FOR THE APRN

The CCCR model presented in this text facilitates the APRN student transition into the role of professional clinician. The model facilitates the collaborative use of nursing models alongside medical models that are essential and unique for the advanced practice nurse. With the significant shortage of primary care physicians expected only to worsen, nurse practitioners (NPs) are expected to fill this gap. One study showed that 83% of faculty physicians believe NPs will improve access to care (Soine, Errico, Redmond, & Sprow, 2013). Most NPs work in the primary care setting after graduation from a nationally accredited graduate education program. These programs educate three nurse practitioner students to every one primary care physician student (Sustaita, Zeigler, & Brogan, 2013). The CCCR model is a way to rapidly process complex cases, which are commonly seen in the primary care setting. The CCCR model aligns well with the essentials of care coordination presented by Lamb (2013). Repeated use of the model's processes and concepts promotes a habitual way of thinking about care coordination. The model's processes can also serve as a talking tool for interprofessional collaboration as they address the concerns of all health care disciplines related to care coordination. The CCCR model is also useful for the experienced advanced practice nurse clinician as it walks the expert clinician through the use of values, network exchanges, and processes of collaborative practice.

SUMMARY

Faculty and students are on the horizon of new and exciting changes in health care as it relates to care coordination. The strategies and worksheets presented in the CCCR model moves the process forward and provides support to reinforce the professional standards and curricula that are being implemented in current professional health care educational programs.

REFERENCES

Allee, V., Schwabe, O., & Babb, M. K (Eds.). (2015). *Value networks and the true nature of collaboration.* Tampa, FL: Megher–Kifer Press ValueNet Works and Verna Allee Associates.

American Nurses Association (ANA). (2013). *ANA Leadership Institute competency model.* Silver Spring, MD: Author. Retrieved from http://ana-leadershipinstitute.org/Doc-Vault/About-Us/ANA-Leadership-Institute-Competency-Model-pdf.pdf

American Nurses Association (ANA). (2015). *Nursing: Scope and standards of practice* (3rd ed.). Silver Spring, MD: Author.

Bartlett, R., Bland, A., Rossen, E., Kautz, D., Benfield, S., & Carnevale, T. (2008). Evaluation of the Outcome-Present State-Test Model as a way to teach clinical reasoning. *Journal of Nursing Education, 47*(8), 337–344.

Bhargava, R., & Johnmar, F. (2013/2014). *15 surprising trends changing health care.* Oakton, VA: Ideapress. Retrieved from epatient 2015.com

Bolick, B. N., Bevacqua, J., Kline-Tilford, A., Reuter-Rice, K., Haut, C., McComiskey, C. A.,…Verger, J. T. (2013). Recommendations for matching pediatric nurse practitioner education and certification to pediatric acute care populations. *Journal of Pediatric Health Care: Official Publication of National Association of Pediatric Nurse Associates & Practitioners, 27*(1), 71–77.

Cabrera, D., & Cabrera, L. (2015). *Systems thinking made simple: New hope for solving wicked problems.* New York, NY: Odyssean Press.

Cronenwett, L., Sherwood, G., Barnsteiner, J., Disch, J., Johnson, J., Mitchell, P., Sullivan, D. T., & Warren, J. (2007). Quality and safety education for nurses. *Nursing Outlook, 55*(3), 122–131.

Ekmekci, O. (2013). Promoting collaboration in health care teams through interprofessional education: A simulation case study. *Clinical Research and Leadership Faculty Publications.* Retrieved from http://hsrc,himmelfarb.gwu.edu/smhs_crl_facpubs/23

Haas, S., Swan, B. A., & Haynes, T. (2013). Developing ambulatory care registered nurse competencies for care coordination and transition management. *Nursing Economics, 31*(1), 44–9, 43.

Haas, S. A. (2014). *Care coordination and transition management core curriculum.* Pitman, NJ: American Academy of Ambulatory Care Nursing (AAACN). Retrieved from www .aaacn.org

Institute for the Future. (n.d.). *Future work skills 2020.* Retrieved from http://cdn.theatlantic. com/static/front/docs/sponsored/phoenix/future_work_skills_2020.pdf

Institute of Medicine (IOM). (2010). *The future of nursing: Leading change, advancing health.* Committee on the Robert Wood Johnson Foundation Initiative on the Future of Nursing, at the Institute of Medicine. Washington, DC: The National Academies Press.

Interprofessional Education Collaborative Expert Panel. (2011). *Core competencies for interprofessional collaborative practice: Report of an expert panel.* Washington, DC: Interprofessional Education Collaborative. Retrieved from https://ipecollaborative.org/uploads/IPEC-Core-Competencies.pdf

Jacobsen, F., & Lindqvist, S. (2009). A two-week stay in an interprofessional training unit changes students' attitudes to health professionals. *Journal of Interprofessional Care, 23*(3), 242–250.

Kautz, D., Kuiper R., Pesut, D., & Williams, R. (2006). Unveiling the use of NANDA, NIC and NOC (NNN) language with the Outcome-Present State Test model of clinical reasoning. *International Journal of Nursing Terminologies Classification, 17,* 129–138.

Kautz, D. D., Kuiper, R., Pesut, D. J., Knight-Brown, P., & Daneker, D. (2005). Promoting clinical reasoning in undergraduate nursing students: Application and evaluation of the Outcome Present State Test (OPT) model of clinical reasoning. *International Journal of Nursing Education Scholarship, 2,* Article 1.

Kuiper, R. A. (2002). Enhancing metacognition through the reflective use of self-regulated learning strategies. *Journal of Continuing Education in Nursing, 33*(2), 78–87.

Kuiper, R., Pesut, D., & Kautz, D. (2009). Promoting the self-regulation of clinical reasoning skills in nursing students. *Open Nursing Journal, 3,* 76–85. Retrieved from http://www .ncbi.nlm.nih.gov/pmc/articles/PMC2771264

Lamb, G. (2013). *Care coordination: The game changer how nursing is revolutionizing quality care.* Silver Springs, MD: American Nurses Association, Nurse Books.

Lamb, G., Zimring, C., Chuzi, J., & Dutcher, D. (2010). Designing better healthcare environments: Interprofessional competencies in healthcare design. *Journal of Interprofessional Care, 24*(4), 422–435.

Morphet, J., Hood, K., Cant, R., Baulch, J., Gilbee, A., & Sandry, K. (2014). Teaching teamwork: An evaluation of an interprofessional training ward placement for health care students. *Advances in Medical Education and Practice, 5,* 197–204. Retrieved from http:// dx.doi.org/10.2147/AMEP.S61189

National Organization of Nurse Practitioner Faculty (NONPF). (2014). Retrieved from http://www.nonpf.org/general/custom.asp?page=14

Phillips, J. M., Stalter, A. M., Dolansky, M. A., & Lopez, G. M. (2015). Fostering future leadership in quality and safety in health care through systems thinking. *Journal of Professional Nursing, 32*(1), 15–24.

Rahim, R. A., & Goolamally, N. (2014). *Pedagogical model to inculcate clinical reasoning skills among nursing students in the open distance learning institution.* Seminar conducted at the Open University Malaysia, Kuala Lampur, Malaysia.

Ritt, E. (2014). Essential analytics in nursing education: Building capacity to improve clinical practice. *Journal of Nursing Education and Practice, 4*(12), 9–16.

Schraeder, C., & Shelton, P. (2013). Effective care coordination models. In G. Lamb (Ed.), *Care coordination: The game changer how nursing is revolutionizing quality care* (pp. 57–79). Silver Spring, MD: American Nurses Association, Nursesbooks.org.

Soine, L., Errico, K., Redmond, C., & Sprow, S. (2013). What do faculty physicians know about nurse practitioner practice? *Journal for Nurse Practitioners, 2*(9), 93–98.

Sustaita, A., Zeigler, V., & Brogan, M. (2013). Hiring a nurse practitioner: What's in it for the physician? *Nurse Practitioner, 11*(38), 41–45.

Thistlewaite, J. (2012). Interprofessional education: A review of context, learning and the research agenda. *Medical Education, 46*(1), 58–70. Retrieved from http://dx.dos .org/10.1111/j1365–2923.2011.04143.x

Topol, E. (2015). *The patient will see you now: The future of medicine is in your hands.* NewYork, NY: Perseus-Basic Books.

GLOSSARY

Care coordination—The deliberate organization of patient care activities between two or more participants (including the patient) involved in a patient's care to facilitate the appropriate delivery of health care services (Agency for Healthcare Research and Quality [AHRQ], 2014).

Care coordination clinical reasoning—The application of critical, creative, systems, and complexity thinking to determine the practice issues, interdependencies, and interconnections of role relationships for collaborative work in service of caring for people to address problems, interventions, and outcomes through time and across health care contexts and services.

Care Coordination Clinical Reasoning systems model—A concurrent iterative model of clinical reasoning that visually represents the complexities and essential care coordination practice issues that need attention so as to organize thinking that focuses on patient's and/or family's priority needs within the context of services provided within and between health care delivery systems.

Clinical judgments—The meaning the provider attributes to the evidence derived from the test or gap analysis of the present state to the outcome state in the Outcome-Present State-Test (OPT) model.

Clinical reasoning—Reflective-, concurrent-, critical-, creative-, systems-, and complexity-thinking processes embedded in nursing practice that nurses use to filter, frame, focus, juxtapose, and test the match between a patient's present state and desired outcome state.

Clinical reasoning web—A graphic representation of the functional relationships between and among competing nursing care issues derived from systems and complexity thinking, which results in a convergence and identification of the central keystone issue that becomes the focus point for organizing nursing care.

Clinical vocabulary—Standardized terminology relevant to nursing practice that pertains to relevant domains of nursing practice.

Comparative analysis—Process of considering the strengths and weaknesses of competing alternatives.

Competence—Ability to do something well (Merriam-Webster.com).

Complexity thinking—Combining all thinking strategies with an understanding of the complexity among relationships embedded in a particular patient story.

Creative thinking—A metacognitive process that supports clinical reasoning by generating associations, attributes, elements, images, and operations to solve problems (Pesut, 2008).

Critical thinking—Purposeful self-regulatory judgment that results in interpretation, analysis, evaluation, and inference as well as the explanation of the evidential, conceptual, methodological, criteriological, or contextual considerations on which that judgment was based (Facione, 1990).

Critical thinking skills—Skills of interpretation, analysis, inference, explanation, evaluation, and self-regulation.

Cue—Sign, symptom, behavior, or characteristic displayed by a person that serves as data for clinical reasoning.

Cue connection—The process of clustering two or more cues to form a pattern to guide framing, outcome specification, and establishment of a test.

Cue/web logic—Consideration of biopsychosocial–spiritual facts, standardized terminologies system data, and functional relationships among diagnostic hypotheses. A reflective decision-making process that refers to inductive, deductive, and retroductive connection of cues and concepts in a clinical reasoning web in order to establish an organizing frame for a clinical reasoning scenario.

Decision making—Considering and selecting interventions from a repertoire of actions that facilitate the achievement of a desired outcome state.

Deduction—Reasoning that moves from the general to the specific.

Deliverable—The specific values or objects that are conveyed from one role or participant to another role or participant (Allee, Schwabe, & Babb, 2015).

Exchange—Two or more transactions between two or more roles or participants that evoke reciprocity. A process in which one role as agent receives resources from another role or agents and provides resources in return (Allee, Schwabe, & Babb, 2015).

Explicit knowledge—The knowledge that is codified and conveyed to others through dialogue, demonstration, or media (Allee, Schwabe, & Babb, 2015).

Feedback—Information returned about the impact of an activity. It can also mean the return of a portion of the output of a process as new input (Allee, Schwabe, & Babb, 2015).

Framing—Mental models that influence and guide our perception and behavior for the process of deriving the theme or meaning of a client-in-context situation. The frame then becomes the lens through which all thinking is viewed.

Human capital/competence—The knowledge, skills, and competencies that reside in individuals who work in an organization or that are embedded in the organization's internal and external social networks (Allee, Schwabe, & Babb, 2015).

Hypothesizing—Determining an explanation that accounts for a set of facts and that can be tested by further investigation.

ICD-10 codes—The tenth version of the coding system (International Classification of Diseases) used to categorize diagnoses that serves as a standard diagnostic tool for epidemiology, health management, and clinical purposes (World Health Organization, 2015).

If–then thinking—A thinking strategy that involves linking ideas and consequences together in a logical sequence.

Impact analysis—An assessment of how an input for a role is handled (Allee, Schwabe, & Babb, 2015).

Induction—Reasoning that moves from specific to general.

Interprofessionality—The development of a cohesive practice among professionals from different disciplines. It is the process by which professionals reflect on and develop ways of practicing that provide an integrated and cohesive answer to the needs of the patient–family–population (D'Amour & Oandasan, 2005).

Judgment—Analysis, evaluation, and conclusions drawn from comparison of the present-state to the desired outcome-state.

Juxtaposing—Side-by-side comparison of specified outcome state criteria with present-state data.

Keystone issue—Central supporting element of the client's story that guides reasoning and care planning based on an analysis and synthesis of concepts and diagnostic possibilities as represented in a clinical reasoning web.

Knowledge-complexity archetype—Knowledge as a complex system that has underlying patterns or basic organizing structures (Allee, 1997).

Knowledge management—The degree to which the team facilitates and supports processes for creating, sustaining, sharing, and renewing organizational knowledge in order to generate social or economic gain or improve performance (Allee, Schwabe, & Babb, 2015).

Metacognitive check—The process one engages in to monitor, correct, reinforce, and evaluate one's own thinking about a specific task or situation.

Nursing—A scientific discipline focused on the protection, promotion, and optimization of health and abilities, prevention of illness and injury, facilitation of healing, alleviation of suffering through the diagnosis and treatment of human response, and advocacy in the care of individuals, families, communities, and populations (American Nurses Association [ANA], 2015).

Nursing analytics—Extensive use of data to describe, predict, prescribe, and compare data that drives decision making with the goal of improving results surrounding patient–family care problems.

Nursing art—Conceptualization of nursing that focuses on caring and respect of human dignity using a compassionate approach to patient care that embrace spirituality, health, empathy, mutual respect, and partnership (ANA, 2015).

Nursing informatics—The science and practice that integrated nursing, its information, and knowledge, with management of information and communication technologies to promote the health of people, families, and communities worldwide (American Medical Informatics Association [AMIA], 2016).

Nursing Minimum Data Set—A set of variables with uniform definitions and categories concerning the specific dimensions of nursing, which meet the information needs of multiple data users in the macro health care system (AMIA, 2015; Nursing

Working Group of the American Medical Informatics Association, 2015; Werley, Ryan, & Zorn, 1995).

Nursing process—A multi-step process that uses assessment, diagnosis, planning, implementation, and evaluation to teach, learn, think, and reason about nursing care situations.

OPT (Outcome-Present State-Test) model—A concurrent iterative model of clinical reasoning that emphasizes reflective self-monitoring while filtering, framing, and focusing the context and content of clinical reasoning and juxtaposing outcome state with present state client data. Clinical decision making in this model relates to choosing nursing actions. Clinical judgment in this model attributes meaning to the results of a test or match between desired criteriological outcome state and present state.

Organization-centered thinking—Thinking intended to transform problems through care coordination activities that considers organizational contexts in order to achieve success.

Outcome-focused thinking—Thinking that emphasizes outcomes or end results.

Outcome specification—Process of determining the desired end state of the client.

Outcome state—The desired condition of the client derived from the frame and initial present-state data as well as criteria that define the desired condition.

Patient-centered thinking—Thinking that transforms problems through care coordination activities that considers the patient and family needs and issues in order to achieve success.

Perceived value—The degree of value participants feel they receive from individual deliverables, which can come from roles, participants, or the networks (Allee, Schwabe, & Babb, 2015).

Present state—The initial condition of the patient derived from cue/web cluster logic that is defined by standardized terminology that changes over time as a result of nursing actions and decisions as well as the current condition of the client at the time of the test.

Prototype identification—Using a model or textbook case as a reference point for comparative analysis.

Reflective thinking—Conscious application of the thinking strategies and functional relationships of self-talk, prototype identification, schema search, hypothesizing, if–then thinking, how-so thinking, juxtaposing, comparative analysis, reflexive comparison, and reframing.

Reflexive comparison—Making a judgment about the state of a situation after gauging the presence or absence of some quality against a standard using the current case as a reference criterion.

Reframing—Attributing a different meaning to the content or context of a situation, given a set of cues, web logic, tests, decisions, or judgments.

Resilience—The degree to which the network is able to reconfigure to respond to changing conditions and then return to original form (Allee, Schwabe, & Babb, 2015).

Retroduction—The process of reasoning using inductive data and deductive premises concurrently.

Scenario—An outline of a hypothesized or projected chain of events.

Scenario development—The process of developing a hypothesized or projected chain of events.

Schema—An organized pattern of thought or behavior that organizes categories of information and the relationships among them (DiMaggio, 1997).

Schema search—Accessing general and/or specific patterns of past experiences that might apply to the current situation.

Scientific method—Problem-solving approach in which a problem is identified, possible solutions to the problem are hypothesized, and experiments are designed to test a proposed solution to the problem.

Self-regulation—Metacognitive process whereby individuals actively pursue and sustain behaviors, cognitions, and emotions geared toward goal attainment (Zimmerman & Schunk, 2001).

Self-talk—Expressing one's thoughts to one's self.

Spinning and weaving a web—The process of using thinking strategies to analyze and synthesize functional relationships among diagnostic hypotheses associated with a client's health status.

Standardized medical languages—Health and biomedical vocabularies and terminologies (Unified Medical Language System [UMLS] of the U.S. National Library of Medicine, 2015).

Structured capital—The infrastructure, routines, concepts, models, information systems, work systems, and business processes that support productivity and sustainability (Allee, Schwabe, & Babb, 2015).

Systems thinking—Attention to distinctions (D), systems rules (S), relationship rules (R), and perspective rules (P) to make distinctions between and among ideas or things to split them into parts, lump them into a whole, or relate them to each other (Cabrera & Cabrera, 2015).

Team-centered thinking—Thinking about transforming problems through care coordination activities that considers the team dynamics and communication in order to achieve success.

Test—The process of juxtaposing the present state and outcome state and evaluating the criteriological match between present-state data and a specified outcome.

Thinking strategies—Specific cognitive and metacognitive techniques and strategies that nurses use when engaged in reflective clinical reasoning.

Value-impact analysis—The analysis of the dynamic exchanges and relationships between individuals that are collaborative, trusting, and interdependent; and that are embedded in the competing values of creating, competing, controlling, and collaborating (Allee, Schwabe, & Babb, 2015).

Value-network analysis—A method to help explain the values added from individuals, groups, and teams as they contribute to a transaction or enterprise (Allee,

Schwabe, & Babb, 2015). In health care, it refers to the tangible and intangible value exchanges between health care providers in the context of care coordination.

Value realization—The degree to which tangible or intangible values turn the input into gains, benefits, capabilities, or assets that contribute to the success of an individual, group, organization, or network (Allee, Schwabe, & Babb, 2015).

REFERENCES

Agency for Healthcare Research and Quality (AHRQ). (2014). Chapter 2. *What is care coordination? Care coordination measures atlas update.* Rockville, MD: Author. Retrieved from http://www.ahrq.gov/professionals/prevention-chronic-care/improve/coordination/atlas2014/chapter2.html

Allee, V. (1997). *The knowledge evolution: Expanding organizational intelligence.* Boston, MA: Butterworth Heinemann.

Allee, V., & Schwabe, O., & Babb, M. K. (Eds.). (2015). *Value networks and the true nature of collaboration.* Tampa, FL: Megher–Kifer Press.

American Medical Informatics Association (AMIA). (2016). *Nursing Informatics working group.* Retrieved from https://www.amia.org/programs/working-groups/nursing-informatics

American Nurses Association (ANA). (2015). *Nursing: Scope and standards of practice* (3rd ed.). Silver Spring, MD: Author.

Cabrera, D., & Cabrera, L. (2015). *Systems thinking made simple: New hope for solving wicked problems.* New York, NY: Odyssean Press.

Competence. (n.d.) In *Merriam-Webster: Dictionary and thesaurus.* Retrieved from http://www.merriam-webste.com/; http://www.learnersdictionary.com

D'Amour, D., & Oandasan, I. (2005). Interprofessionality as the field of interprofessional practice and interprofessional education: An emerging concept. *Journal of Interprofessional Care, 19*(1), 8–20.

DiMaggio, P. (1997). Culture and cognition. *Annual Review of Sociology, 23,* 263–287.

National Library of Medicine. (2009). *UMLS reference manual.* (2015). Retrieved from http://www.ncbi.nlm.nih.gov/books/NBK9676

Nursing Working Group of the American Medical Informatics Association. (2015). Retrieved from http://www.amia.org/programs/working-groups/nursing-informatics

Pesut, D. J. (2008). Thoughts on thinking with complexity in mind. In C. Lindberg, S. Nash, & C. Lindberg (Eds.), *On the edge: Nursing in the age of complexity* (pp. 211–238). Bordentown, NJ: Plexus Press.

U.S. National Library of Medicine (2015). *Unified medical language system.* Bethesda, MD: U.S. Author. Retrieved from htps://www.nlm.nih.gov/research/umls

Werley, H. H., Ryan, P., & Zorn, C. R. (1995). The NMDS: A framework for the organization of nursing language. In *An emerging framework: Data system advances for clinical nursing practice.* Silver Spring, MD: American Nurses Association.

World Health Organization (WHO). (2015). *Manual of the International Classification of Diseases and related health problems* (10th rev. ed.). Geneva, Switzerland: Author. Retrieved from http://www.icd10data.com

Zimmerman, B., & Schunk, D. S. (2001). *Self-regulated learning and academic thought.* Mahwah, NJ: Lawrence Erlbaum.

INDEX

Printed in the United States
By Bookmasters